Back Care

For Churchill Livingstone:

Editorial Director: Mary Law
Project Development Manager: Mairi McCubbin
Project Manager: Jane Shanks
Design Direction: George Ajayi

Back Care

A Clinical Approach

Sheila Braggins MCSP SRP

Chartered Physiotherapist, London, UK

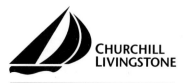

CHURCHILL
LIVINGSTONE

EDINBURGH LONDON NEW YORK PHILADELPHIA ST LOUIS SYDNEY TORONTO 2000

CHURCHILL LIVINGSTONE
An imprint of Harcourt Publishers Limited

© Harcourt Publishers Limited 2000

⟋⟋ is a registered trademark of Harcourt Publishers
Limited

First published 2000

ISBN 0 443 06488 1

British Library Cataloguing in Publication Data
A catalogue record for this book is available from the British
Library.

Library of Congress Cataloging in Publication Data
A catalog record for this book is available from the Library
of Congress.

Note
Medical knowledge is constantly changing. As new
information becomes available, changes in treatment,
procedures, equipment and the use of drugs become
necessary. The author and the publishers have, as far as it is
possible, taken care to ensure that the information given in
this text is accurate and up-to-date. However, readers are
strongly advised to confirm that the information, especially
with regard to drug usage, complies with the latest
legislation and standards of practice.

The
publisher's
policy is to use
**paper manufactured
from sustainable forests**

Printed in China

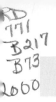

Contents

Preface

Since 1994 and the publication of my first book, *The Back: Functions, Malfunctions and Care*, research has broadened therapeutic horizons in two important areas: it has provided a greater understanding of the complexities of acute and chronic pain and it has demonstrated the importance of dynamic muscle stabilization in the recovery from acute pain and possibly in the prevention of recurrent pain.

The broadening of these concepts has expanded the scope of clinical reasoning. Pain can no longer be considered as a clearcut localized tissue injury sensation. We need to accept the multifactorial nature of pain and to think laterally about every presentation or symptom. We can no longer accuse the psyche of fabricating the soma – they are neurally and chemically inseparable. Similarly, we can no longer continue along the road of traditional, set exercises whilst ignoring the poor performance of everyday patterns of movement. The new approach demands an adaptability of thought and poses a challenge to our ingenuity.

Chronic pain with disability has become an important economic issue for health service resources throughout Europe and North America and needs to be addressed by all medical professions. I firmly support the hypothesis that if acute back pain is resolved with function and stability restored, chronic pain may be avoided. As there is a growing incidence of disabling back pain sufferers, the need to remedy pain in the early stages becomes all the more urgent. In addition, the treatment of acute pain involves not solely dealing with tissue damage but also educating the patient in relation to pain management, which includes the need for paced activity.

We shall never know how many sufferers years ago stuck a nutmeg in their pocket to relieve the 'rheumatism' (as my grandfather did) and got on with normal activities in spite of 'sciatica'. They instigated their own pain management. What is clear is that expectation is greater now. People expect to be pain free and quite rightly so in most cases. We can now consistently treat and clear many vertebral conditions (for example, disc lesions and facet joint referral) as never before. But with the heightened expectations comes the snag that people are more ready to complain and some conditions cannot be completely cleared by magic hands or scalpels. Hence the endless search adopted by chronic pain sufferers for someone to provide a 'cure'. We must take on the responsibility of preventing this at the acute pain stage.

Our present lifestyle is also very different from that of our ancestors, whose everyday activity was part of living. Movement was inevitable. Today, unless exercise is specifically undertaken, many people lead a sedentary and statically provocative lifestyle. So, did our grandparents, by spontaneously moving and continuing the practice of good functional activities, actually help to reduce their pain, either because they ignored the stimulus or because the physical activity promoted healing?

My previous book was primarily on back care and was addressed to professional readers, aiming to raise their own physical self-awareness before passing this on to their patients. The book has been used in nurses' manual handling training, in physiotherapy departments and training schools, and, as it is easy to read, it is also popular with the lay population.

Now, with physical therapy's growth and development in the past 5 years into a more specialized and sophisticated profession, I felt the need to write a book that was a clinical approach to back pain, rather than on back care *per se*. I wanted to incorporate an approach to acute pain which recognized the negative results of merely treating local tissue pain, ignoring the frequent widespread neurogenic elements and the possibility of dysfunctional stabilization; an approach founded on positive, accurate clinical diagnosis and thorough treatment, on reeducation and rehabilitation. As therapists, we must teach our patients to understand their pain, to pace their activity in relation to it, in the knowledge that activity is essential, and to work with pain in the right way, implementing back care but without back fear. In accepting responsibility for their pain, patients may help to clear the pain and manage any repeating episodes which may occur. This book, then, is more about treating pain and preventing recurrence than about pain prevention alone.

There are many excellent books on examination and assessment in physical therapies, books that are the baseline of our profession. I have therefore avoided this detailed and very specialist field. However, I felt there was a need to gather together the revolutionary thoughts on back pain and place them in a clinical setting for all therapists, osteopaths, chiropractors, orthopaedic nurses, general practitioners or anyone in contact with back pain and pain referral. Hopefully, if we all work towards understanding and shortening the period of acute pain, the number of chronic pain sufferers can be reduced.

In writing this book, I have had some invaluable help from specialists in their fields. It is impossible to say whose help was the greatest, so I shall mention everyone in order of the chapters in which they were involved.

I am eternally grateful to: Nicholas Goddard, orthopaedic consultant at the Royal Free Hospital and the Royal Free Hospital Medical School, for providing the X-rays that I needed; Mark Comerford for his detailed help and advice and hours of telephone discussions about Chapter 5, together with Kinetic Control's permission to use their material throughout the book, both in references and diagrams; Louis Gifford for reading Chapter 7, offering his expert advice and encouragement for me to make my own position clear; John Altree for his advice on pain and acupuncture; Desley Kettle for her ongoing, brilliant clinical advice and for lending me the diagrams she uses in lecturing; Geraldine Turner for thrashing out points and difficult paragraphs as the book progressed; and last but by no means least, Colin for the hours he has spent chasing up articles in the British Library, Belinda for being my tireless guinea-pig reader and Martha for being there at the end of the phone to lend an ear to my stress.

Finally, when treating a patient, I must admit that I frequently feel like a detective searching for clues that will lead to a criminal – except that most of the time there is not one criminal, there is a gang. I hope that this book passes on the excitement felt when one manages, with the patient's help, to solve an intricate puzzle.

London, 2000

Sheila Braggins

Abbreviations

AHCPR	Agency for Health Care Policy and Research	IP	interphalangeal
AMT	adverse mechanical tension	ITB	iliotibial band
ANT	adverse neural tension	ITT	iliotibial tract
A–P	anterior–posterior	IVD	intervertebral disc
AS	ankylosing spondylitis	IVF	intervertebral foramen
ASIS	anterior superior iliac spines	LBP	low back pain
BMD	bone mineral density	LM	lumbar multifidus
CAT scan	computed axial tomography	MOM	(the) mature organism model
CCI	chronic constrictive injury	MRI	magnetic resonance imaging
CHD	coronary heart disease	MSD	musculoskeletal disorder
CLBP	chronic low back pain	MTP	metatarsophalangeal
CNS	central nervous system	NBF	National Bed Federation
CSA	cross-sectional area	NBPA	National Back Pain Association (newly renamed Back Care)
CSAG	Clinical Standards Advisory Group	NN	nervi nervorum
CT	computed tomography	NS (neurones)	nociceptive specific
CTD	cumulative trauma disorders	NSAIDs	non-steroidal antiinflammatory drugs
DH	dorsal horn	OA	osteoarthritis
DOMS	delayed onset muscle pain	PAG	periaqueductal grey matter
DRG	dorsal root ganglion	PEME	pulsed electromagnetic energy
EMG	electromyography	PICR	path of instantaneous centre of rotation
EO	external oblique (muscles)		
EPSP	excitatory postsynaptic potential	PID	prolapsed intervertebral disc
		PKB	prone knee bend
ES	erector spinae	PMH	post medical history
HEA	Health Education Authority	PNF	passive neck flexion
HLA	human leucocyte antigen	PNS	peripheral nervous system
HRT	hormone replacement therapy	PSIS	posterior superior iliac spine
HSC	Health and Safety Council	RA	rheumatoid arthritis
HSE	Health and Safety Executive	RCP	Royal College of Physicians
IAP	intraabdominal pressure	RAb	rectus abdominis
IDD	internal disc disruption	RCGP	Royal College of General Practitioners
IO	internal oblique (muscles)		

RCN	Royal College of Nursing
RICE	rest, ice, compression and elevation
ROM	range of movement
RSI	repetitive strain injury
RTA	road traffic accident
SI (joint)	sacroiliac
SLR (test)	straight leg raise (test)
SNS	sympathetic nervous system
SRT	spinoreticular tract
STT	spinothalamic tract
SWD	short wave diathermy
TA	transversus abdominis

TENS	transcutaneous electrical nerve stimulation
TFL	tensor fascia latae
ULTT	upper limb tension test
VAS	visual analogue scale
VDU	visual display unit
VEP	vertical endplate
WDR	wide dynamic range
WMSD	work related musculoskeletal disorders
WRLUD	work related upper limb disorders

Introduction

As early as 400 BC Hippocrates wrote about treating 'hyboma' or acute lumbar kyphosis (McKenzie 1987) but low back disability is now an ongoing Western epidemic. Hard work and excessive lifting strains must have caused injury through the millennia (how many back pains resulted from the building of the pyramids or Stonehenge?) but today, in spite of sophisticated tools to lessen the toil of labour, disability resulting from simple low back pain (LBP) is a growing problem, engendering considerable health care use and societal costs (Waddell 1998).

In the UK and USA, back pain accounts for the greatest loss of work hours and 60–80% of the population will experience back pain at some time in their lives, with 5% of those in the US impaired or disabled. It is this degree of chronic pain and disability that is causing the greatest concern. In the Saskatchewan Health and Back Pain Survey, 11% of the adult population studied had been disabled by LBP in the previous 6 months (Hurwitz & Morgenstern 1997, Cassidy et al 1998).

Today's lifestyle, more than any other in history, creates an insidious strain on the back, stressing the soft tissues and predisposing them to injury. As described throughout this book, all static postures, sitting or standing, are detrimental. The back is at its most vulnerable in flexion and this is the bane of present society; a greater number of sedentary workers are presenting with back pain than ever before (Refshauge & Gass 1995, HSE 1998) and back pain is occurring more frequently in children who are less fit than they were 10 years ago (CSP 1995).

Motorized transport not only replaced the horse and cart; more damagingly, it replaced human legs. People no longer walk. Cars, buses, trains and planes provide hours of stressful accommodation for the back. The seats into which people drape their bodies may add to the aesthetics of the sitting room, the appearance of a car or the accommodation of an aeroplane, but they too frequently do very little to support the back correctly. This has not always been the case: the craftsmen of William and Mary, Queen Anne and the early Georgians made furniture to show a closeness of functional relationship with the human body which has never been surpassed (Pheasant 1988).

Ergonomics, the study of the often complex interrelationship between people and their occupational, domestic and leisure activities (Hayne 1984), is at last having an effect on the designs of objects in many areas of life. Office furniture is being constantly updated in design to fit the body, especially in the realm of computer work. However, workers need to be taught how to use it all. Car seats are improving in supportive shape and adjustability but again, people need education in their correct use. The industrial environment is being scrutinized, not only from the safety angle but also in relation to back health, with laws and guidance from the EEC (1990) and the HSE (1992, 1998). In an effort to avoid 80 000 back injuries to nurses each year, nursing policy has replaced 'lifting' with 'manual handling', combined with careful assessment of each move and examination of the surrounding environment (HSC 1998, NBPA/RCN 1999). The domestic workplace is an area which seems to be lagging behind: in the easy chair industry luxury is still the overriding criterion, except in rare and specialist designs, and far too many tools in daily use are still overweight (for example, vacuum cleaners).

Standing, sitting, stooping, lifting, pulling, pushing and carrying are the everyday activities of life. When performed with no regard to body mechanics, stress is placed upon the soft tissue

structures of the vertebral column. Poor performance or maintained positions may lead to change in length of these tissues, which in turn can lead to dysfunction. Dysfunction and alteration of the patterns of movement may predispose to injury and pain. Most back pain results from abuse, new use or a culmination of constant overuse and misuse which stress and strain the soft tissues (Maitland 1986) and now 'disuse' needs to be added to this list (Lee 1995).

As medical workers attending to patients, it is important that we realize how devastating back pain can be. In its most minor form, it can be irritating and frustrating; in its more major manifestations the gripping, crippling pain can be of such dimensions that, for the patient, images of permanent disability, wheelchairs and paralysis are all quite common and the possibility of recovery can seem remote. Yet, complete recovery takes place in the majority of cases providing that the damage is not too great, that self-treatment or therapeutic treatment is started early and that function is restored with back care education and pain management implemented.

The medical worker and the patient both bear a responsibility for achieving recovery from simple low back pain and preventing chronicity. The following points appear to be vital.

1. Early pain reduction in the acute stage in the form of advice, medication and pain modulation, possibly with manipulation or mobilization (CSAG 1994, RCGP 1999).
2. Treatment for dysfunction affecting range of movement, neural mobility, dynamic stability and muscle balance. Finally restoring function.
3. Reeducation socially: teaching back care, relating it to the patient's work, home and leisure activities.
4. Reeducation emotionally: simplifying the complexities of pain and teaching pain management; pain *must* be respected but '*hurt does not necessarily harm*' (Gifford 1999).
5. Reeducation physically: describing the body's need for movement, stressing the importance of correct movement, regular movement and regular exercise, especially aerobic activity.

Possibly starting with children in school, the general population should be taught the essential requirements of back care.

1. An awareness of the mechanical function of the healthy back.
2. A knowledge of the structures most at risk and a recognition of the forces that are a danger to those structures.
3. An understanding of the predisposing and precipitating causes of vertebral pain, especially the risk situations.
4. An understanding of the physiological changes that take place during injury and during the healing process.
5. An understanding of pain with the ability to interpret and listen to its messages.
6. An awareness of self-imposed back care at work and at leisure.
7. A sense of responsibility for avoiding injury and pain.

Confidence and reassurance play a major role in recovery. Attitudes to pain are shrouded in too many misconceptions, archaic rules and advice which, far from providing help, often lead to further misinterpretation and mishandling of many signs and symptoms.

With 40 years of 'patient mileage' behind it, this book is intended as a guide for medical workers/therapists in relation to their patients. It is the responsibility of the medical profession to listen, to treat, to rehabilitate and to reeducate. The last point is of major importance and explains the reason for some of the more colloquially descriptive passages in the book.

REFERENCES

Cassidy J D, Carroll L J, Cote P 1998 The Saskatchewan Health and Back Pain Survey. The Prevalence of Low Back Pain and Related Disability in Saskatchewan Adults. Spine 23(17): 1860–1867

CSP 1995 Press release: physiotherapists concerned about unfit, fat, flabby young people. Chartered Society of Physiotherapy, London

Clinical Standards Advisory Group (CSAG) 1994 Back pain. HMSO, London

EEC 1990 Official Journal of the European Communities, No. L 156/17 and 18, 21 June

Gifford L 1999 Tissue and input related mechanisms. In: Gifford L (ed) Topical issues in pain. Physiotherapy Pain Association Year Book 1998–1999. NOI Press, Falmouth, Adelaide

Hayne C 1984 Ergonomics and back pain. Physiotherapy 70(1): 9–13

Health and Safety Commission (HSC) 1998 Manual handling in the health services. HMSO, London

Health and Safety Executive (HSE) 1992 Manual handling – guidance on regulations. HMSO, London

Health and Safety Executive (HSE) 1998 A pain in your work place? HMSO, London

Hurwitz E L, Morgenstern H 1997 Correlates of back problems and back-related disability in the United States. Journal of Clinical Epidemiology 50(6): 669–681

Lee M 1995 Biomechanics of joint movement. In: Refshauge K, Gass E (eds) Musculoskeletal physiotherapy. Clinical science and practice. Butterworth Heinemann, Oxford

McKenzie R 1987 Mechanical diagnosis and therapy for low back pain. In: Twomey L T, Taylor J R (eds) Physical therapy for the low back. Churchill Livingstone, New York

Maitland G D 1986 Vertebral manipulation, 5th edn. Butterworths, London

National Back Pain Association (NBPA)/Royal College of Nursing (RCN) 1999 The guide to the handling of patients. NBPA, Teddington

Pheasant S 1988 Body space. Anthropometry, ergonomics and design. Taylor & Francis, London

Refshauge K M, Gass E M 1995 The context of musculoskeletal physiotherapy practice. In: Refshauge K, Gass E (eds) Musculoskeletal physiotherapy. Clinical science and practice. Butterworth Heinemann, Oxford

Royal College of General Practitioners (RCGP) 1999 Clinical guidelines for the management of acute low back pain. Royal College of General Practitioners, London

Waddell G 1998 The back pain revolution. Churchill Livingstone, Edinburgh

Function and dysfunction

1

The human back

FORM AND MOVEMENT

As the central pivot of the body, the back needs to be strong and stable. It is symbolically recognized as the strength of the body; 'put your back into it' means that there is heavy work to be done. However, the back may run into trouble if this saying is actually carried out. The back is not designed to *perform* the work, it is designed to act as a strong adaptable base while the arms and legs execute the activities. The back muscles and the abdominal muscles provide the source for this stabilization (Richardson et al 1992, Sahrmann 1993, Jull & Richardson 1994, Comerford & Kinetic Control 1998). This will be discussed throughout the following chapters.

Because of the engineering skill of its design, the back's solidity and strength in no way inhibit its mobility. Its flexibility means that its shape can be adapted to withstand changing forces, thus ensuring stability (Aspden 1989, Panjabi 1992). The back allows for movement in all directions: forward flexion, extension, side flexion and rotation. Combined movements are used many times a day in common activities, often while performing lifting tasks, for example in the act of picking up a heavy suitcase.

Before looking at the biomechanics of the back, it is important to look at the overall shape of the spine and the way in which this shape has developed.

THE SHAPING OF THE CURVES

At birth, after lying in the fetal position in the womb, the baby's back is curved with only slight cervical extension. As the baby learns to hold its head up, the cervical spine changes, and by the time the baby is sitting up the **cervical lordosis** is an established spinal curve (Fig. 1.1). Later, when the toddler stands, the spine adapts still further, forming the **lumbar lordosis** (Fig. 1.2). The result is a prolonged 'S' shape, concave at the top and bottom and convex in the middle, the thoracic **kyphosis**.

The 'S' shape with its alternating curves is a valuable characteristic of the overall mechanism, giving the spine a spring-like action, with a bounce and recoil that a straight rod of bone could never provide, adding strength to adaptability. The curvature of the spine is essential for its load-bearing function (Aspden 1989). The lumbar curve is the strongest section, taking the greatest postural strain and burden of activity. Aspden (1989) compares the lumbar spine to a masonry arch, which is supported strongly on the convex side by the abdominal muscles and intraabdominal pressure (see Chapter 14). All three curves and their relationship to each other play an integral part in the function of the healthy back.

In daily living, whether standing or sitting, constantly maintained postures influence the curves, either increasing or flattening them. Alteration of one curve affects the others (Kendle et al 1993). Changes in the curves correspondingly alter the surrounding structures and permanent adaptation takes place, forcing soft tissues into new shapes and new roles. Lack of the right exercise with inappropriate patterns of movement may lead to muscle imbalance and dysfunction while insufficient activity with maintained positions may lead to alteration of tissue length, with some tissues becoming longer and weaker while others shorten and stiffen.

Permanent changes in soft tissue may lead to a decrease in mobility and/or stability. The 'springy' facility no longer remains intact and the overall mechanism ceases to be as efficient. The three curves need to be preserved with care, neither exaggerated nor diminished, the shape maintained with constant stabilizing correction and the flexibility maintained with movement. The back then retains its essential characteristics of strength with mobility.

This is why posture is so important to back care. 'Habitual movement can **induce** pathology, not just be a result of it – musculoskeletal pain syndromes are seldom isolated events' (Sahrmann 1993). Much of the literature discounts the link between posture and pain. There is no proof that good posture will prevent pain (Refshauge & Gass 1995). People with bad posture are frequently pain free but clinically, dysfunction and loss of mobility are the main precursors for musculoskeletal pain.

However, the literature does not support clinical observations. Pain is subjective and dysfunction is objective, something that can be measured with ensuing poor movement, weak-

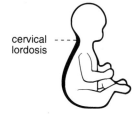

Figure 1.1 The first spinal curve.

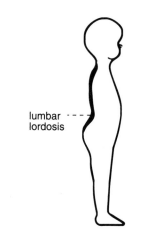

Figure 1.2 The S-shaped spine.

ness and muscle changes in length, stiffness and inhibition. Very little research has tried to measure the clinical observation that poor posture may lead to dysfunction which may in turn lead to pain (M Comerford, personal communication, 1999). This is questioned and discussed by Bookhout (1996) and Herbert (1995), who hopes that in the coming years it will be researched and finally better understood.

The connection between altered posture and pain is not an easy subject to research as dysfunction may never cause pain unless it is compromised in some way. So a good posture may have a hidden dysfunction that is never exposed and a poor posture with obvious dysfunction may never be stressed. In clinical practice the relationship between poor posture and dysfunction and dysfunction and pain is common, and frequently merely postural correction, for example around the shoulder girdle area, will actually eliminate pain.

Not only are the three curves interrelated but pelvic position and limb position have an effect on the back. Pronated feet, medially rotated femurs, knee flexion or hyperextension in standing and hamstring length all affect the position and shape of the pelvic musculature and the function of the lumbar spine (Kendle et al 1993). Similarly, arm movements are stabilized by upper quadrant musculature. Maintained postures with stressful arm activity, prolonged inactivity or functionally inaccurate activity can generate alteration of the muscle balance around the shoulder girdle, affecting

joint structure and neural tissue (Mottram 1997). The body is a whole and, especially with regard to the skeletal structures, each part must be considered in relation to the rest. So although the curves are a component of the back, they must be viewed as a part of the entire body shape from the feet upwards.

Panjabi (1992) describes the basic biomechanical functions of the spinal system (Box 1.1). Alteration of spinal shape, injury or disease can all affect the mechanisms involved with movement. Disturbance of function may lead to pain.

Box 1.1   The basic biomechanical functions of the spinal system

1. To allow movements between body parts
2. To carry loads
3. To protect the spinal cord and nerve roots

Key points

- The three spinal curves maintain the springy adaptability of the vertebral column.
- The abdominal muscles provide vital support for the lumbar arch.
- Altered posture affects the curves and their relationship with each other.
- Maintained poor posture may lead to dysfunction which may lead to pain.
- Stabilization of the upper and lower quadrants is essential for good arm and leg movement.

REFERENCES

Aspden R M 1989 The spine as an arch, a new mathematical model. Spine 14(3): 266–274
Bookhout M R 1996 Exercise and somatic dysfunction. Physical Medicine and Rehabilitation Clinics of North America 7(4): 845–862
Comerford M, Kinetic Control 1998 Dynamic stability and muscle balance. Course notes. Kinetic Control Ltd, Harrow
Herbert R 1995 Adaptations of muscle and connective tissue. In: Refshauge K, Gass E (eds) Musculoskeletal physiotherapy: clinical science and practice, Butterworth Heinemann, Oxford
Jull G A, Richardson C A 1994 Rehabilitation of active

stabilisation of the lumbar spine. In: Taylor R J, Twomey L T (eds) Physical therapy of the low back. Churchill Livingstone, New York
Kendle F P, McCreary E K, Provance P G 1993 Muscle testing and function, 3rd edn. Williams and Wilkins, Baltimore
Mottram S L 1997 Dynamic stability of the scapula. Manual Therapy 2(3): 123–131
Panjabi M M 1992 The stabilizing system of the spine. Part 1. Function, dysfunction, adaptation, and enhancement. Journal of Spinal Disorders 5(4): 383–389
Refshauge K M, Gass E M 1995 The context of musculoskeletal physiotherapy practice. In: Refshauge K,

Gass E (eds) Musculoskeletal physiotherapy: clinical science and practice. Butterworth Heinemann, Oxford

Richardson C, Jull G, Toppenberg R, Comerford M 1992 Techniques for active lumbar stabilisation for spinal protection: a pilot study. Australian Physiotherapy 38(2): 105–112

Sahrmann S 1993 Course study notes. Washington University School of Medicine

2

The vertebral column

THE STRUCTURE OF BONE

Bone is a uniquely versatile tissue combining strength with adaptability. It moulds its structure to accommodate long-term stress and is continually modelling and remodelling itself:

- by the control of hormones which stabilize blood calcium
- in response to long-term changes of force patterns (strains and stresses) acting on the bone.

Growth and remodelling, regulating both the size and shape of bone, depend on balanced activity between two cell types: **osteoclasts** (which remove bone tissue) and **osteoblasts** (which lay down new tissue) (Palastanga et al 1991).

Daily usage provides the loads that cause strains and stress in bone. Strains are the forces that tend to deform bone and stress the internal force that resists them (Frost 1995). Modelling can add to and strengthen bone under strain and remodelling can remove bone when the mechanical need for it ceases.

Most bones consist of two definite types: **compact** bone and **cancellous** bone (Table 2.1). Bones are enclosed by a tough outer covering, the **periosteum**, containing nutrient arteries which nourish the bone cells.

BONY ANATOMY

The vertebral column

As all therapists are familiar with the anatomy

11

Table 2.1 The difference between compact and cancellous bone

Type of bone	Structure	Area found
Compact bone	Thousands of Haversian systems, composed of four parts: lamellae, lacunae (small cavities filled with osteocytes), canaliculi and the Haversian canal (a channel containing blood vessels). Held together by interstitial tissue	Shaft of long bones Outer layer of vertebral bodies
Cancellous or spongy bone	A web of trabeculae running in many directions, arranged to resist compressive, tensile and shearing stresses. Spaces between filled with red marrow	At the ends of long bones Vertebral bodies

of the vertebral column, only those aspects relevant to biomechanics will be discussed.

The vertebral column consists of 33 **vertebrae**, 24 of which are individual, jointed bones placed one above the other starting from the sacrum as the base (Fig. 2.1). Between each vertebra is the **intervertebral disc**.

The seven cervical vertebrae are the smallest and the most mobile, having only the head to support. In the atlantooccipital region (between the skull and the atlas) flexion is 20° but side flexion is limited to 8°. The suboccipital region (C1 and C2) is especially designed to give 15° of rotation in both directions, with flexion/extension of only a few degrees (Palastanga et al 1991). In the lower cervical region (C3–T1), side flexion and rotation occur as linked movements, flexion being about 25° with extension 85°, side flexion about 40° to each side, rotation 50° in each direction (Palastanga et al 1991).

The 12 thoracic vertebrae are larger than the cervical. They are attached to the ribs and are adapted for this purpose. The combined range of flexion/extension is between 50° and 70° with flexion much greater than extension. Side flexion

has a range of 20–25°, being greater in the lower half of the region. In spite of possible rib restriction, thoracic rotation is surprisingly large, 35° in each direction. This is due to the special orientation of the facet joints.

The five lumbar vertebrae are the largest and toughest, designed to bear the full weight of the upper body. Flexion and extension are relatively free, with flexion about 55° and extension 30°. Side flexion varies with age from a large 60° in youth to a grossly limited range. Rotation is limited by the orientation of the facet joints, being only a few degrees, slightly greater in flexion than in extension (Palastanga et al 1991).

The five sacral vertebrae are fused together to form the triangular **sacrum**. The upper surface of S1 bears the full weight of the trunk. This would tend to rotate the sacrum forwards were it not for strong controlling ligaments (Taylor & Twomey 1994). The sacrum joins the ilium of the two innominate or hip bones on either side, forming the **sacroiliac joint** (Fig. 2.2).

The **coccyx** is composed of four rudimentary vertebrae which lie below the sacrum. Their only articulation is with the apex of the sacrum. The bones are directed downwards and forwards (Fig. 2.1).

The pelvis

The pelvis consists of the sacrum, the coccyx and the two innominate bones. The innominate bones consist of three areas: the **ilium**, the **ischium** and the **pubis**, all uniting around the **acetabulum**, the recess for articulation with the head of the **femur** (Fig. 2.2). The **greater trochanter** of the femur is palpable as a large bony knob at the top of the thigh. Patients are often confused about pain in the area of the iliac crest/greater trochanter and worry because a hip replacement is obviously imminent (Patient advice 2.1).

The **ilium** is the large portion above the acetabulum. It has an extended crest which runs from the **anterior superior iliac spine** (ASIS) at the front to the **posterior superior iliac spine** (PSIS) at the rear (Fig. 2.2). The landmarks are easily palpable by placing the fingers and thumb

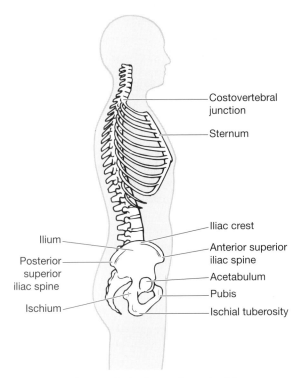

Figure 2.1   The vertebral column, ribs and pelvis.

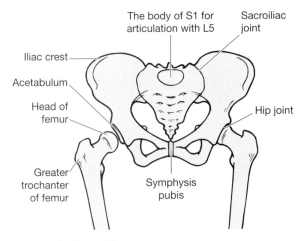

Figure 2.2   The pelvis.

around the waist and pressing down onto the **iliac crest**. The anterior superior iliac spine is the bony prominence palpable on each side in the front while at the back the two dimples by the sacrum clearly denote the two posterior superior iliac spines (Figs 2.1 & 2.2).

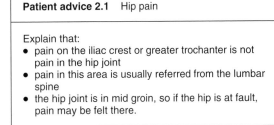

> **Patient advice 2.1**   Hip pain
>
> Explain that:
> * pain on the iliac crest or greater trochanter is not pain in the hip joint
> * pain in this area is usually referred from the lumbar spine
> * the hip joint is in mid groin, so if the hip is at fault, pain may be felt there.

The **ischium** is the lower part of the innominate surrounding the posterior part of the acetabulum. The most obvious landmark is the **ischial tuberosity** which is palpable in the sitting position (Fig. 2.1).

The **pubis** is the most anterior portion, the two pubic promontories coming together to form the **symphysis pubis** which can be palpated below the abdomen (Fig. 2.2).

The vertebral column and pelvis provide the body with two contradictory needs: rigidity and mobility (Kapandji 1974) (Box 2.1).

A typical lumbar vertebra

It is beyond the scope of this book to provide detailed anatomy of each vertebral type but although they vary considerably in size and architecture, the overall principles are the same.

A typical lumbar vertebra can be divided into anterior and posterior elements united by a bridge of bone called the **pedicle**. The anterior element is made up of the vertebral body and the posterior element consists of the neural arch, laminae, spinous process, transverse processes and articular processes (Figs 2.3 & 2.4). The two sections play very different functional roles, hence the complete contrast of design.

Box 2.1 Two seemingly opposing functions of the vertebral column	
Rigidity	Tough bones, giving strength and support as well as protection for soft tissue within and around them
Mobility	Provided by the presence of many small-jointed bones rather than one long pole

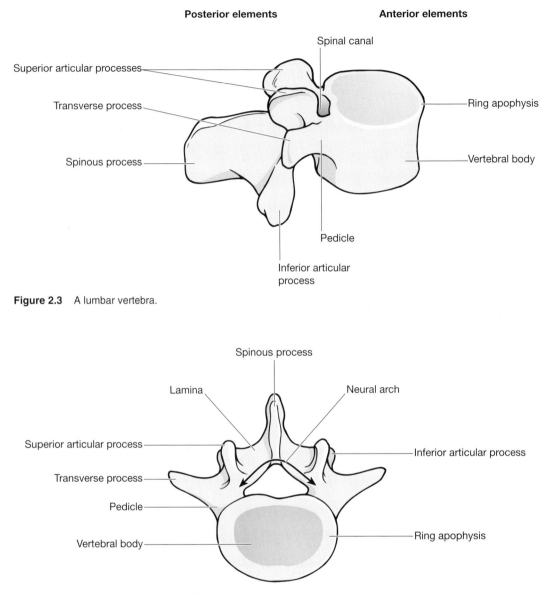

Figure 2.3 A lumbar vertebra.

Figure 2.4 Lumbar vertebra viewed from above.

The **vertebral body** resembles a kidney-shaped drum. It is designed to sustain immense vertical loads, the whole weight of the trunk being transmitted through the solid structures. Although solid, vertebral bodies are not heavy. They are constructed of vertical and transverse beams of cancellous bone trabeculae, surrounded by a shell of cortical bone. The space between the trabeculae forms convenient channels for the blood supply and venous drainage of the vertebral body and even for the making of blood cells. When filled with blood, the area appears like a sponge and is referred to as the vertebral **spongiosa**. This structure forms a rigid, lightweight cylinder, able to sustain huge longitudinal pressures as weight is transmitted from one body to another (Bogduk & Twomey 1991). The central area of the upper surface of the vertebral body is perforated with minute holes and surrounded by a small rim of smoother bone on the perimeter, the **ring apophysis** (Figs 2.3 & 2.4). The perforations at the top, as well as others visible on the posterior body wall, are openings for the transmission of tiny blood vessels to the vertebral body.

The **pedicles** (Figs 2.3 & 2.4) are the connecting link between the vertebral body and the posterior elements. They are subjected to considerable bending force when the muscles of the back, attached mainly to the posterior elements, exert a downward pressure on the rear of the spine (Bogduk & Twomey 1991). It is worth examining a vertebra with a patient in order to visualize these forces when the back is functioning, especially in moments of heavy lifting.

The **neural arch** is the semicircle of bone from pedicle to pedicle which, together with the posterior border of the vertebral body, forms the circumference of the vertebral or **spinal canal** (Fig. 2.4). The role of the spinal canal is to give solid protection to the sensitive structures inside the canal: the spinal cord and its meninges, the nerve roots and blood vessels.

The **laminae** are two leaves of bone on the posterior border of the neural arch that eventually join together to form the spinous process. As the spinous process is an area of considerable muscular attachment, any force exerted upon it must be transmitted through the lamina.

The **spinous process** is the rounded projection that is palpable from one vertebra to another down the back (Fig. 2.3).

The **transverse processes** project laterally on either side from the junction of the pedicle and lamina. Together with the spinous process, they provide areas for muscular and ligamentous attachments.

The **articular processes** – superior and inferior – are the joint-forming elements of the vertebrae. The inferior articular processes of one vertebra lock onto the superior articular processes of the vertebra below to form the **zygapophyseal** or **facet** joints (see Chapter 3).

The **intervertebral foramen** (IVF) is an opening which only becomes apparent when two vertebrae are articulated (see Fig. 3.2). On an individual vertebra the upper and lower halves of the foramen appear merely as two unnamed notches between the articular processes and the vertebral body. As soon as the motion segment is articulated, they form the pear-shaped circumference of the IVF. The IVF is the vital and important passageway for the spinal nerve, the sinuvertebral nerve and blood vessels entering and leaving the canal. Each IVF is narrowed by rotation of the spine towards it and enlarged with rotation away from it. The IVF can be narrowed by the formation of osteophytes.

BONY DISORDERS

Trauma, disease and deformity are the three main bony disorders.

Trauma

Trauma to bone is usually related to an accident in sport or transport, falls or assault of one kind or another. Direct trauma to bone can result in damage at the point of impact or take the form of force thrust through the bony structure. Mourad (1991) gives very clear descriptions of types of fractures and the complications which may ensue.

Vertebral fractures

Microdamage. Repeated loading and deloading as in running cause microscopic damage which can weaken bone sufficiently to allow normal usage to cause stress fractures or spontaneous fractures. Small amounts of microdamage seldom cause pain but pain can result if there is enough microdamage to result in a fracture. This can affect aggressive athletes or those with conditions such as osteoporosis (Frost 1995).

Avulsion fractures. Sudden twisting movements with thrust or great pressure behind them, as in road accidents or whiplash injuries, can avulse small particles of bone at the junction of ligamentous or muscular attachments on any of the vertebral processes.

Compression fractures. Compression fractures of the vertebral body can be sustained by a fall from a height, perhaps landing on the base of the spine, or by a weight falling onto the shoulders or as a result of vertical force such as ejection from a pilot's seat (Porter 1986). Such fractures can occur in youth and may not be discovered until later in life when for one reason or another X-rays of the spine are taken. They sometimes result in the vertebral body becoming wedge shaped which may in turn lead to deformity (see 'Scoliosis' and 'Thoracic kyphosis', pp. 20 and 23).

The danger of spinal fracture lies in the possible damage to neural tissue in both the vertebral canal and the IVF. If the spinal canal is already narrow (see 'Spinal stenosis', p. 50), a flexion deformity which follows a compression fracture may cause critical compression of the spinal cord with resulting paraplegia (Porter 1986). Neurological damage is lessened if the posterior elements avoid injury. Generally a compression fracture without bony injury to pedicles, facet joints or lamina is not considered to be a serious injury (Porter 1986). A simple fracture with no displacement should heal well with little resulting discomfort.

The process of injury and healing in fractures

The process of injury and healing in a fracture can be divided into three phases: inflammatory, repair and remodelling (Box 2.2) (Mourad 1991, Thomas 1992).

In the repair phase, callus is made of immature woven bone and does not have the sophisticated structure of mature bone. As the purpose of callus is to prevent relative movements of bone ends, it continues to form until it is strong enough to prevent movement. Production of callus is therefore initiated and maintained by movement. If there is no movement at all, then no callus will form; if there is too much movement it will continue to grow in an attempt to stop it. Callus is a 'one-off' response. If it does not occur within a few weeks of injury it will not occur at all (Thomas 1992).

There is no definite moment of fracture union.

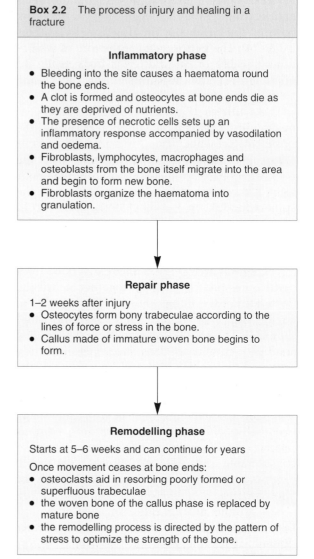

Box 2.2 The process of injury and healing in a fracture

Inflammatory phase

- Bleeding into the site causes a haematoma round the bone ends.
- A clot is formed and osteocytes at bone ends die as they are deprived of nutrients.
- The presence of necrotic cells sets up an inflammatory response accompanied by vasodilation and oedema.
- Fibroblasts, lymphocytes, macrophages and osteoblasts from the bone itself migrate into the area and begin to form new bone.
- Fibroblasts organize the haematoma into granulation.

Repair phase

1–2 weeks after injury
- Osteocytes form bony trabeculae according to the lines of force or stress in the bone.
- Callus made of immature woven bone begins to form.

Remodelling phase

Starts at 5–6 weeks and can continue for years

Once movement ceases at bone ends:
- osteoclasts aid in resorbing poorly formed or superfluous trabeculae
- the woven bone of the callus phase is replaced by mature bone
- the remodelling process is directed by the pattern of stress to optimize the strength of the bone.

The clinician uses the X-ray appearance, professional experience, the extent of the original injury and the presence or absence of pain to decide when weight bearing can take place (Thomas 1992).

All fractures are extremely painful and movement can be excruciating. In certain fractures, for example those of the pelvis, blood loss can be significant. In cases of multiple fractures metabolic changes can take place which can cause the patient to enter a catabolic state for several days. Psychologically, fractures can be an alarming experience. Apart from the shock of injury, fear over the prognosis and bewilderment because of the new experience of plasters and crutches can be quite overpowering. Patients need great support and reassurance (Thomas 1992).

Disease

Persistent pain evokes a nagging fear that something 'nasty' is happening within the body, even if it is obvious that the pain started after tripping over a stone. As therapists, one of our priorities must be to eliminate fear. To do this, we have to be confident in our first assessment and diagnosis. If the patient has been referred full investigations may have been made but any doubtful signs or symptoms should be rechecked with the referring practitioner. If the patient is self-referred and if we feel that there is evidence of some serious structural change, then further investigation should be requested.

X-rays are often taken quite unnecessarily before commencing any physical treatment. They show no soft tissue injury and in most cases give no clue to the cause of pain but they do serve to discount the presence of bony disease or deformity.

Describing the possible bony diseases, for example tumour, tuberculosis, Paget's disease, osteomalacia, etc., serves no purpose in this book, particularly as physical exercises can be entirely contraindicated in certain cases. Porter (1986), Mourad (1991) and Tidswell (1992) all give excellent information on this subject. However, it is important to mention two conditions that are extremely relevant to back care: osteoporosis and ageing in bone.

Osteoporosis

Characteristics. Osteoporosis occurs when the process of bone resorption and new formation breaks down; the balance is disturbed, with resorption becoming more extensive than bone deposition: osteoclast activity outpaces osteoblast activity. The marrow spaces are enlarged, the medullary trabecular bone is sparse and the cortical bone thin from loss of bone mineral and collagenous protein mix. There is a tendency for the more horizontal trabeculae to disappear and the vertical trabeculae to be preserved (Mourad 1991, Darby 1992, Dixon 1996).

Osteoporosis is now recognized to be a disease of major importance, affecting 40% of women over 70 years of age (RCP 1999). Its major consequences – wrist, vertebral and hip fractures – are associated with significant morbidity (RCP 1999).

Diagnosis. Ordinary X-rays are inefficient for detecting early osteoporosis as 30% of bone mineral density (BMD) must be lost before it shows with certainty. A screening test, single-energy X-ray absorptiometry, provides a simple method of assessing bone density at specific sites and dual-energy X-ray absorptiometry measures more precise bone density in vulnerable sites such as the lumbar spine and femoral neck (Silver & Einhorn 1995, Dixon 1996, RCP 1999).

Bone loss rate can also be measured biochemically. Two thresholds of BMD have been defined by the World Health Organization on the basis of the relationship of fracture risk to BMD (Table 2.2) (RCP 1999).

Cause. Although osteoporosis can be the consequence of ageing, the three most influential factors are hormonal, mechanical and nutritional. If there is a deficiency in any of these areas, bone loss is likely to occur. The disease is five times more common in women, especially postmenopausal women, but it also occurs in men and in fact can affect people of all ages, although

Table 2.2 The classification of osteoporosis based on BMD thresholds

Definition	BMD value
'Osteoporosis'	T-score –2.5
Low bone mass or osteopenia	T-score between –1 and –2.5
'Severe' or 'established' osteoporosis	Osteoporosis as defined above plus one or more documented fragility fractures

T-score is the young adult mean for BMD

it is still more common after the age of 50 (Grieve 1989, Drinkwater 1995, Silver & Einhorn 1995, Rollo 1996, National Osteoporosis Society 1997). Osteoporosis can occur in pregnancy but it is uncertain whether pregnancy is the causative factor or the highlighting event (Dunne 1994). However, there could be a link with lactation and the fetal demand for calcium (Khastigir & Studd 1994, Rizzoli & Bonjour 1996).

Hormonal. Mature bone requires the normal function of parathyroid hormones and the sex hormones oestrogen and androgen. The decrease in oestrogen in the menopause is one of the most discussed areas of hormonal change but recent studies of athletes have disclosed a complicated picture with regard to exercise and hormonal changes. It appears that despite vigorous activity, oligo/amenorrhoeic athletes have lower BMD than women with normal menses and some studies have reported a low BMD in male runners. In fact, excessive exercise can result in low testosterone levels in men and low oestrogen levels, amenorrhoea and subsequent decrease in vertebral BMD in women (Drinkwater 1995, Swezey 1996).

Mechanical. Because of the beneficial effect of strains and stress on bone tissue, it is not surprising that osteoporosis is linked to immobility and lack of exercise; it is easier to lose bone through inactivity than to gain it through functional loading. Immobilization for whatever reason leads to a decrease in BMD, for example long-term bed rest or immobilization in plaster, or just lack of daily activity and exercise. Rollo (1996) suggests that the inability to rise from a chair without using one's arms can be a risk factor for a fractured femur.

Nutritional and other factors. Nutritionally, a decrease in dietary protein, calcium, phosphorus and vitamins C and D predisposes to osteoporosis. Metabolically, there is a negative calcium balance and an increase in bone collagen breakdown in the urine (Dixon 1996).

People on long-term, high-dose corticosteroids, high doses of thyroxin and those with certain chronic illness states are all at risk. Heavy smoking, heavy drinking, a lack of sunshine and a familial record of osteoporosis are all factors which may contribute (Dixon 1996, RCP 1999).

Presentation. Osteoporosis can be localized or general. It manifests in the frequent femoral neck fractures of the older age group and in the 'dowager's hump' found in the lower cervical spine of office workers who maintain poor static postures of the C6–C7 area. It is responsible for considerable vertebral pain, often manifesting as a persistent, deep bony ache in the lower thoracic area, sometimes with girdle pains. This vertebral pain is often ascribed to trabecular buckling or trabecular fractures but may also be due to venous stasis in the spongiosa of the vertebral bodies (Grieve 1989).

LBP can be a frequent symptom with radiation into the buttocks and upper thighs. There is shortening of stature, increased thoracic kyphosis, with the lower ribs settling on the iliac crests in severe cases, and a possibility of vertebral fractures as a result of minor trauma, such as a cough or sneeze (Grieve 1989, Twomey & Taylor 1994). Following hip fractures, one in five patients with osteoporosis will die within 6 months and half will be unable to live independently afterwards (National Osteoporosis Society 1997, RCP 1999).

Treatment and prevention.

Medication and nutrition. Hormone replacement therapy (HRT) will stop or slow bone loss at any age, although the longer after the menopause, the less is the effect. Other medication can include thyroparathyroid agents (calcium regulators), bisphosphonates and calcitonin, anabolic steroids, fluoride, vitamin D and calcium supplements (Dixon 1996, RCP 1999).

Adequate calcium, which is found in milk products, water, pulses and vegetables, is essential for bone health, together with a balanced diet. Sunshine also plays an important role in activating vitamin D, providing, of course, that all precautions are taken with regard to skin protection.

Exercise. Recently, considerable attention has been given to the important role of exercise in the prevention of osteoporosis (Taylor & Twomey 1994). However, research is identifying the effects of specific forms of exercise as well as of exercise in general. Weight-bearing exercises such as walking and jogging, which play an important role in aerobic conditioning, seem to have only a modest benefit in the prevention and treatment of osteoporosis, whereas site-specific isometric and resistive exercises appear to have a more consistent effect on BMD. In other words, skaters develop a greater leg and pelvic BMD than non-athletes but less in the arms and/or spine; tennis players have greater BMD in their dominant hands and forearms, as do weight lifters, rowers and labourers, compared to office workers. Lumbar-spine BMD and whole-body BMD are significantly higher in gymnasts (Drinkwater 1995, Smith 1995, Swezey 1996, RCP 1999).

Drinkwater (1995) suggests that one of the best ways to exercise all the major muscle groups is to incorporate 'bone building' as well as aerobic activities into one's daily living: walk instead of drive, climb stairs instead of using elevators, go backpacking, go cross-country skiing, use a rowing machine and use weight training for different areas. Rollo (1996) adds that women over 65, who are able, should walk for exercise and spend a minimum of 4 hours a day on their feet. Women must commit themselves to a lifetime of exercise.

In children longitudinal bone growth adds new trabecular bone and length to cortical bone. Modelling can thicken and strengthen both, while remodelling can conserve or remove them. As adults no longer have longitudinal bone growth and effective cortical bone modelling, remodelling mostly maintains the bone mass and strength they accumulated during growth. For this reason children should aim to achieve and maintain a high peak bone mass so that despite the inevitable later age-related bone loss, there is always enough reserve bone strength to resist trivial trauma (Frost 1995, Dixon 1996, Swezey 1996).

One of the reasons why astronauts must exercise regularly in space is that a few days of gravitational weightlessness can cause them to lose massive amounts of bone density (Twomey 1989).

Box 2.3   Treatment for osteoporosis

Treatment should be based on:
- postural correction and exercises to maintain flexibility and aerobic activity
- exercises to improve balance, to diminish the risk of falling
- site-specific exercises with care, recommended by Robert Swezey:
  - lifting free weights or pulley-attached weights
  - combination of minimally expandable elastic strap stretching and inflatable ball squeezing.

These exercises should be applied to the key areas, e.g. neck, back and upper and lower extremities, two to three times per week for 10–45 minutes (depending upon the length of the warm-up periods). When properly performed, these exercises are safe, convenient and economical and have been demonstrated to have a strengthening effect.

(Reproduced with permission from Swezey 1996)

Physical therapy. Osteoporosis is a contra-indication to vigorous manual therapy as there is a risk of fracture and so any manual treatments should be applied with very gentle forces (Refshauge & Latimer 1995). Therapists need to be aware that in cases of severe osteoporosis, lumbar flexion-abdominal crunching exercises can predispose the back to spinal compression fractures. Any overstressful exercise with no proper conditioning, even in healthy adults, can also lead to stress fractures (Swezey 1996) (Box 2.3).

Age changes in bone (Box 2.4)

Peak bone mass is obtained by the age of 30, after which individuals lose a small amount

---

Box 2.4   Age changes in bone

1. Overall decrease in bone density and bone strength.
2. Loss of support in horizontal beams of bone in the vertebral body which leads to buckling of the vertebra.
3. Risk of stenosis and osteoporosis.
4. Formation of osteophytes.
5. These changes accent the need for exercise for the trunk and arms and constant use of full-range leg movements to be continued well into old age.

each year. In young people, the load-bearing capacity of the vertebral body is 1000 kg which reduces to 80–150 kg in an elderly person (Zipnick et al 1996).

Vertebrae may widen, become wedge shaped or collapse with loss of mass. The increase in width is caused by the addition of new consolidated layers at the periosteal surface while removal of bone occurs at the centre of the vertebra. **Osteophytes** are formed by bone seemingly in a protective attempt to increase the surface area to support loads.

Spinal stenosis (see p. 50) and osteoporosis are the two most common results of ageing. Bone disease can cause considerable spinal pain and can also lead to deformity.

Deformity

Deformity is more common than disease but is often misleading in relation to pain. Many people with deformities live completely pain-free lives, unaware of anything amiss. However, deformity does provide a dysfunction which may cause structures to succumb to stress more easily than a perfect mechanism, thus becoming an indirect cause of pain.

Deformity of bone can occur during fetal development (Taylor & Twomey 1994), during the later growth period or as a result of accident at any age. It can also be the result of disease. It can take the form of an alteration of vertebral body shape, an inequality in the shape of the facet joints, a variation in the size of the vertebral canal or any bony irregularity of any part of the vertebra, even to the fusion of two vertebrae. The following are some of the more common vertebral anomalies.

Unilateral hemivertebra

A unilateral hemivertebra is a fault in fetal development. When one side of the vertebral body fails to develop, a congenital scoliosis results. Developmental failure of the anterior area of the body leads to a congenital kyphosis.

Scoliosis

Seen from the rear, the normal vertebral column appears straight and symmetrical with sometimes a slight thoracic curve to the right, possibly due to the arch of the aorta.

Scoliosis is defined by the Scoliosis Research Society as a structural lateral curve of the spine exceeding 10°. A non-structural scoliosis is a problem of right–left symmetry but a structural scoliosis is combined with a front–back asymmetry, a complex three-dimensional deformity involving all planes (Banks & Garvey 1994, Millner & Dickson 1996). There are several types of scoliosis.

Osteopathic or structural scoliosis. This can be created by a vertebral asymmetry which can be congenital or acquired. The wedge-shaped bone in Figure 2.5 can result from a failure of bony development, a vertebral fracture sustained in childhood or from bone disease.

Neuromuscular scoliosis. The spine may be normal at birth but any neuromuscular condition, for example cerebral palsy or one of the muscular dystrophies, can affect the stabilizing spinal musculature with resulting alteration in spinal shape (Eisenstein & Draycott 1992).

Idiopathic scoliosis (ISc). Also called 'cause unknown', this is the most common type. The spine is usually normal at birth but deforms

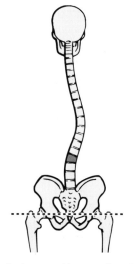

Figure 2.5 Scoliosis caused by a wedge-shaped vertebra.

with rapid growth for reasons not understood. It develops most often in adolescent girls from age 10 to the end of skeletal growth, although infantile and juvenile ISc do exist (Kisner & Colby 1990, Banks & Garvey 1994).

There is usually an element of structural abnormality which results in a lateral bending (coronal plane), associated with axial rotation (transverse plane) and increased or decreased flexion/extension (sagittal plane). The rib 'hump', particularly evident on flexion, occurs because of rotation in the thoracic spine. This buckling develops during the growth phase and tends to occur more in taller adolescents. The curve can be associated with a decrease or increase of thoracic kyphosis or lumbar lordosis and an inequality of shoulder levels. With increasing curvatures there can be some pulmonary compromise (Eisenstein & Draycott 1992, Banks & Garvey 1994, Millner & Dickson 1996)

Some reports show that there is a correlation between handedness and spinal configuration. Goldberg & Dowling (1991) believe that idiopathic scoliosis, which can be a hereditary trait, is possibly an expression of cerebral organization, which is itself a genetically influenced asymmetry of form and function (Hansen et al 1994).

Non-structural scoliosis. Spasm in the back muscles in acute back pain can elicit a temporary scoliosis, as can habitual asymmetric postures.

Another of the more common causes is an alteration of the base level from which the spine grows: either an irregularity of pelvic symmetry or a difference in leg length which causes the pelvis to tip to one side, both altering the level of the sacrum (Fig. 2.6). There need only be a difference of half a centimetre to induce a scoliosis. Leg length difference can be checked in standing either by looking at the horizontal positioning of the posterior superior iliac spines or by placing both hands along the iliac crests which should be level with each other. If there is a true leg length difference, the spine should straighten in sitting. Leg length can also be ascertained in lying, measuring from the ASIS to

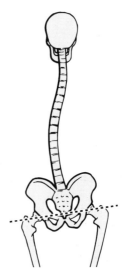

Figure 2.6   Scoliosis caused by a difference in leg length.

the medial malleolus; however, pelvic symmetry must be checked first (Kendal et al 1993).

Difference in leg length is extremely common but the cause is often unknown. Before the advent of poliomyelitis vaccine, shortening due to the muscle paralysis of one leg used to be a common cause (Specht & De Boer 1991, Evans & Draycott 1992). Congenital abnormality, infection of bone and joint, fractures of long bones or overgrowth of one limb can all cause inequality of leg length.

Treatment. There is no statistical increase in the incidence of low back pain in scoliotic backs but disc degeneration at the apex of the curve does occur (Wiltse 1971, Dieck et al 1985). There is some doubt as to whether exercises are of help in controlling idiopathic scoliosis but it is reasonable to incorporate exercise to improve general fitness (Banks & Garvey 1994).

Bracing should be considered for curves over 20°, with operative procedures considered for curves over 40° (Kisner & Colby 1990). In some centres bracing has been abandoned, not only because it is unacceptable for sensitive teenagers but because recent studies have raised doubts about its efficacy. The non-bracing philosophy leaves the scoliosis to halt its progression spontaneously or prove its need for surgical intervention if it progresses beyond 35–40°

(Eisenstein & Draycott 1992). However, a recent survey in the US for structural idiopathic scoliosis advocates early screening of school children, with bracing for curves of 25–30°, which reduces the need for surgery by 81% (Roubal et al 1999).

Orthotic treatment may be the only therapy that favourably influences the outcome of scoliosis with leg length difference (Banks & Garvey 1994). Correction can be made by a heel raise, although there is a difference of opinion about the time to do this or its advisability altogether.

Correction of a severe scoliosis is highly desirable from the cosmetic and psychological point of view as the condition can be an upsetting one for adolescents, especially if there is a thoracic deformity. They require considerable encouragement and support (Mourad 1991).

Thoracic kyphosis

Thoracic kyphosis is a gross increase in thoracic flexion. It occurs in Scheuermann's disease (see p. 44), from an infection or spinal injury causing vertebral wedging, from biochemical changes (osteoporosis), from congenital abnormalities or from degenerative changes of the discs.

Spina bifida

Spina bifida is a developmental anomaly in which the neural tube fails to fuse along its length, most commonly at its lower end. The laminae of the vertebra usually close over the cord at 11 weeks of embryonic life. Failure to unite occurs most frequently at L5. Spina bifida varies in complexity from a simple deformity which causes little problem to a major disrup-tion including splitting of the skin, vertebral arch and underlying neural tube with associated neurological deficits (Wiltse 1971, Taylor & Twomey 1994, Pountney & McCarthy 1998).

In more minor cases, known as **spina bifida occulta**, the defect may be covered by skin. If skin, bone and dura meninges become involved a **meningocoele** occurs but in **spina bifida cystica** the skin, dura and spinal cord are all affected, called a **myelomeningocoele**. This occurs in 80% of spina bifida lesions. The neural tissue can also be displaced and exposed on the surface of the lesion, called a **rachischeisis** (Fig. 2.7). Other abnormalities include an **encephalocoele**, if the tube fails to fuse at a higher level, or **hydrocephelus**, if there is an obstruction of cerebral spinal fluid outflow from the cerebral ventricles.

Folic acid has been shown to be of benefit in preventing the occurrence of neural tube defects during pregnancy (Pountney & McCarthy 1998). Because of the possible connection between folate deficiency and dementia and other central nervous system disorders (Walton 1982), Wald & Bower (1995) have suggested that flour should now be regularly fortified with folic acid.

Transitional vertebra

A transitional vertebra is a fusion, in varying degree, of the transverse processes on one or both sides of two adjoining vertebrae, usually of L5 and S1. This in itself does not give rise to pain.

Back pain may be a feature of the anomalies and deformities listed here, mainly because of the resulting stress on other tissues; on the other hand, the conditions may remain pain free and often undetected throughout life.

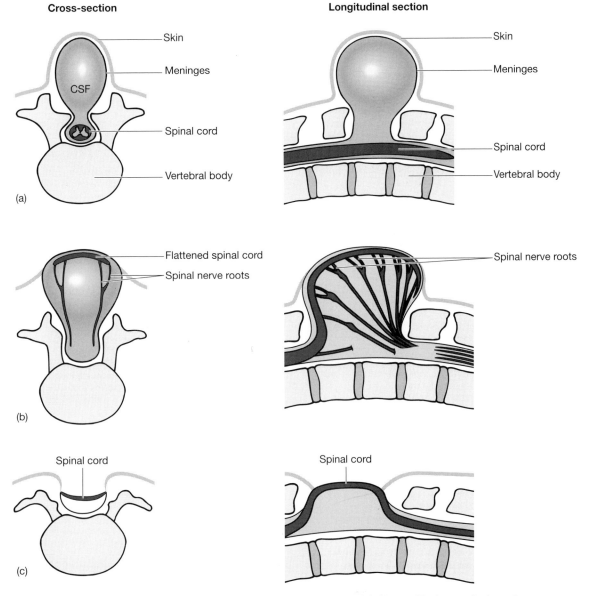

Cross-section

Longitudinal section

- Skin
- Meninges
- CSF
- Spinal cord
- Vertebral body

(a)

- Skin
- Meninges
- Spinal cord
- Vertebral body

- Flattened spinal cord
- Spinal nerve roots

(b)

- Spinal nerve roots

Spinal cord

(c)

Spinal cord

Figure 2.7 Types of spinal lesion in spina bifida. (a) Meningocoele: no neural tissue outside the vertebral canal. (b) Myelomeningocoele: neural tissue and nerve roots may be outside the vertebral canal. There may be fatty tissue or a bony spur present. (c) Rachischeisis: there is no sac and the neural tissue lies open on the surface as a flattened plaque. (Reproduced with permission from McCarthy G T 1992 Physical disability in childhood. Churchill Livingstone, Edinburgh.)

Key points

- The vertebral column provides both rigidity and mobility.
- Bone can be affected by trauma, disease or deformity.
- Bone is constantly modelling and remodelling itself in response to activity or inactivity.
- Exercise, both aerobic and site specific, is necessary for bone health and should be continued well into old age.

REFERENCES

Banks G M, Garvey T A 1994 The non-operative treatment of idiopathic scoliosis. Physical Therapy Practice 3(3): 136–147

Bogduk N, Twomey L T 1991 Clinical anatomy of the lumbar spine, 2nd edn. Churchill Livingstone, Edinburgh

Darby A J 1992 Bone and joint pathology. In: Tidswell M E (ed) Cash's textbook of orthopaedics and rheumatology for physiotherapists, 2nd edn. Mosby Year Book Europe, London

Dieck G S, Kelsey J L, Goel V K et al 1985 An epidemiologic study of the relationship between postural asymmetry in the teen years and subsequent back and neck pain. Spine 10(10): 872–877

Dixon A St J 1996 Osteoporosis and the family doctor. In: Butler R C, Jayson M I V (eds) Collected reports on the rheumatic diseases. Arthritic and Rheumatism Council for Research, Chesterfield

Drinkwater B L 1995 Weight-bearing exercise and bone mass. Physical Medicine and Rehabilitation Clinics of North America 6(3): 567–577

Dunne F 1994 Idiopathic osteoporosis occurring in pregnancy. Journal of the Association of Chartered Physiotherapists in Gynaecology 75: 18–20

Eisenstein S, Draycott V 1992 Spinal deformities. In: Tidswell M E (ed) Cash's textbook of orthopaedics and rheumatology for physiotherapists, 2nd edn. Mosby Year Book Europe, London

Evans G A, Draycott V 1992 Childhood disorders of the hip and inequality of leg length. In: Tidswell M E (ed) Cash's textbook of orthopaedics and rheumatology for physiotherapists, 2nd edn. Mosby Year Book Europe, London

Frost H M 1995 Bone: recent concepts important to musculoskeletal physiotherapy. In: Refshauge K, Gass E (eds) Musculoskeletal physiotherapy. Clinical science and practice. Butterworth Heinemann, Oxford

Goldberg C J, Dowling F E 1991 Idiopathic scoliosis and asymmetry of form and function. Spine 16(1): 84–87

Grieve G P 1989 Common vertebral joint problems. Churchill Livingstone, Edinburgh

Hansen P D, Woods L, Blaszcyk J W 1994 A model for neurological findings in idiopathic scoliosis. Physical Therapy Practice 3(3): 148–155

Kapandji I A 1974 The physiology of the joints, the trunk and the vertebral column, vol. 3. Churchill Livingstone, Edinburgh

Kendal F P, McCreary E K, Provance P G 1993 Muscle testing and function, 3rd edn. Williams and Wilkins, Baltimore

Khastigir G, Studd J 1994 Pregnancy-associated osteoporosis. British Journal of Obstetrics and Gynaecology 101: 836–838

Kisner C, Colby L A 1990 Therapeutic exercise. Foundations and techniques, 2nd edn. F A Davis, Philadelphia

Millner P A, Dickson R A 1996 Idiopathic scoliosis: biomechanics and biology. European Spine Journal 5: 362–373

Mourad L A 1991 Orthopaedic disorders. Mosby Year Book, St Louis

National Osteoporosis Society 1997 Osteoporosis: are you at risk? Nation Osteoporosis Society, Radstock

Palastanga N, Field D, Soames R 1991 Anatomy and human movement. Heinemann Medical Books, Oxford

Porter R W 1986 Management of back pain. Churchill Livingstone, Edinburgh

Pountney T, McCarthy G 1998 Neural tube defects: spina bifida and hydrocephalus. In: Stokes M (ed) Neurological physiotherapy. Mosby International, London

Refshauge K M, Latimer J 1995 The history. In: Refshauge K, Gass E (eds) Musculoskeletal physiotherapy. Clinical science and practice. Butterworth Heinemann, Oxford

Rizzoli R, Bonjour J P 1996 Pregnancy-associated osteoporosis. Lancet 347: 1274–1275

Rollo V J 1996 Osteoporosis: the silent condition. New Zealand Journal of Physiotherapy. April: 11–12

Roubal P J, Freeman D C, Placzek J D 1999 Costs and effectiveness of scoliosis screening. Physiotherapy 85(5): 259–268

Royal College of Physicians (RCP) 1999 Osteoporosis. Clinical guidelines for prevention and treatment. Royal College of Physicians, London

Silver J J, Einhorn T A 1995 Osteoporosis and aging. Clinical Orthopaedics and Related Research 316: 10–20

Smith E L 1995 The role of exercise in the prevention and treatment of osteoporosis. Topics in Geriatric Rehabilitation 10(4): 55–63

Specht D L, De Boer K F 1991 Anatomical leg length inequality, scoliosis and lordotic curve in unselected clinic patients. Journal of Manipulation and Physiological Therapeutics 14(6): 368–375

Swezey R L 1996 Spine update. Exercise for osteoporosis – is walking enough? Spine 21(23): 2809–2813

Taylor J R, Twomey L T 1994 The lumbar spine from infancy to old age. In: Twomey L T, Taylor J R (eds) Physical therapy of the low back. Churchill Livingstone, New York

Thomas P B M 1992 Fractures – clinical. In: Tidswell M E (ed) Cash's textbook of orthopaedics and rheumatology for physiotherapists, 2nd edn. Mosby Year Book Europe, London

Tidswell M E 1992 Cash's textbook of orthopaedics and rheumatology for physiotherapists. Mosby Year Book Europe, London

Twomey L T 1989 Physical activity and ageing bones. Patient Management 'Focus' 27–34

Twomey L T, Taylor J R 1994 Lumbar posture, movements and mechanics. In: Twomey L T, Taylor J R (eds) Physical therapy of the low back. Churchill Livingstone, New York

Wald N J, Bower C 1995 Folic acid and the prevention of neural tube defects. British Medical Journal 310: 1019–1020

Walton J 1982 Essentials of neurology, 5th edn. Pitman Books, London

Wiltse L 1971 The effect of the common anomalies of the lumbar spine upon disc degeneration and low back pain. Orthopedic Clinics of North America 2(2): 569–582

Zipnick R I, Gorek J, Kostuik J P et al 1996 The aging spine. Spine 10(3): 467–488.

FURTHER READING

Clinical Guidelines Care Development Group 1999 Physiotherapy guidelines for the management of osteoporosis. Chartered Society of Physiotherapists, London

Drinkwater B L 1995 Weight bearing exercise and bone mass. Physical Medicine and Rehabilitation Clinics of North America, Vol. 6, No. 3, August 1995

Millner P A, Dickson R A 1998 Idiopathic scoliosis: biomechanics and biology. European Spine Journal 5: 362–372

Palastanga N, Field D, Soames R 1998 Anatomy and human movement, 3rd edn. Butterworth Heinemann, Oxford

Royal College of Physicians 1999 Osteoporosis, clinical guidelines for prevention and treatment. Royal College of Physicians, London

Silver J J, Einhorn T A 1995 Osteoporosis and aging. Clinical Orthopaedics and Related Research 316: 10–20

Stokes M 1998 Neurological physiotherapy. Mosby International, London

3

The motion segment

JOINT ANATOMY

Joints are classified by the type of material between them and they are of three kinds: synovial, cartilaginous and fibrous. Fibrous joints are immobile. The joints of the spine are of two types: synovial and cartilaginous.

Synovial joints

Cartilage

The bone ends of a synovial joint are covered in a layer of cartilage, a smooth, resilient layer of dense connective tissue which varies in size and importance depending upon the stress imposed on the joint.

Capsule

Surrounding and enclosing the whole structure is a fibrous capsule which is lined by a **synovial membrane**. The synovial membrane secretes a thick **synovial fluid** into the joint which is important for the health of the joint tissues

---

Box 3.1   The role of synovial fluid in maintaining joint health

- Reduces friction.
- Provides lubrication and nourishment of the cartilage.
- Provides nutrients and oxygen for all tissues.
- Carries out phagocytic and other immunological functions within the joint.

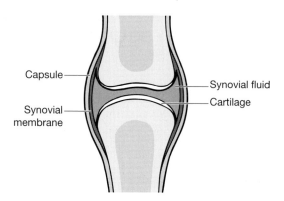

Capsule

Synovial membrane

Synovial fluid

Cartilage

Figure 3.1 A basic synovial joint.

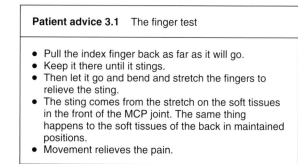

Patient advice 3.1   The finger test

- Pull the index finger back as far as it will go.
- Keep it there until it stings.
- Then let it go and bend and stretch the fingers to relieve the sting.
- The sting comes from the stretch on the soft tissues in the front of the MCP joint. The same thing happens to the soft tissues of the back in maintained positions.
- Movement relieves the pain.

(Mourad 1991) (Fig. 3.1). Exercise stimulates its flow and the secretion tends to lessen with inactivity, another reason for continuing exercises into old age (Twomey 1991). Injury causes the synovial fluid to increase, hence the swelling of any damaged joint.

Ligaments

A joint is surrounded at strategic places by ligaments – tough, inelastic fibrous bands. Ligaments can be compared to rubber bands in that they resist stretching and buckle when released. They are sometimes incorporated into the capsule or they may cross the joint quite independently. Ligaments have a static and dynamic function.

Static. The static role is to prevent excessive movement and keep the joint compact. For this reason they are placed at positions of greatest stress in order to control undesirable movement and prevent dislocation. In normal movement the capsule and ligaments tighten and slacken around a joint depending upon the accent of direction. Forced joint dislocation invariably damages restraining tissues, causing tears or ruptures.

Dynamic. The dynamic role of ligaments is related to a proprioceptive function, a sensory feedback of muscle and joint information (Macleod et al 1987). Thus passive ligamentous stretching and reflex muscle control are closely linked and finely balanced.

It is important for patients to understand ligamentous strains of the back and the reaction of pain when the ligaments are put under stress. The 'finger test' is one of the best ways to explain joint stress (Patient advice 3.1).

Cartilaginous joints

Cartilaginous joints have no capsule or synovial fluid. The cartilage is in the centre of the joint, attached to the bone on either side. The symphysis pubis (see Fig 2.2) and the joint of the intervertebral disc, discussed below, are examples of cartilaginous joints.

VERTEBRAL JOINTS

Each of the vertebral joints has a small range of movement but their combined movement throughout the spine creates a large range overall. The mechanism is intricate but extremely effective.

The three vertebral joints form a triad: a large simple joint of the **intervertebral disc** and two small, more complicated **zygapophyseal** joints or **facet** joints. All three work together at all times.

The joints of the triad

The intervertebral disc

The intervertebral disc (IVD), placed between the two vertebral bodies, acts as a shock absorber transmitting the forces of weight bearing down through the tough bones of the vertebral bodies. It is connected to the vertebral bodies above and below by a layer of cartilage, the **vertebral endplate** (VEP) (see 'Intervertebral disc structure', p. 31). The whole mechanism forms a cartilaginous joint.

The zygapophyseal or facet joints

As two adjacent vertebrae meet, the facet joints are formed by the inferior articular processes of the top vertebra overlapping and locking onto the superior articular processes of the vertebra below. Each forms a synovial joint, enclosed by a fibrous capsule, with a layer of cartilage on the adjoining bony surfaces. The capsule is thickened by strong controlling ligaments with the ligamentum flavum forming its anterior aspect (see 'Spinal ligaments' below).

The shape and orientation of the joint surfaces on the articular processes vary in the different regions of the vertebral column. This is to enable the vertebrae to meet their varying mobility requirements.

The sacroiliac joints

The sacroiliac is a synovial joint between the sacrum and the ilium (see Fig. 2.2). The wedge shape of the sacrum is stabilized by the innominate bones, with an irregular-shaped cartilage in the joint. The joint has minimal movement, mainly allowing for a rotational 'give' as the weight of the spine tends to rock the sacrum between the innominates and a glide as the ilium lifts during one-sided pelvic raise as in single-leg lifting. During the latter part of pregnancy the joint is affected by the increase in diameter of the pelvic inlet and outlet to accommodate the fetal head.

Everyday movements of the joint occur during weight transference as in walking, climbing stairs or dancing, in turning to look behind whilst both feet remain stationary and in stooping forwards whilst sitting.

THE MOTION SEGMENT

Two vertebrae and the structures around them form a motion segment of the spine, a duo that is repeated with relevant variations of shape in each vertebral group throughout the spine. The meeting of the two vertebrae creates the **intervertebral foramen** (IVF), an exit for any structures entering or leaving the spinal canal (Fig. 3.2).

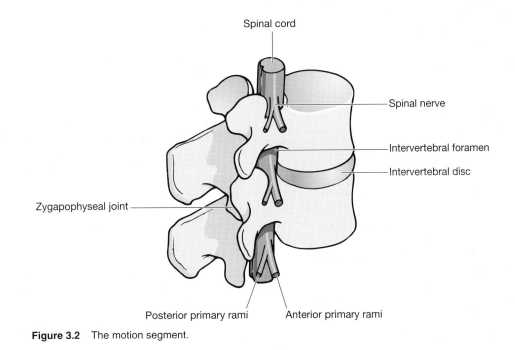

Figure 3.2 The motion segment.

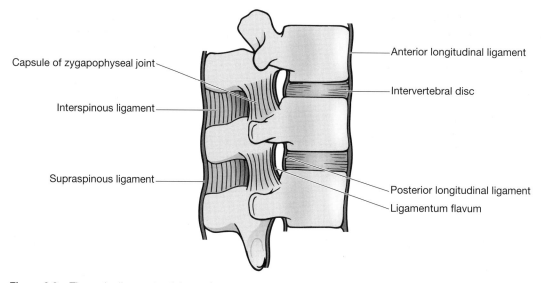

Figure 3.3 The major ligaments of the motion segment.

The spinal cord descends through the centre of the spinal canal, giving off two nerve roots on either side which join to form the spinal nerve. The spinal nerve exits from the spinal canal through the IVF, to supply the relevant body areas. Blood vessels also enter and exit through the IVF.

SPINAL LIGAMENTS

For the purpose of description, the vertebrae are divided into anterior and posterior elements (Fig. 3.3).

Ligaments of the anterior elements

The ligaments of the anterior elements of the vertebrae are the **anterior** and **posterior longitudinal ligaments** which are attached to the front and rear of each vertebral body and disc. These ligaments regulate stretch and separation between two adjacent vertebral bodies. The annulus of the disc itself forms a ligamentous structure with its attachment to the ring apophysis of the vertebra above and below (Bogduk & Twomey 1991) (Fig. 3.4).

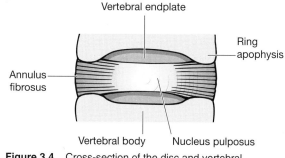

Figure 3.4 Cross-section of the disc and vertebral endplate.

Ligaments of the posterior elements

The ligaments of the posterior elements, the **ligamentum flavum**, the **supraspinous** and **interspinous ligaments**, are related to functional control of spinal movements as they stretch during flexion. The ligamentum flavum forms the anterior part of the facet joint capsule and is the most elastic of all body ligaments (Panjabi & White 1980). It lines the back of the spinal canal and maintains the smooth contour of the canal in all postures. It stretches in flexion and contracts and thickens in extension without buckling. With age, however, it become more fibrous and may buckle on extension, narrowing the spinal canal (Taylor & Twomey 1994).

Ligaments of the lumbosacral area

Iliolumbar ligaments

The iliolumbar ligaments join the transverse processes of L5 to the ilium, forming a strong bond between them and acting to prevent L5 slipping forwards on the sacrum.

Ligaments of the sacroiliac

The sacroiliac is surrounded on both sides of the joint by a strong mass of ligamentous structures which are normally firm and tight. However, during pregnancy hormonal changes induce a laxity in the ligaments of the sacroiliac and of the lumbar spine, allowing for greater range of movement. This creates a vulnerability to stress which can in turn lead to pain. A similar situation arises during menstruation with the same tendency towards sacral and lumbar pain. Sacroiliac pain during pregnancy can be successfully treated with physiotherapy but in most cases it is relieved immediately after delivery. There may be remaining uncertainty in the joint for at least 4 months postpartum, necessitating a great deal of back care, especially as the state of motherhood requires an increased amount of bending (see Chapter 9).

A considerable amount of pain in the area of the sacroiliac which is ascribed to the joint is, however, often misdiagnosed and is instead referred pain from the lumbar spine.

THE INTERVERTEBRAL DISC: STRUCTURE AND NUTRITION

A normal, healthy disc is a symmetrical kidney shape. In the average adult male discs of the lumbar spine are about 1 cm thick and the vertebral bodies above and below are about 2.5 cm thick. Female sizes average some 15% smaller (Taylor & Twomey 1994).

The IVD is composed of three parts: the nucleus pulposus in the centre, surrounded by the annulus fibrosus, with the vertebral endplate separating the structure from the vertebral bodies above and below (Fig. 3.4). The ability of the disc to act as a hydrostatic 'cushion' depends on the high water content of its tissues, in particular the nucleus pulposus ((Markolf & Morris 1974, Palastanga et al 1991, Adams et al 1996).

The nucleus pulposus

The nucleus pulposus is an oval-shaped gelatinous mass, a soft toothpaste-like substance which is made up of a certain amount of cartilage cells and collagenous fibres in a water-bound medium, 75–90% of its weight being fluid content (Markolf & Morris 1974). The nucleus is indistinctly separated from the surrounding annulus fibrosus by a thin transition zone between them but the two disc components have no obvious boundary. Because of its fluid nature, the nucleus does not resist deformation in the way that rubber can but is deformed under pressure like a water-filled balloon, the displaced pressure being transmitted in all directions towards the perimeter of the annulus. The fluid pressure rises substantially when the volume of fluid is increased and falls when it is decreased (Bogduk & Twomey 1991, Buckwalter 1995, Adams et al 1996).

The annulus fibrosus

The annulus fibrosus is also made up of collagen fibres packed in a gel-like substance, with water amounting to 60–70% of its weight (Bogduk & Twomey 1991). The outer layer of the annulus is made up of a ring of highly orientated, densely packed collagen fibril lamellae which acts as a tensile skin for the rest of the disc (Buckwalter 1995, Adams 1996). The inner fibres are arranged in layers of concentric circles, not unlike an onion. They surround the nucleus, with their fibres melding into the transition zone where they meet. The fibres of each layer run in obliquely opposite directions but as the layers are bound together by a cement-like substance, the overall effect is of a lattice-like structure. The anterior and lateral portions of the disc are thicker than the thinner posterior part where the layers are more tightly packed (Markolf & Morris 1974).

The vertebral endplate

The VEP is a layer of cartilage covering the whole area of the vertebral body apart from the ring apophysis (Fig. 3.4). It is attached to three-quarters of the disc surface, covering the nucleus entirely but leaving an area of annulus at the perimeter which is embedded in the ring apophysis of the vertebral body.

Disc nutrition

The disc receives its nourishment from a limited blood supply of two arterial sources: a group of small arteries forming a fine network on the very periphery of the annulus and from a capillary plexus beneath the VEP (Urban et al 1977). As there is no arterial supply within the disc, nutrients are passed through the matrix of the VEP and through the annulus fibrosus by the process of diffusion and varying osmotic pressures (Bogduk & Twomey 1991).

However, the distance from the blood cells to the nucleus is large and it is believed that nutrient absorption is aided by a 'pumping action' which occurs with changing loads to the disc. Compression of the IVD tends to squeeze water out of it and when the compression is released, the water returns. This water is capable of carrying nutrients with it. So, it is believed that there is a link between posture, fluid flow within the disc and nutrition (Adams & Hutton 1983). This is why movement is so important to the health of the disc.

Factors affecting the blood supply seem to have an effect on nutrient concentration in the tissues. Both vibration and smoking lead to a rapid fall in oxygen concentration in the nucleus and a rise in lactate concentration which take several hours to reverse (Buckwalter 1995, Urban & Roberts 1995) (see 'Disc mechanisms' below).

Diurnal variation

During an average day, the disc loses fluid which reduces its thickness by 20%. At night when the body is at rest, often lying curled up in flexed, unloaded postures, the discs absorb fluid. This is why the back feels stiff on rising

from sleep. The disc spaces are packed tight and there is less room for manoeuvre. As a result, there is a height gain of 1% during the night.

During the day moisture is squeezed out of the disc and height is lost again. The greatest loss of fluid takes place in the first half-hour of being upright and in 4 hours fluid content is down to the daily average. In view of this the advisability of exercising immediately on rising from bed is questionable. A more sensible regime, especially for backs that are potentially at risk or recovering from pain, would be to delay exercise for at least half an hour, preferably longer, after rising (Adams & Hutton 1983, Adams 1996).

By the afternoon, disc height loss leads to increased vertical loading of the facet joints, while on the other hand, the intervertebral ligaments and the posterior annulus fibres are slacker and resist bending movements less (Adams 1996).

The disc has certain qualities which enhance its shock absorbing function (Box 3.2).

MECHANISM OF MOVEMENT OF THE TRIAD

The mechanism of movement of the triad is intricate and when examined in detail, it varies from group to group in the different spinal vertebrae, but the basic mechanism is similar throughout. The disc joint is the major member of the triad, taking 80% of the weight-bearing force (Twomey & Taylor 1994), but the facet joints play an essential role of stabilization.

At each level the range of movement of the triad is very small but the overall range of spinal

---

Box 3.2 Special qualities of the IVD

The IVD:
- is malleable and adaptable to change of movement, yet able to resume its form at rest
- is strong enough to sustain weight, as load is transmitted from one vertebra to the other during weight-bearing activities
- remains uninjured by this normal dynamic activity
- acts as a hydrostatic cushion, depending upon its water content
- loses fluid in maintained positions
- needs movement to provide nourishment.

movement is achieved by a spiral staircase effect with each vertebra contributing a few degrees to the combined range.

As the three joints of the triad are inseparably linked, a faulty performance in either one of them can cause disruption in the function of the others, so not only can a faulty disc cause strain on a facet joint but a faulty facet joint can equally well create stress on a disc with resulting degenerative wear (Vernon-Roberts 1992). The balanced interplay between disc and facet joint is crucial to perfect spinal coordination and function.

Facet joint mechanism

During movement of the vertebral bodies on each other, the facet joints to the rear stabilize and control any tendency of the bodies to slide or glide excessively or to become unstable horizontally (Bogduk & Twomey 1991).

The vertical orientation of the lumbar facet joints favours flexion/extension; they restrict side flexion and rotation and thus protect the annular fibres of the disc from excessive stress during these movements (Cailliet 1995).

In flexion, the vertebrae tilt forward on each other, so that there is both a forward rotation and a forward translation of the top vertebral body on the lower. This forward translation is known as the **shear force**. The inferior articular process rises upwards and forwards on the one below, impacting on it and so resisting the slide. The greatest restraining factors of flexion appear to be the opposed articular surfaces of the facet joints, the joint capsule and posterior ligament, in that order (Adams et al 1980, Twomey & Taylor 1994).

The facet joints thus provide a protection from the shearing forces applied to the IVD. If the vertebral arches break, instability results with danger of damage to the disc and the neural tissues in the vertebral canal (see 'Spondylolisthesis', p. 52).

End-of-range extension is limited by bony contact as the inferior joint facet impacts on the lamina of the vertebra below or as the spinous processes meet. The interspinous ligament can be pinched in extreme hyperextension. Extreme extension does not often happen in everyday life but it occurs in whiplash injuries or sporting activities (see Chapter 4).

Intervertebral disc mechanism

Functionally, the IVD separates the two adjacent vertebrae due to the intrinsic internal pressure of the nucleus pulposus. This internal pressure not only separates the vertebral endplates but causes increased tension in the annular fibres and ligaments of the motion segment (Cailliet 1995).

The lattice-like construction of the annulus gives the disc its strength and ability to resist deformation from both pressure within the nucleus and load from the vertebral body. Although compressive forces descend through the vertebral bodies in all upright postures, straight compression has been found to be the least damaging force for the disc, compared to sustained flexion and rotation (Markolf & Morris 1974, Panjabi & White 1980). However, all upright postures decrease disc height by driving water out of the disc, which is replaced when recumbent.

As movement takes place between the vertebrae in daily activity, the disc's qualities are put to the test. Each change of direction causes pressure within the nucleus to be dispersed into the fibres of the annulus and out towards the periphery. In flexion the disc is compressed anteriorly and pressure is exerted towards its stretched posterior annular boundary (McKenzie 1981) (Fig. 3.5) The opposite pressure is exerted in extension. It is thought that these *repetitive* deformations may lead to failure of the matrix which can appear as fissures or degeneration and eventually compromise function (Buckwalter 1995).

Considerable research has been done on measurement of intradiscal pressures in order to validate theories regarding the effect of postural change on disc function. Intradiscal pressure is least in lying and greatest when stoop lifting (Fig. 3.6) (Nachemson & Morris 1964, Nachemson & Elfstrom 1970, Andersson et al 1974, 1976). It is less in lordotic postures than in straight or kyphotic ones, increased with passive lumbar flexion of more than 20°, further increased by repeated active flexion and greatest with heavy

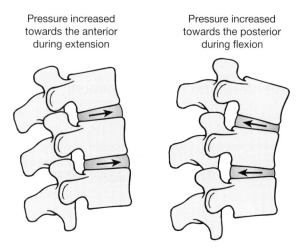

Pressure increased towards the anterior during extension

Pressure increased towards the posterior during flexion

Figure 3.5 Movement of the nucleus under pressure.

lifting, especially using the Valsalva manoeuvre (Twomey & Taylor 1994)

Merriam et al (1984) showed that degenerated discs behave in an inconsistent way which does not necessarily conform to the pressure changes of normal discs. All these facts provide a valid scientific backing to the theories of postural care (Nachemson 1992).

In *any* sustained position, the load to the disc results in loss of disc fluid and height.

Motion segment mechanism

In maintained standing the body weight applies an axial load to the disc, with resulting fluid loss. Fatigue tends to decrease the abdominal support for the lumbar spine and the lordosis may increase. With increased extension, pressure is increased on the posterior fibres of the annulus fibrosus which is the narrowest part of the disc and least designed for compressive stress. The supply of nutrients to the disc is impaired, the volume of the intervertebral canal is reduced and the vertical loading is increased on the facet joints.

In sustained flexion under load (5–10 minutes or more in stoop or slouch sitting) fluid is squeezed out of all tissues: the disc (compressed anteriorly), the articular cartilage (compressed) and the spinal ligaments (put on stretch). The tissues adjust by redistributing the remaining fluid within them and **creep** takes place. Creep is the progressive deformation of a structure under constant load when the forces are not large enough to cause permanent damage and flexion slowly increases beyond the endpoint of normal range (Twomey & Taylor 1994, Adams et al 1996).

There is loss of fluid from all the soft tissues and they are deprived of nutrition. It takes some

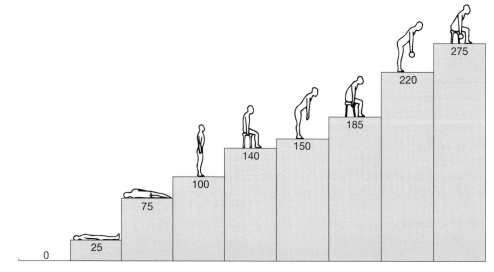

Figure 3.6 Relative increase and decrease in intradiscal pressure in different postures compared with 100% pressure in upright standing. (Reproduced with permission from Nachemson 1992.)

time for this fluid to return once more into the disc but movement helps and enhances the process. Movement activates synovial fluid and increases the circulation in the soft tissues, restoring their fluid loss. Creep is greater in the elderly than in the young and the rate of recovery is slower (Twomey & Taylor 1987).

Torsional strain is one of the greatest causes of annular damage (see Chapter 4). In flexion the potential for torsional damage is increased as the rotational control exerted by the facet joints is less effective in this position (Panjabi & White 1980, Twomey & Taylor 1994).

So, thinking in terms of back care, turning becomes an especially stressful and potentially harmful movement if performed in flexion, even more so when combined with holding an extra weight. High-velocity torsional forces, such as whiplash injuries sustained in a rotated position, often result in tears of the annulus (Twomey & Taylor 1994) (Table 3.1).

It is important to remember that the disc forms one of the anterior boundaries of the inter-vertebral foramen and as the spinal nerve passes through the IVF, it lies directly behind the disc (Palastanga et al 1991) (Fig. 3.2). The disc also forms part of the anterior wall of the spinal canal so a posterior bulge could compromise the contents of the spinal canal as well as the spinal nerves (Patient advice 3.2) (see Chapter 4).

INNERVATION OF THE MOTION SEGMENT

There has been great controversy regarding the innervation of the disc but recent findings have proved that there are abundant nerve endings in the outer fibres of the annulus which can be the source of severe pain (Bogduk & Twomey 1991). There appears to be no nerve supply within the inner annular layers or in the nucleus. The vertebral column is surrounded by a vast net-work of nerve plexuses, description of which is beyond the scope of this book. The nerve supply of the motion segment is abbreviated in Table 3.2 (Bogduk & Twomey 1991, Palastanga et al 1991, Adams 1996).

Table 3.1 The structures most affected by postural stress

Movements or positions	Structures affected
• Flexion	• Interspinous ligament • Facet joints: opposed articular surfaces and capsule stretch • Posterior ligament • Posterior disc
• Torsion in flexion	• Facet joint surfaces • Annulus of disc
• Asymmetrical flexion/side flexion, • Sustained/sudden flexion	• Discs – possible injury
• Extension	• Impact of facet joints on lamina • Spinous processes approximated • Vertebral canal narrowed
• Sustained standing	• Facet joint surfaces • Posterior annulus – fluid loss, nutrition impaired
• Torsion in extension	• Facet joint surfaces
• Compression	• Vertebral body and VEP • Facet joints • Disc injury after damage to vertebral body
• Repetitive high-velocity forces in any position	• Annular tears
• Trauma	• VEP fractures • Vertebral body compression fractures

---

Patient advice 3.2 Posture

1. Avoid sustained standing.
2. Avoid maintained flexion in stoop or slouch sitting.
3. Avoid twisting in stoop, especially when holding a weight.
4. Keep a rhythm of activity and rest during work.
5. Movement is good and necessary.
6. Rest in bed every 24 hours is essential.
7. Try to avoid exercising immediately on rising.

The VEP has previously been described as having no nerve supply but Adams (1996) has found that immunoreactive nerve endings in rats are innervated by substance P; if this is so in humans, they may have the potential to cause pain.

Table 3.2 The nerve supply of the motion segment

Nerve	Branch	Area supplied
Spinal nerve	Dorsal rami: lateral branch	• The skin • Iliocostalis lumborum muscle
	Intermediate branch	• Longissimus muscle • Lateral aspect of facet joints capsule
	Medial branch (hooks round base of superior articular process)	• Facet joints • Interspinous ligament • Interspinous muscle • Lumbar multifidus muscle (with individual segmental innervation)
Spinal nerve	Ventral rami and grey rami communicantes	• Psoas major muscle and quadratus lumborum • Medial aspect of facet joints • Posterior longitudinal ligament • Anterior longitudinal ligament • Posterior and lateral surfaces of IVD
Sinuvertebral nerve	Within the spinal canal	• Posterior annulus fibrosus • Posterior longitudinal ligament • Periosteum • Blood vessels • Anterior aspect of the dura • IVD above and below each level of its entry into the spinal canal

BLOOD SUPPLY OF THE VERTEBRAL COLUMN

The vertebral column receives a liberal blood supply from branches of the arteries and veins which lie adjacent to it, apart from the intervertebral discs which have only an anastomosis of small blood vessels on the outer surface of the annulus fibrosus (Bogduk & Twomey 1991).

A network of blood vessels enmeshes the rest of the whole motion segment, providing nutrients to the vertebral body, the facet joints and all surrounding soft tissues, including branches that enter the intervertebral foramen supplying the spinal cord and all structures within the spinal canal (Bogduk & Twomey 1991). The brain, spinal cord and neural tissue consume 20% of the available oxygen in the circulating blood (Dommisse 1995).

The veins of the spinal column form an external plexus, which lies superficial to the vertebra, and an internal plexus within the spinal canal. The internal plexus, together with the epidural fat, occupies the space in the spinal canal between the vertebral bodies and the meninges, anastomosing through the IVF with the external vertebral plexus. The vertebral veins throughout the length of the whole vertebral column form a valveless venous pathway providing an alternative venous channel which can bypass the normal system. Blood can flow in any direction in the plexus, according to regional differences in pressure, and with every rise of pressure in the trunk, as in coughing, sneezing, lifting, holding one's breath or any increase of intraabdominal pressure (IAP), venous blood is actually shunted

---

Key points

1. Sustained loading leads to loss of disc fluid and height and stress on facet joints.
2. Sustained flexion: 'creep' or loss of tissue fluid takes place in the disc and all soft tissues.
3. Synovial fluid lessens with inactivity and is activated with movement, as is the general blood supply to the whole area.
4. Alternating periods of activity and rest with postural change tend to boost fluid exchange which increases nutrition.
5. Torsional stress is the greatest cause of annular damage.
6. Flexion in the lying or unloaded position allows the disc to take in nutrients.

---

into the vertebral system. In this situation the system seems to act as a 'pressure absorber' for venous flow when the IAP is increased. Circumstantial evidence suggests that distension of epidural veins can cause pain (Bogduk 1994, Twomey & Taylor 1994) and back pain, for example in osteoporosis, may be due to venous stasis in the vertebral body spongiosa (Grieve 1989). So the venous blood supply may play quite an important role in back pain.

REFERENCES

Adams M 1996 Biomechanics of low back pain. Pain Reviews 3: 15–30

Adams M, Hutton W C 1983 The effect of posture on the fluid content of the lumbar intervertebral discs. Spine 8(6): 665–671

Adams M, Hutton W C, Stott M A 1980 The resistance to flexion of the lumbar intervertebral joint. Spine 5(3): 245

Adams M, McMillan D W, Green T P, Dolan P 1996 Sustained loading generates stress concentrations in lumbar intervertebral discs. Spine 21(4): 434–438

Andersson B J B, Ortengren R, Nachemson A et al 1974 Lumbar disc pressure and myoelectric back muscle activity during sitting. Scandinavian Journal of Rehabilitation Medicine 6: 104

Andersson B J B, Ortengren R, Nachemson A 1976 Quantitative studies of back loads in lifting. Spine 1(3): 178

Bogduk N 1994 Innervation, pain patterns, and mechanisms of pain production. In: Twomey L T, Taylor R T (eds) Physical therapy of the low back, 2nd edn. Churchill Livingstone, New York

Bogduk N, Twomey L T 1991 Clinical anatomy of the lumbar spine. Churchill Livingstone, New York

Buckwalter M D 1995 Spine update: aging and degeneration of the human intervertebral disc. Spine 20(11): 1307–1314

Cailliet R 1995 Low back pain syndrome, 5th edn. F A Davis Company, Philadelphia

Dommisse G F 1995 The blood supply of the spinal cord and consequences of failure. In: Boyling J, Palastanga N (eds) Grieve's modern manual therapy, 2nd edn. Churchill Livingstone, Edinburgh

Grieve G P 1989 Common vertebral joint problems. Churchill Livingstone, Edinburgh

McKenzie R 1981 The lumbar spine: mechanical diagnosis and therapy. Spinal Publications, Waikanae, New Zealand

Macleod D, Maughan R, Nimmo M, Reilly T, Williams C 1987 Exercise: benefits, limits and adaptations. E & F N Spon, London

Markolf K L, Morris J M 1974 The structural components of the intervertebral disc. Journal of Bone and Joint Surgery 56-A(4): 675–687

Merriam W F, Quinnell R C, Stockdale H R et al 1984 The effect of postural changes on the inferred pressures within the nucleus pulposus during lumbar discography. Spine 9(4): 406

Mourad L A 1991 Orthopedic disorders. Mosby Year Book, St Louis

Nachemson A 1992 Lumbar mechanisms as revealed by lumbar intradiscal pressure measurements. In: Jayson M I V (ed) The lumbar spine and back pain, 4th edn. Churchill Livingstone, Edinburgh

Nachemson A, Elfstrom G 1970 Intravital dynamic pressure measurements in lumbar discs. Scandinavian Journal of Rehabilitation Medicine 1(1)

Nachemson A, Morris J M 1964 In vivo measurements of intradiscal pressure. Journal of Bone and Joint Surgery 46-A(5): 1077–1092

Palastanga N, Field D, Soames R 1991 Anatomy and human movement. Butterworth Heinemann, Oxford

Panjabi M M, White A A 1980 Basic biomechanics of the spine. Neurosurgery 7(1): 76–93

Taylor J R, Twomey L T 1994 The lumbar spine from infancy to old age. In: Twomey L T, Taylor J R (eds) Physical therapy of the low back. Churchill Livingstone, New York

Twomey L T 1991 Musculoskeletal physiotherapy: the age of reason. Proceedings of the 11th Congress of the World Confederation for Physical Therapy, 343–347

Twomey L T, Taylor J R 1987 Age changes in the lumbar vertebrae and intervertebral discs. Clinical Orthopaedics and Related Research 224: 97–103

Twomey L T, Taylor J R 1994 Lumbar posture, movement, and mechanics. In: Twomey L T, Taylor J R (eds) Physical therapy of the low back. Churchill Livingstone, New York

Urban J P, Roberts S 1995 Chemistry of intervertebral disc in relation to functional requirements. In: Boyling J, Palastanga N (eds) Grieve's modern manual therapy, 2nd edn. Churchill Livingstone, Edinburgh

Urban J P, Holm S, Markoudas A, Nachemson A 1977 Nutrition of the intervertebral disc. Clinical Orthopaedics and Related Research 129: 101–114

Vernon-Roberts B 1992 Age-related and degenerative pathology of the intervertebral discs and apophyseal joints. In: Jayson M I V (ed) The lumbar spine and back pain, 4th edn. Churchill Livingstone, Edinburgh

FURTHER READING

Bogduk N 1997 Clinical anatomy of the lumbar spine and sacrum. Churchill Livingstone, Edinburgh

Boyling J, Palastanga N 1995 Grieve's modern manual therapy, 2nd edn. Churchill Livingstone, Edinburgh

Low J, Reed A 1996 Basic biomechanics explained. Butterworth Heinemann, Oxford

Palastanga N, Field D, Soames R 1998 Anatomy and human movement, 3rd edn. Butterworth Heinemann, Oxford

Trew M, Everett T (eds) 1991 Human movement, 3rd edn. Churchill Livingstone, New York

White A A, Panjabi M M 1990 Clinical biomechanics of the spine, 2nd edn. J B Lippincott, Philadelphia

4

Disorders of the motion segment

MISCONCEPTIONS

Back pain has been discussed throughout history with reasons given for its onset ranging from punishment from heaven to 'just a muscle strain'. Fortunately, our understanding of the mechanisms involved has become more scientific although the precise cause of pain is still often obscure, mainly because of the number and complexity of structures which can be implicated. In the search for knowledge certain myths have been invalidated; we must pass on these corrections to our patients and be sure not to create new myths as we try to explain the possible sources of their pain.

One of the more controversial claims used by some manipulators is that a vertebra is 'out', waiting to be dramatically 'put back'. This idea needs to be firmly refuted. A spinal dislocation would only occur after a major accident such as a bad road traffic accident or an airplane crash. Perhaps the error of diagnosis results from a misunderstanding of the postural deviation evoked by protective muscle spasm. The strong contraction can cause an artificial scoliosis, producing a kink at one particular vertebra with some vertebral rotation, giving the appearance of a spinous process being out of alignment. Depending upon the cause of pain, manipulation could have a curative effect, possibly by releasing a locked joint, but not because a bone has been 'put back' in place.

The second myth in need of clarification is one concerning draughts. Patients often miss the true aggravating factor of their pain because they associate its origin with sitting in a draught. It is necessary to explain that if pain is the aftermath of being in a draught it is not because of the breeze but as a consequence of muscular tension, for example tightening the upper trapezius or side flexing the neck, in an attempt to protect against discomfort.

The third and perhaps most common misconception is the idea of a 'slipped disc'. The diagnosis is often pronounced during any acute attack of back pain, especially if spinal X-rays have shown a narrowing or irregularity in the disc space. We need to explain that X-rays show only bone, the condition of the bone, the spinal alignment and the shape of the disc spaces between the vertebral bodies. If there is alteration in the disc space it is probable that the disc is worn or even destroyed in some way which may or may not be relevant to the particular pain. Discs narrow, bulge, herniate, degenerate, disrupt, become deranged and suffer degradation but they do not slip.

DISORDERS OF THE DISC, THE VERTEBRAL ENDPLATE AND THE FACET JOINTS

Daily abuse

A young healthy intervertebral disc is strong, resilient and elastic, able to accept both deformation, followed by return to its former shape, and dehydration, followed by its own speedy process of rehydration. However, throughout the course of normal active life, even discounting the more noticeable traumatic events, the disc suffers constant abuse.

Loading in flexion, side flexion, extension and rotation repeatedly pressurizes the nucleus into the annulus, eventually giving rise to areas of wear in the inner annulus. These will not in themselves generate pain unless they spread in the form of radial fissures into the outer, innervated annular layers. Disc lesions will remain undetected providing the disturbance remains within the inner annulus, the outer layers do not become involved and the disc in no way compromises

the sensitive structures within the spinal canal or IVF (Markolf & Morris 1974, Panjabi & White 1980, Adams & McMillan 1996).

The potential for damage lies in the disc's reaction to progressive deformation or creep, that is, loss of fluid content. As described in Chapter 3, deformation occurs in any maintained position: sustained standing and sustained flexion. Although sustained flexion is a more common posture in daily activity, with intradiscal pressure increased and exerted towards a stretched posterior annulus, Adams (1996) found that the greatest nuclear fluid loss occurs in maintained, lordotic postures. When a disc is compressed, the pressure in the nucleus initially causes the VEPs to bulge into the vertebral bodies. The inner and middle annulus also resists compression and the disc bulges radially outwards. If the volume of fluid in the nucleus then reduces, the hydrostatic pressure within it falls and the inner annulus resists more compression, bulging outwards to the perimeter like a 'flat tyre' (Adams 1996) (Patient advice 4.1).

All sustained postures squeeze fluid not only from the discs but also from the articular cartilage of the facet joints and the spinal ligaments and distort and reshape the soft tissues by redistributing the remaining fluid in them. The longer the static hold, the longer the recovery period and the greater the potential disc damage (Twomey et al 1988).

Repetitive high-velocity forces or any repetitive movement, especially when associated with rotation, can initiate annular tears or extend

---

Patient advice 4.1 The disc mechanism

- Describe a water-filled balloon.
- Imagine pressure being place on it from above and below – the inner pressure would bulge out towards the perimeter in all directions.
- Relate this to sustained standing.
- If pressure is exerted on one side, the pressure is forced to the other.
- Relate this to positions of flexion and extension, side flexion.
- Then describe the balloon if pressed in one direction and rotated – relate this to rotation in flexion.

Patient advice 4.2   Movement is good

- Avoid stressed movements in stoop.
- Avoid turning while bending forwards; always turn by moving the feet.
- Avoid twisting while reaching up.
- Avoid all sustained postures, even good ones.
- In sustained sitting, shift position frequently, get up and walk around whenever possible.
- In sustained standing, support the lordosis with strong abdominal holds, try to keep moving, shifting the weight from leg to leg, rock the pelvis backwards and forwards, and sit for 5 minutes whenever possible.

lines of wear already present. Of the three most potentially damaging forces of compression, flexion and torsion, the last two are more likely to cause failure of the annulus into a posterior protrusion, while compression is more likely to affect the vertebral endplate and vertebral body (Hickey & Hukins 1980, Adams & Hutton 1985) (Patient advice 4.2).

Back care tends to concentrate on the lumbar spine but clinically patients present with as many cervical spine problems as those of the lower back. In fact, because of the different orientation of the cervical facet joints, compared with the lumbar, the cervical spine incurs greater translation during movement, with more shearing than in the lumbar spine. Much greater forward slide in the cervical spine results in a greater number of fissures in the cervical discs (Taylor & Twomey 1994).

Disc derangement

Characteristics

Disc derangement is a mechanical disturbance of the disc which can occur in stages or as a result of sudden trauma (Adams & Hutton 1982). The process of disc derangement from normal healthy disc through wear and continued pressure to herniation was described as long ago as 1934 by Mixter & Barr and by others since, including McKenzie (1981), Adams & Hutton (1985) and Adams & McMillan (1996) (Fig. 4.1).

Diagnosis

The diagnosis of disc protrusion or prolapse can only be made accurately by MRI scan, CT scan, myelogram or discography. Normal radiography will show nothing conclusive (Fig. 4.2).

Cause

Prolonged abuse of sustained and repetitive postures causes the disc to develop the lines of wear described above (Fig. 4.1b). The lines extend into radial fissures of the inner annulus, becoming an **internal disc derangement**. Pain will be experienced if the fissures extend into the perimeter of the disc. Recovery can be spontaneous at this stage and can be complete if full movement is regained with treatment and back care education.

With repetitive abuse or poor recovery, the weak lines of stress in the annulus cannot with-

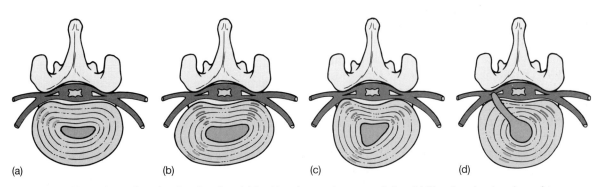

(a)   (b)   (c)   (d)

Figure 4.1   Lines of wear in a deteriorating disc. (a) Looking down onto a normal disc. (b) The disc showing signs of wear. (c) A line of wear starts to become a bulge. (d) A herniating disc with extrusion onto the nerve root.

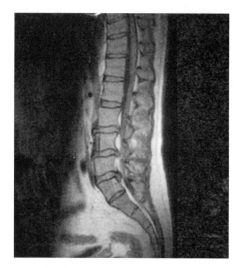

Figure 4.2 Disc protrusions at L3–4 and L4–5.

stand the continued pressure and the annulus bulges, becoming a protruding disc (Fig. 4.1c). Areas of weakness can occur at any point on the perimeter but the most common site is a posterolateral bulge, towards either side, the area most pressurized by forward bending in rotation (Hickey & Hukins 1980). Again, this stage can recover, with the protrusion retracting and the tissues healing.

In a protrusion that has not resolved, any sudden, possibly small movement can cause the bulge to weaken and become a **disc herniation** (Fig. 4.1d). When the nucleus pulposus breaks through the annulus fibrosis but remains confined by the posterior longitudinal ligament, it is considered to be a **disc extrusion**. A **disc sequestration** occurs if the herniated material penetrates the posterior longitudinal ligament and lies freely in the epidural space or if a disc fragment migrates beneath the posterior longitudinal ligament. The extruded material may have to be removed from the surrounding areas by operative procedure but it is possible for it to be absorbed naturally and for the disc to heal (Markolf & Morris 1974).

The processes shown in Figure 4.1 can occur at any age but disc herniation is unlikely to occur in the older disc as the nucleus is less fluid.

The above anatomic concept of gradual nuclear herniation, accepted as the only form for a long time, has been shown to represent only one facet of the true biological model. Protrusion or prolapse need not involve the nucleus pulposus but can occur with degeneration of the annulus fibrosus with the annular fibres protruding or prolapsing into the vertebral canal, while compressive loading applied to the discs, as above, creating stress peaks in the annulus, may cause the lamellae of the annulus to collapse into the nucleus (Lipson 1988, Yasuma et al 1988, 1990, Adams & McMillan 1996). Rauschning (1998) found that the dense layer of the outer annulus offered the only barrier to free dislocation of annular fragments.

Presentation

To the rear of the disc lie all the pain-sensitive structures of the spinal canal (see Chapter 6). Pressure or irritation of these structures can cause symptoms of pain in the back or pain, paraesthesia and anaesthesia in a limb.

The clinical picture which accompanies any gradual mechanical derangement of a lumbar disc is one of repetitive incidents of low back pain, with or without referral of pain into the buttocks and legs, each incident increasing in severity and length of time for recovery. Depending upon the amount of soft tissue involvement, the pain can be constant but more often it is relieved by certain positions or movements and aggravated by others. This is an occasion when the patient's analysis of the pain and understanding of the process of injury and healing can make all the difference between success and failure of recovery (Patient advice 4.3).

Treatment

Assess and treat using the McKenzie principle (McKenzie 1981).

It is important to remember that thousands of cadavers have shown disc bulges in spines that have been known to be pain free, so once again changed pathology does not necessarily lead to pain.

Patient advice 4.3   Possible disc lesions

Initially
- Teach the timescale of healing: 3–6 weeks for deep tissues is quite normal. Discs can take up to a year to recover.
- Give exercises for self-treatment, using the McKenzie analysis (McKenzie 1981).
- Teach back care in all situations, stressing the need for day-long awareness.
- Encourage early return to work but discuss environmental issues at home and in the workplace.

When limb referral is centralizing
- Encourage fast walking and swimming as soon as possible.
- In time, restore full ROM, with care in lumbar flexion.

Internal disc disruption

Characteristics

Internal disc disruption (IDD) is a condition in which a chemical destruction or degradation of the nucleus takes place, which causes the nucleus to discolour (Crock 1986, Vernon-Roberts 1992).

Diagnosis

Although this is normally evident on MRI or CT scan, patients with this syndrome can have normal X-rays, normal spinal scans and normal neurological findings. The only accurate diagnosis can then be made through discography (Crock 1986).

Cause

It is usually the result of trauma to a disc from heavy lifting or from the high-speed application of force, for example the compressive thrust of a heavy fall, which can damage the disc or fracture the VEP; but it can also be associated with inflammatory conditions such as osteomyelitis (Liston 1994). Inflammatory nuclear material may advance along radial fissures, causing erosion of the annulus. The result can be the production of noxious substances which may either drain into the spinal canal, irritating nerves in the vicinity, or pass into the vertebral body through the capillaries of the vertebral endplate (Crock 1986,

Bogduk & Twomey 1991). Crock (1986) has put forward a hypothesis suggesting that the irritating substances that enter the circulation via the vertebral endplate or that drain into the spinal canal can set up an autoimmune reaction.

Presentation

Internal disc disruption can present a syndrome of intractable pain, increased considerably on movement, leg pain, loss of energy, marked weight loss and profound depression. Reviewing the anatomy and pathophysiology of whiplash, Bogduk (1986) describes many similar symptoms relating to the cervical spine and upper limbs. Clinically this may be significant, especially in relation to the prolonged symptoms of pain, anxiety and depression in whiplash sufferers (see p. 54), who are often wrongly classed as malingerers, and in the repetitive 'unwell' reactions of some patients after extensive spinal surgery.

Treatment

The condition may require only medication until the inflammatory reaction has completely subsided.

Disc narrowing and disc degeneration

Research recorded by Twomey & Taylor (1987, 1991) and Bogduk & Twomey (1991) has shown that although disc narrowing is seen mostly in elderly people, possibly because they are more frequently investigated radiologically, it is not a phenomenon of ageing. With ageing, the vertebral endplates collapse and the discs tend to 'balloon' into the vertebral bodies (Fig. 4.3). Disc narrowing and degeneration are a consequence of wear and tear or injury during maturation, with reduction in the water content, especially of the nucleus pulposus. They occur mainly at discs which incur the greatest shearing strain of weight bearing, especially L5–S1, but can be more general. The loss of height can compromise the mechanics of the motion segment, causing increasing wear on the facet joints and the surrounding soft tissue.

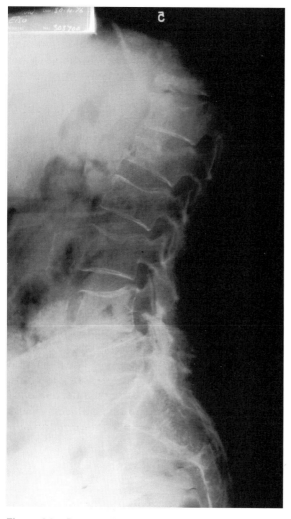

Figure 4.3 Degenerative and age changes showing disc ballooning and wedge-shaped L5.

Box 4.1   The causes of disc narrowing
• Mechanical early changes as in disc derangement. • Nuclear degradation as in IDD. • Annular collapse into the nucleus. • Loss of disc material from herniation or dehydration.

It is not a syndrome on its own and occurs in many associated presentations. Treatment relates to the presentation and not to the pathology (Box 4.1).

Disorders of the vertebral endplate

The VEP is the weakest part of the motion segment. Fractures can occur in compression and torsional injuries such as a fall from a height, explosion blasts, road accidents and rugby-type assaults. The injuries are usually asymptomatic. They can heal with no ill effects but changes may result if healing is incomplete (Bogduk & Twomey 1991). Endplate fractures can evoke an inflammatory repair response that can extend beyond the fracture site and invade the nucleus, leading to nuclear degradation and protrusion of the nucleus into the vertebral body. Nuclear extrusion into the vertebral body can form **Schmorl's nodes**.

Schmorl's nodes

The VEPs of infants have an excellent blood supply from the adjacent vertebral periosteum which brings nutrition to the growing IVDs. The disappearance of these vascular canals from the VEP of the developing vertebrae leaves weak areas which are the sites of potential prolapse of disc material into the vertebral bodies. In a variety of conditions which weaken the cartilaginous VEP, including trauma, disc degeneration, rheumatoid arthritis, osteoporosis and Scheuermann's disease (see below), the disc material prolapses into the VEP and forms cartilaginous nodes in the vertebral body above or below. The nodes can be centrally placed or towards the periphery and can be asymptomatic (Vernon-Roberts 1992, Taylor & Twomey 1994, Bigg-Wither & Kelly 1995).

Scheuermann's disease

Characteristics. Scheuermann's disease or vertebral osteochondrosis is a condition which occurs in adolescence, usually between the ages of 10 and 15, causing an exaggeration of the normal thoracic kyphosis, though it can affect any part of the spine.

Diagnosis. Radiographs can show any of the following: irregularity of the VEP, detached epiphyseal ring, multiple Schmorl's nodes, irregular or narrow disc spaces, anterior vertebral

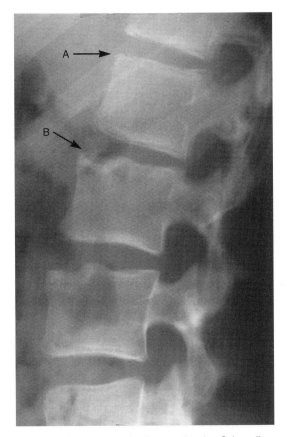

Figure 4.4 Scheuermann's disease showing Schmorl's nodes. (A) Normal ring epiphysis and VEP. (B) Abnormal, with the Schmorl's node interfering with the anterior half of the ring epiphysis. The anterior part of the vertebral body may then grow less than the posterior part, with the vertebra becoming wedge shaped.

body wedging, increased A–P vertebral body diameters with blurring and fuzziness of the bone (Bigg-Wither & Kelly 1995) (Fig. 4.4).

Cause. The cause is unknown but there may be an associated trauma or osteoporosis predisposing to VEP weakness. There is a relationship between lumbar Scheuermann's disease and hard physical labour in teenagers and it occurs more commonly in young athletes (Galasko 1992, Taylor & Twomey 1994).

Presentation. Although less severe cases may be symptom free, some teenagers present with intermittent back pain and stiffness, often in the dorsolumbar area, aggravated by contact sports

and sustained flexion. There can be a pronounced kyphosis and difficulty in maintaining good posture. The increased stiffness in one area can cause a hypermobility in another. Although there is usually no limb referral, on examination neural structure biomechanics may be altered, with positive slump tests and positive cervical spine flexion in standing forward bend, due to the increased resting length of the spinal canal (Grieve 1989).

Treatment. Treatment consists of improving the mobility of stiff segments and reducing irritability of painful ones (Grieve 1989). Check hamstring length because of the relationship between tight hamstrings and thoracic stress on forward bend. Give postural correction and advice about the need for active non-aggressive sports, like swimming, whilst avoiding contact sports. Teach gentle stretching exercises and spine stabilization of relevant areas. Persistent pain usually responds to rest and, if necessary, immobilization or bracing (Galasko 1992).

Deformity can continue until growth ceases, when the symptoms usually subside, but pain can recur in later life, presenting as insidious LBP or thoracic spine pain and stiffness. These conditions usually respond to mobilization and postural advice.

Disorders of the facet joints

Characteristics

In their stabilizing role as part of the vertebral triad, the facet joints are under constant stress. Not only do they control the shear force in flexion but they control all movements. For many years the disc was considered to be the main source of back pain but later investigations of the facet joints revealed that they too could be the culprits and the term 'facet syndrome' was coined (Mooney & Robertson 1976). Clinically, we now rarely isolate this syndrome as it is usually part of a more generalized presentation, but therapists are very aware of the important role dysfunction of these joints plays in the search for the source of pain (see 'The clinical picture', Chapter 9).

Diagnosis

X-rays may be normal or they may show narrowing of the joint space, some subchondral sclerosis and osteophytes at the joint margins (see 'Spondylosis', p. 48).

Cause

The facet joints, apart from the cartilage, have a liberal nerve supply and pain can originate from various sources (Box 4.2). The facet joint osteophytes are accompanied by enlarged synovial fat pads which form cushions between the osteophytes and the inferior articular process. The fat pads are innervated vascular structures, connected to the joint capsule and if they become trapped between the articular surfaces, pain can result. Pain may be due to either stimulation of the trapped tissue or the resulting traction on the capsule (Taylor & Twomey 1986, Vernon-Roberts 1992). Taylor & Twomey (1994) also suggest that a 'locked joint' could be the result of part of the cartilage, still attached to the capsule, being trapped in the same way.

Presentation and treatment

There can be vertebral pain with limb referral and limitation of function, both spinal and neural. Assessment should define and treat these reasonably accurately with mobilization and relevant movement. The action of the multifidus

---

muscle (see Chapter 5) in controlling accurate apposition of the joint surfaces would be important to assess and treat.

Tropism

Tropism is an asymmetry of the facet joints which leads to vertebral imbalance of the triad and therefore stress on structures. It is always associated with IVD problems because the facet joints are unable to protect the discs during rotation (Twomey 1998).

GENERAL VERTEBRAL DISORDERS

Certain disorders of the spine have, in the past, been considered to be 'diseases' but they are now accepted as degenerative changes which may or may not be part of the pain syndrome presented.

Some of the most commonly encountered terms are 'arthritis', 'degenerative joint disease', 'spondylosis' and 'spondylitis'. They are, unfortunately, often thrown at patients as a diagnosis which seems to imply: 'you have a whole lot of arthritic and degenerative disease in your spine, nothing can be done about it and you must expect to have pain'. The effect on patients is often distressing, partly because the word 'arthritis' in itself conjures up pictures of total disability with the use of aids and wheelchairs and partly because of the insinuation that there is no cure. As one of our roles is to teach and to reassure, it is important to explain the differences, especially those between osteoarthritis and rheumatoid arthritis.

The word 'arthritis' is derived from the Greek word *arthron* meaning 'joint'. So, arthritis means 'inflammation of a joint' but this term covers a number of disorders. It is important clinically to be able to differentiate between:

- rheumatoid arthritis (RA)
- osteoarthritis (OA)
- the 'seronegative' patterns of arthritis associated with ankylosing spondylitis, Reiter's disease (reactive arthritis), psoriasis, ulcerative colitis and Crohn's disease (enteropathic arthritis)

Box 4.2   The causes of facet joint pain

- An inflammatory capsular or ligamentous reaction to trauma.
- A mechanical incompetence of the joint in response to stress, possibly due to scarring from previous injury or shortening of tissue from maintained, immobile posture.
- A 'locked joint' or trapped fat pads between the articular surfaces.
- From degenerative conditions of the joint, which are often a sequel to disc degeneration altering the triad balance and throwing excessive stress on the joints.
- From occupations involving postural stress in sustained or repetitive stoop or sustained standing, especially with increased loading.

Table 4.1 A comparison between osteoarthritis and rheumatoid arthritis

	Osteoarthritis	Rheumatoid arthritis
Characteristics	• Hyaline cartilage damage • Changes in subchondral bone • Osteophyte formation	• Chronic systemic autoimmune inflammatory polyarthritis • Thickening and inflammation of synovial membrane, infiltrated with lymphocytes • Leads to cartilage degeneration and bone erosion
Diagnosis	• Exclude other disease • X-ray • Exclude pain from vertebral referral	• Blood tests: ESR, serum rheumatoid factor, plasma viscosity, C-reactive protein • X-ray
Cause	• Abnormal metabolic and physiological factors • Joint's inadequacy to meet mechanical stress of gait, weight, injury, occupational stresses • Possible impaired proprioception • Possible genetic basis	• Aetiology unknown • Genetic and microbiological factors
Presentation	• Joint pain and hard knobbly swelling • Stiffness after any period of rest • Heberden's nodes on distal IP joints • Can be inflamed with effusion	• Joint swelling, often soft, boggy texture • Stiffness am & pm • Shiny skin • Synovitis of tendon sheaths • Rheumatoid nodules • Episodes of acute pain and inflammation
Joints affected	• Joints under stress • Usually large weight bearing or small overused • Can occur in one or more joints but occurrence unrelated	• Symmetrical peripheral joints • Often starts in joints of hands and feet • Can progress to vertebrae • Several joints systemically affected
Musculature	• Weakened through disuse: lack of use or pain inhibition	• Weak and wasted around joints
Age group	• Most people over 30	• Any age, mainly 20–55 years. Known as Still's disease in children
Treatment	• Treat vertebrae if any referral • Rest and treat symptoms of swelling, inflammation, pain • Mobilize in pain-free ROM • Strengthen muscles • Encourage all activity, especially aerobic • Encourage weight loss if excessive • Educate for prevention rather than cure • Analgesics or NSAIDs • Local steroid injections but can lead to cartilage damage if overdone • Joint replacement	• Rest in acute phase • Splinting if necessary in position of function • Exercise using maximum range and minimal weight bearing • Encourage swimming • First-line drugs: analgesics and NSAIDs. Second-line drugs: corticosteroids, gold, drugs aimed at the immune system • Joint replacement

Compiled from Mourad 1991, Butler & Kerr 1992, Grennan & Jayson 1984, Hutton 1995, Walker 1995, Spector 1996

• postviral or post-streptococcal arthritis (rheumatic fever)
• systemic lupus.

It is beyond the scope of this book to describe all these but see *Collected reports on the rheumatic diseases* in Further reading.

Osteoarthritis and rheumatoid arthritis

Although all therapists are well aware of the differences between OA and RA, Table 4.1 clarifies the various points. It is important to explain the major differences to patients with OA and to reassure them they have not got an incurable 'disease' which travels round the body. The most important issue to emphasize is that, like so many structural and pathological changes, OA in itself need not give pain, although a number of factors in its complicated tissue involvement can contribute towards an inflammatory reaction and pain. An OA joint is possibly dysfunctional, less adaptable to change and so vulnerable to minor injury and overuse.

Interesting new research is reexamining connections between impaired proprioception and OA (Sharma & Yi-Chung Pai 1997, Gill & Callaghan 1998, Sims 1999). The question left unanswered is: does decreased proprioception lead to inappropriate movement and then OA or does OA cause a loss of proprioception? The first part of the question requires more research but in the meantime we can perhaps think in these terms: people's reaction to new stiffness is generally to avoid movement. Perhaps the opposite should be the case (Patient advice 4.4). Disuse can also result from natural inactivity or inactivity in pain avoidance from referred pain – perhaps leading to loss of proprioception. If this is so, how many hip replacements have been done that might have been saved by treating the lumbar spine initially? Maintenance of joint movement range and muscle balance could be one of the most important safeguards against OA.

Patient advice 4.4 Stiffness

1. Avoid stiffness by keeping a full ROM; for example:
   - if the neck feels stiff when turning in the car, don't avoid turning, push into the stiffness, slowly and repeatedly until it goes. Do not push into it if there is sharp pain
   - use every opportunity to stretch the hip joint in walking
   - use every opportunity to bend the knees during everyday activities; for example, squat when reaching into a low cupboard or picking up even a small object from the floor
   - don't be frightened of slight pain; for example, if the knee feels stiff, don't limp around on a bent knee – try to straighten it and move it as normally as you can until it eases.
2. Encourage an analytic, confident approach to stiffness and pain.

Spondylosis and degenerative joint disease

Although the word 'disease' occurs here, these are degenerative conditions of the vertebral column which most people have and which can be asymptomatic. In all degenerative disorders adaptive changes take place when the stressed tissues are capable of remodelling and opposing the applied stress, but if the stresses are severe or repetitive, destructive features may develop (Bogduk & Twomey 1991) (Fig. 4.5).

Spondylosis

Spondylosis describes disc narrowing and osteophytic formation along the junction of the vertebral bodies and their intervertebral discs, with irregularity of vertebral bodies and vertebral lipping (Nathan & Israel 1962, Bogduk & Twomey 1991, Vernon-Roberts 1992). As mentioned in

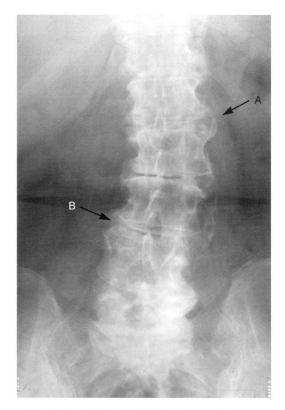

Figure 4.5 Spondylosis and spinal degeneration. (A) Pointed curved osteophyte. (B) Disc space narrowing.

Chapter 2, osteophytes are beak-like outgrowths composed of dense bone, more compact and stronger than the vertebral bodies (which are often osteoporotic). They can be viewed as a reactive and adaptive change that seeks to compensate for biomechanical failure. As the vertebrae become more osteoporotic with age the osteophytes become larger and more numerous. They can grow from the vertebral bodies until they meet, forming the vertebrae into a pillar-like shape which acts as a support against increased pressure. By growing onto the disc surfaces of the vertebral bodies, they can double the size of the original body, thus reducing pressure by dispersing it. Where there is gross disc narrowing, the facet joints become approximated and the IVF can be narrowed. Any of these changes can compromise neural tissue (Nathan & Israel 1962, Bogduk & Twomey 1991).

Cervical spondylotic myelopathy

Characteristics. This is an age-related degenerative condition occurring in people over 50. IVD deterioration and loss of disc height approximates the vertebral bodies; ligamentous laxity leads to vertebral body subluxation; disc herniation frequently occurs. Osteophytes may compress the blood vessels and neural tissue of the spinal canal. Facet joints degenerate and further osteophytes compress the spinal nerve roots. The ligamentum flavum becomes inelastic, bulging into the spinal canal and compressing the cord.

Diagnosis. Diagnosis is by MRI scan.

Presentation. Loss of dexterity in the upper extremities, abnormal hand sensations, diffuse non-specific weakness and a broad-based, jerky gait.

Treatment. Physical therapy to improve function. Collar/brace immobilization, NSAIDs, muscle relaxants, epidural steroids. If severe, operative decompression (Zipnick et al 1996).

Degenerative joint disease or osteoarthrosis

Osteoarthrosis is extensive OA of the facet joints. The discs and vertebral bodies are relatively normal. There are synovial changes, cartilage destruction with subchondral sclerosis, loss of joint spaces and osteophytic formation at the joint margins. The condition can be symptom free or can cause severe nerve root irritation on certain movements. In the cervical spine, osteophytes can impinge on the vertebral artery or in the thoracic spine they can cause irritation of the sympathetic chain. The problem with all degenerative conditions is that the joint is no longer able to withstand stress.

Spondylitis

Spondylitis is a group of diseases in which an inflammatory arthritis accompanies persistently negative tests for the rheumatoid factor.

Ankylosing spondylitis

Characteristics. Ankylosing spondylitis (AS) is an inflammatory disease of the spinal column affecting young adults; the sex prevalence in males becomes less marked over the age of 16. It affects the synovial and cartilaginous articulations in which ossification of the spinal ligaments and bony ankylosis occurs. It is a progressive disease of the spine and larger joints, such as the hips and shoulders. It is usually self-limiting but may result in complete fusion of the spinal column, giving rise to the term 'bamboo spine' (Grieve 1989, Mourad 1991).

Diagnosis. Diagnosis is by clinical examination showing limitation of spinal movement, sacroiliac stiffness and sharp pain on testing (providing it has not yet fused), flexion contractures of the hip, limitation of bilateral leg abduction and gross limitation of lateral flexion (often a clinical sign of an inflammatory vertebral disease). Blood tests are sometimes unreliable and HLA B27 tissue typing is not always dependable. X-ray can show the typical 'bamboo' spine (Grieve 1989, Rai 1995) (Fig. 4.6).

Cause. The cause of AS is uncertain. It is one of the seronegative spondyloarthritides. The majority of patients are HLA B27 positive and the risk of passing the same antigen onto a child is 1 in 2. Certain populations have a predisposition towards it and there is possibly an environmental or bacterial trigger.

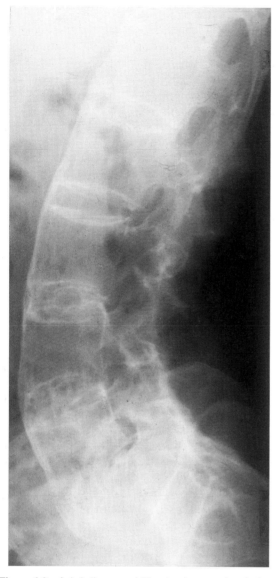

Figure 4.6 Ankylosing spondylitis, showing complete fusion.

Presentation. Insidious onset of LBP and stiffness. Morning back ache and sacroiliac pain are early symptoms (Mourad 1991, Gass 1995). There can be pain referral into both buttocks and posterior thighs. Fatigue is often present. Thoracic spine involvement often introduces reduced chest expansion and respiratory problems. Achilles tendonitis and plantar fasciitis may also be present. Asymptomatic prostatitis may be evident in the majority of males. Recurrent iritis and conjunctivitis can occur early in the disease. Cardiac involvement may be clinically silent or may be significant with an aortic murmur from postinflammatory scarring (Rai 1995). Examination can reveal those points mentioned in the diagnosis.

Treatment.

Medication. NSAIDs and medication to relieve pain and stiffness: possibly phenylbutazone and sulphasalazine.

Therapy. A rigorous exercise routine with diligent postural correction to try to delay, and possibly stop, the progression of the disease. Spinal extension exercises are the key component and exercise should be done twice daily. Education in self-management is vital, with 'doctor dependence' discouraged. These often young patients need a great deal of encouragement and support as self-worth understandably diminishes with the progression of postural deformity (Dixey & Kerr 1992, Rai 1995, Gass 1995).

Reiter's syndrome

This is an aseptic reactive arthritis which means that a local infection at one site may initiate development of a synovitis at a distant site. With Reiter's syndrome there are clinical features of lower limb joint effusion, ocular inflammation, urethritis, heel pain, MTP joint synovitis and thickening on the soles of the feet. There is an association with sexually transmitted disease (Keat 1996).

Psoriatic arthritis

Psoriatic arthritis is a distinct clinical entity as one of the seronegative group. It is a peripheral polyarthritis, frequently symmetrical, with a history of psoriasis, sacroiliitis and asymmetrical spondylitis. It usually responds to NSAIDs and analgesics for pain and dithranol and coal tar for psoriasis (Wright 1996).

OTHER VERTEBRAL ANOMALIES

Spinal stenosis

Characteristics

Spinal stenosis is a narrowing of the spinal canal,

the nerve root canals (see Chapter 6) or the IVF, or all of these structures. It may be localized to one vertebra or be more generalized. The effects range from minor irritation to major neurological or vascular changes.

Diagnosis

Diagnosis is by plain radiographs or MRI scan.

Cause

The narrowing may be caused by bony deformity or soft tissue deformation which could be congenital/developmental, degenerative/acquired (often associated with spondylolisthesis) or a combination of these, with or without disc herniation (Arnoldi et al 1976, Crock & Yoshizawa 1976, Kirkaldy-Willis & McIvor 1976). Morphologically, lumbar stenosis (Fig. 4.7) can be divided into central stenosis, involving the nerve roots and cauda equina, and lateral stenosis, disturbing the spinal nerve in the lateral recess, the nerve root canal or IVF. However, these can occur together.

In congenital and developmental stenosis, the anterior/posterior dimensions can be narrowed from about 20 mm (normal) to less than 12 mm; the laminae are thicker and the pedicles shorter (Fig. 4.7b). In degenerative or acquired stenosis, narrowing can occur because of large disc protrusion or herniation, ligamentum flavum thickening, neural arch thickening, facet joint arthrosis or degenerative spondylolisthesis. The canal is trefoil shaped, with less room in the lateral recess (Fig. 4.7c).

Because of the movement of the spinal cord and cauda equina within the canal, there is less space in the normal canal during lumbar extension than in flexion, with the narrowing possibly increased by the normal relaxation of the ligamentum flavum, with or without any degenerative thickening. With structural narrowing of the canal, extension becomes even more restrictive.

Presentation

The patient can present with some LBP, unilateral or bilateral buttock pain and leg pain. Leg pain is increased with walking and any lumbar extension and relieved by sitting or forward bending, such as leaning on a shopping trolley. Patients often report 'drop attacks' where their legs suddenly give out while walking. Peripheral vascular disease and neuropathy must be excluded as they both mimic neuroclaudication, so there should be a careful search for vascular insufficiency or any neural deficiency. For example, vascular claudication is relieved by merely ceasing activity while neuroclaudication requires the addition of postural alteration into flexion; lower extremity pulses are diminished in vascular claudication but not with neuropathy. Cauda equina symptoms need further investigations and referral to a consultant neurosurgeon. The pain complaint should be activity related and those with pain at rest should be evaluated for other aetiologies (e.g. tumour) (Herkowitz 1995).

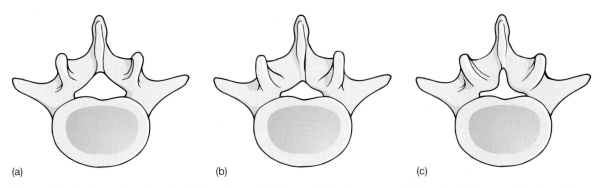

(a)   (b)   (c)

Figure 4.7 Lumbar spinal stenosis. (a) Normal canal. (b) Congenital or developmental stenosis. (c) Degenerative stenosis. (Reproduced with permission from Arnoldi et al 1976.)

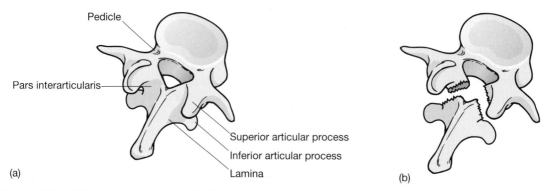

Figure 4.8   (a) Normal lumbar vertebra. (b) Bilateral pars defect in spondylolysis.

Treatment

Treatment is symptomatic and includes NSAIDs and avoidance of aggravating factors. If acute, bed rest for only 2–3 days should be prescribed or a short-term corset if it reduces pain, but a corset tends to maintain extension and may not be of help. Later, therapy should include trunk dynamic stabilization with transversus abdominis and multifidus reeducation. Extension exercises should be avoided. Aerobic activities such as swimming and static bike work should be encouraged. Surgical decompression with or without fusion may be necessary (Schonstrom 1994, Zipnick et al 1996).

Spondylolysis and spondylolisthesis

Spondylolysis

Characteristics. Spondylolysis is a bony defect in the vertebral pars interarticularis (Fig. 4.8). It is a common failure which may be bilateral or unilateral, occurring mainly in the mid or lower lumbar spine.

Diagnosis. Diagnosis is by plain radiographs or MRI scan. Oblique radiological views show a lucent line through the pars region, which is traditionally likened to a collar round the neck of a Scottie dog (Fig. 4.9).

Cause. Although the pars defect is not a congenital lesion there appears to be a familial tendency. The aetiology is thought to be an acquired fracture occurring in infancy or early childhood, often between 5 and 6 years of age

(Grieve 1989). It occurs also in early adulthood, most often seen as a stress-type fracture of the pars following repeated trauma. Spondylolysis is often found in athletes and gymnasts after repeating movements in lumbar extension or extension and rotation. Unlike other fractures, it tends to heal with fibrous union, with or without a pseudoarthrosis. If pseudoarthrosis occurs, hypertrophic changes can develop around the pars which can entrap the nerve root or spinal nerve as it runs under its pedicle (Bigwither & Kelly 1995). A bilateral spondylolysis can lead to a spondylolisthesis (see below).

Presentation. Spondylolysis can be asymptomatic or cause local pain and radicular pain, sometimes with symptoms severe enough to warrant fusion.

Treatment. Treatment is entirely related to symptoms and severity of the condition, with therapy mainly based on lumbar stabilization exercises (O'Sullivan et al 1997).

Spondylolisthesis

Characteristics. Spondylolisthesis is the forward slip (**olisthesis**) of a vertebral body on the one below. Normally, this slip is resisted by:

- the bony block of the facet joints with their normal coronal orientation in the lower lumbar spine (Herkowitz 1995)
- the intact neural arch and pedicle
- the intervertebral discs bonding together with the vertebral bodies

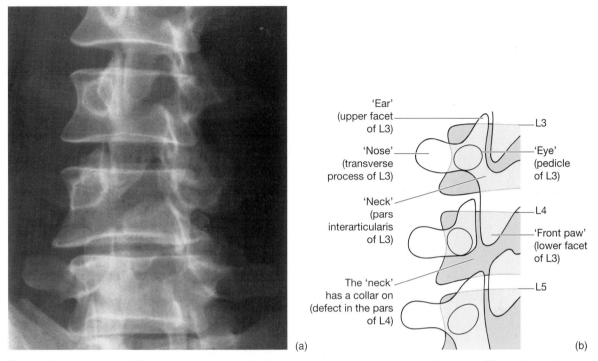

(a)   (b)

Figure 4.9   (a) Fracture of the pars interarticularis. (b) Diagram to illustrate the fracture and the 'collar of the scottie dog'.

- the normal bony plasticity preventing stretch of the pedicles.

Articular defects and defects of the neural arch break down this mechanism and forward slip occurs.

A **retrolisthesis** (backward slip) of L4 on L5 is common in the lumbar spine when there are degenerative changes of the motion segment (Twomey 1998).

Diagnosis. The degree of slippage can be measured on X-ray, usually expressed in quarters of the A–P dimensions of the vertebral body. A first-degree listhesis is equal to the first quarter, a second-degree is equal to half the sagittal diameter, a third-degree slip is a displacement equal to three-quarters. Further slippage is known as **spondyloptosis** (Grieve 1989).

Cause. According to Wiltse et al (1976), there are five clinical groups of spondylolis-thesis:

1. *Congenital*: rare. Usually combined with multiple anomalies, such as spina bifida, often with congenital scoliosis. Usually becomes apparent during the growth spurt.

2. *Isthmic or spondylolytic*: an alteration of the pars interarticularis, most frequently at L5. The pars can be elongated without bony discontinuity, often as a result of microtrauma, or it can be fractured, known as a lytic

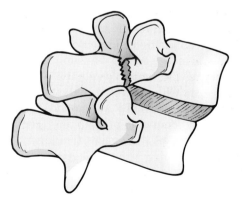

Figure 4.10   Lytic spondylolisthesis with forward slip of upper vertebra.

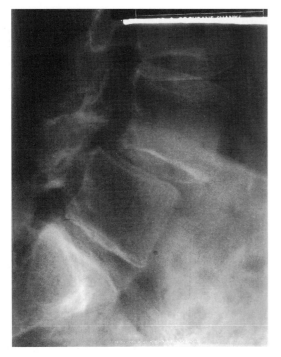

Figure 4.11 Degenerative spondylolisthesis L4–5.

spondylolisthesis (Fig. 4.10). This type of spondylolisthesis can occur in youth, with a high incidence of occurrence in athletes. Extension, extension in rotation or a flexion overload can all cause stress.

3. *Degenerative*: often associated with spinal stenosis. OA of the facet joints plays a major role in increasing a more sagittal facet joint orientation, decreasing the normal resistance to shear forces and predisposing to slippage when other factors are present. The problem often starts with disc degeneration and 'settling' of the motion segment, which leads to buckling of the ligamentum flavum; microinstability of the segment follows with stretching of the hypertrophic facet joint capsules and ultimately slippage. It occurs most commonly at L4–5 and tends to be greater in females than males (Herkowitz 1995) (Fig. 4.11).

4. *Traumatic*: dislocation of the facet joints or fracture of the spinous process which extends into the lamina, or a fracture of the pars. These can be reduced and maintained.

5. *Pathological*: this occurs generally as a result of bone disease, for example osteomalacia.

Presentation. Symptoms of spondylolisthesis can be varied. Typical of lytic spondylolisthesis is sudden LBP, rigid spine, spastic or functional scoliosis, flat sacrum and hamstring spasm. Degenerative spondylolisthesis can give LBP, facet joint pain with relevant referral, root entrapment from disc bulge, stenotic signs from the buckling ligamentum flavum (see 'Spinal stenosis' above) and signs of instability (the loss of spinal ability to maintain the relationship between vertebrae without damage). Cauda equina symptoms must always demand further investigation. Although spondylolisthesis presents a dramatic picture on X-ray, it can be asymptomatic for a lifetime.

Treatment. Treatment is related to symptoms and assessment. Severe pain may require short-term bed rest, with antiinflammatory medication. Once the symptoms are under control, LBP and non-stenotic symptoms should be treated in the normal manner, with pain-reducing modalities, mobilization of relevant stiffness and stabilizing exercises, especially for transversus abdominis and multifidus. If the pattern of abdominal activation has changed in the presence of chronic LBP, rectus abdominis may substitute during attempts to preferentially activate the deep abdominals (O'Sullivan et al 1997). Active flexion exercises and general aerobic exercises, such as a static bike, can be added when appropriate (Herkowitz 1995).

For those with stenosis, see above. If leg pain persists, epidural steroids can be considered. The majority of patients respond to conservative treatment but if there is a neurological deficit or a significant reduction in quality of life, further investigations should be made, with possible surgical intervention (Herkowitz 1995).

INJURY

Whiplash

Characteristics

The most common 'sprain' is the whiplash injury. It involves not only the cervical spine but also the upper thoracic spine and can embroil the whole vertical column, compromising ligamentous, capsular, cartilaginous, discogenic, muscular, vascular and nervous tissue, leading to pathodynamics of the peripheral nervous system, even to implicating the sympathetic nervous chain (Butler 1991).

Diagnosis

By history and report of accident, as radiography does not necessarily show any injury. MRI, CT scans or discography are needed to show any soft tissue lesions.

Cause

Whiplash injuries from road traffic accidents (RTAs) were thought to be hyperflexion/hyperextension injuries but Panjabi et al (1998) propose that there is a more complicated picture. Their research shows that during the first phase of injury there is an S-shaped curvature, with flexion of the upper cervical spine and extension in the lower cervical; during the second phase the entire cervical spine bends into extension (Fig. 4.12).

In forced flexion, the facet joints reach the end of range with capsular ligament elongation and stretch of the posterior ligaments, together with violent disc anterior compression. End-of-range extension can tear the discs anteriorly and the synovial folds within the facet joints and can cause approximation of the spinous processes. The entire

list of possible injuries, which are often multilevel, is extensive: posterior muscle tears, facet joint dislocations, extensive bruising in the facet joints, disc ruptures with posterior herniation, disc rim lesions, anterior tears of the annulus, bleeding in the spinal canal, damage to spinal nerves and a high risk of spinal cord lesions. Injury to the spinal cord and hindbrain or vertebral artery lesions initiated by its stretch may be associated with symptoms of dizziness, nausea and muscle weakness. In less severe injuries there can still be transverse tears at the discovertebral junction, with ligament, muscular and capsular strains (Twomey & Taylor 1993, Panjabi et al 1998, Rauschning 1998, Twomey 1998).

In the lumbar spine fractures of the facet joints are more common, causing wedge compression fractures of the lumbar bodies, intradiscal bleeding or compression of the disc itself (Taylor & Twomey 1994).

Whiplash-type injuries can also occur in sport, for example in diving, in the sudden explosive movement of a tennis serve or in the same flexion/extension action of bowling in cricket. Constant loading of the spine in extension can affect the point of impact of the extended facet joints, giving rise to sclerosis and thickening of the compact bone of the lamina that is often observed in young adult spines (Twomey et al 1988).

Presentation

Varying degrees of cervical, thoracic and/or

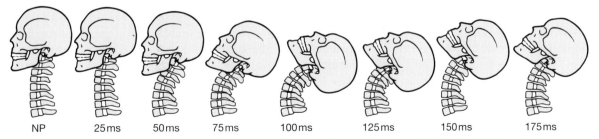

| NP | 25ms | 50ms | 75ms | 100ms | 125ms | 150ms | 175ms |

Figure 4.12 The proposed injury mechanism in whiplash. Starting with neutral posture (NP), it takes 50–75 ms for the neck to form an S-shaped curvature. During this phase, the lower cervical spine intervertebral joints exhibit hyperextension, exceeding their physiological limits. This is the phase of injuries to the lower cervical spine. In the later phase, the entire spine goes into extension but the intervertebral joints do not exceed their physiological limits and therefore there is no potential for injury. (Reproduced with permission from Grauer et al 1997 Spine 22: 2489–2494.)

lumbar pain are experienced immediately or sometimes delayed by 24 hours after injury or can appear some time later with unprovable connections. Other symptoms can include limb pain referral, paraesthesia and anaesthesia, weakness, severe headaches, nausea and dizziness. It is worth remembering IDD described by Crock (1986) above. Any cord signs must be immediately referred to a consultant.

Treatment

X-rays should be made after any RTA as a safeguard in case of severe bony injury, for example a fractured odontoid process, and for a report, as litigation frequently follows.

Advice for treatment of whiplash varies considerably from the need to start immediately, within the first few hours (Harding 1998), to the preference for complete immobilization in a hard collar for 4 weeks (Twomey 1998). Clinically, a mixture of the original Twomey & Taylor (1993) and the recent Harding (1998) advice seems to be most appropriate. However, this decision should rest entirely on the severity of the condition and the initial assessment.

Initial treatment consists of ice and inflammatory medication with a brief period of collar immobilization to ensure that bleeding into the area ceases. Encourage frequent, short periods of rest and relaxation with the head supported in the most pain-free position, possibly supine. Encourage intermittent gentle, small-range active movement – lying supine in severe cases or merely encouraging the small nods and turns of 'yes', 'no' and 'maybe' of flexion, rotation and lateral flexion. Encourage normal general body activities with free active leg movements. Avoid large, rapid, tense, frequent cervical movements and complete rest of the whole body (Harding 1998).

A slow, gentle programme based on the patient's response to movement should be progressed over many weeks. Under no circumstances should these joints be forced or manipulated in the early recovery from whiplash. Cervical manipulation places considerable strain on the annulus fibres, which are slow to heal (Twomey & Taylor 1993). Thacker (Thacker & Butler 1997) agrees with the completely 'hands off' regime but Butler (Thacker & Butler 1997) points out that with whiplash-associated disorders, mobilization may be necessary at a later date.

Whiplash injuries are not to be taken lightly; in fact, Twomey & Taylor (1993) condemn any view that considers patients with whiplash injuries to be hysterical, neurotic or dishonest. In its simplest form the whiplash can equate to 14 'sprained' joints with the normal inflammatory changes.

In January 1995, the Société de l'Assurance Automobile du Quebec (SAAQ) published a text entitled 'Whiplash-associated disorders (WAD): redefining whiplash and its management (Spitzer et al 1995), authored by the Quebec Task Force on Whiplash-Associated Disorders. The Task Force consisted of an eminent panel of experts in different fields and their mandate was to address a variety of issues concerning whiplash injuries. The Task Force has been severely criticized by Freeman et al (1998) for their lack of thorough examination of all aspects of the injury and for their underplaying of the consequences that result. Freeman et al report that the Quebec Task Force conclusion was that whiplash injuries result in 'temporary discomfort', they have a 'favorable prognosis' and the 'pain (resulting from whiplash injuries) is not harmful'. They vehemently question the validity of these conclusions.

Whiplash is a traumatic event, especially in an RTA, and there will inevitably be symptoms of shock and emotional trauma with feelings of anger, frustration, fear of the future, uncertainty and victimization. However, maintained pain is in no way the 'psychosomatic' picture described by the courts; it is intensely more complicated. During the last 15 years of clinical experience, I have never failed to reproduce signs on testing which corroborate the symptoms reported by the patient, which also fit the picture of possible pathological injury, even when litigation is in progress.

The crucial points in avoiding chronic pain are as follows.

Box 4.3 Age changes in the motion segment (compiled from Vernon-Roberts 1987 and Taylor & Twomey 1994)

Disc	• Collagen content greater but less distinction between nucleus and annulus • Loss of fluid content and fall in nuclear pressure – less elastic • Less easily deformed but recovers more slowly • Narrowing usually because of degeneration rather than ageing, greatest in L4–5 disc • Ballooning into vertebral body above and below because of osteoporotic changes in the bone and collapse of the VEP (Fig. 4.3) • Fissures in the annulus but as nucleus has less fluid, less risk of it flowing into the annulus • Increased stiffness and decreased ROM

Vertebral body	• Loss of bone density
	• Loss of horizontal bony trabeculae leading to buckling and fractures of unsupported vertical trabeculae, leading to:
	  • Loss of height
	  • Increase in width – 'thickening of the waist'

VEP	• Cartilage thins • Tiny microfractures can appear • Bows into the vertebral body (Fig. 4.3)
Facet joint	• Degeneration of cartilage – irregular thickness • Splits in cartilage and shearing from subchondral bone. Fat pads can become trapped between bony surfaces • Thickening of capsule, less elastic • Synovial fluid more viscous • Loss of movement because of increased stiffness
Bone	• Osteophytes at joint margins, with enlarged synovial fat pads as cushions between osteophytes and inferior articular process • Shortening of vertebral column with possible 'kissing spines', leading to: • Formation of adventitious joints between them
Soft tissues	• Stiffness due to lack of movement and alteration of fibres • Buckling of the ligamentum flavum

• Early practical advice for the patient to understand the type of injury (often the comparison with a sprained ankle can be helpful).
• Reassurance and instruction about the timescale of healing.
• Thorough treatment, including reeducation on pain management and the need to introduce gradually increased movement.
• Early restoration of normal activities and return to work as tissue healing permits, in spite of some remaining discomfort.

We must give confidence that, in time, activity is the greatest healer.

AGE CHANGES IN THE MOTION SEGMENT

Age changes may take place in any of the tissues of the motion segment. They may be minimal, both in degree and effect, especially if ROM and good activity is maintained. Box 4.3 describes the changes which may occur.

Key points

1. Altered pathology does not necessarily give pain.
2. X-rays can be misleading; the pain may be entirely related to soft tissue dysfunction and unrelated to anything shown.
3. A thorough assessment is essential.
4. Treatment aims should be to explain the problem in a positive way, to reduce pain and restore function, to educate in back care and self-responsibility, to restore confidence and return to normal work and activities.

REFERENCES

Adams M A 1996 Biomechanics of low back pain. Pain Reviews 3: 15–50

Adams M A, Hutton W C 1982 Prolapsed intervertebral disc: a hyperflexion injury. Spine 7(3): 184–191

Adams M A, Hutton W C 1985 Gradual disc prolapse. Spine 10(6): 524–531

Adams M A, McMillan D W 1996 Sustained loading generates stress concentrations in lumbar intervertebral discs. Spine 21(4): 434–438

Arnoldi C C, Brodsky A E, Couchoix J 1976 Lumbar spinal stenosis and nerve root entrapment syndromes. Clinical Orthopaedics 115: 4–5

Bigwither G, Kelly P 1995 Diagnostic imaging in musculoskeletal physiotherapy. In: Refshauge K, Gass E (eds) Musculoskeletal physiotherapy. Butterworth Heinemann, Oxford

Bogduk N 1986 The anatomy and pathophysiology of whiplash. Clinical Biomechanics 1(2): 92–101

Bogduk N 1992 The sources of low back pain. In: Jaysen M I V (ed) The lumbar spine and back pain, 4th edn. Churchill Livingstone, Edinburgh

Bogduk N, Twomey L T 1991 Clinical anatomy of the lumbar spine, 2nd edn. Churchill Livingstone, Edinburgh

Butler D 1991 Mobilisation of the nervous system. Churchill Livingstone, Edinburgh

Butler R C, Kerr M 1992 Rheumatoid arthritis and juvenile chronic arthritis. In: Tidswell M E (ed) Cash's textbook of orthopaedics and rheumatology for physiotherapists. Mosby Year Book Europe, London

Crock H V 1986 The presidential address: ISSLS. Internal disc disruption: a challenge to disc prolapse fifty years on. Spine 11(6): 650–653

Crock H V, Yoshizawa H 1976 The blood supply of the lumbar vertebral column. Clinical Orthopedics 115: 6–21

Dixey J J, Kerr M 1992 The spondyloarthropathies. In: Tidswell M E (ed) Cash's textbook of orthopaedics and rheumatology for physiotherapists, 2nd edn. Mosby Year Book Europe, London

Freeman D F, Croft A C, Rossignol M R 1998 'Whiplash associated disorders: redefining whiplash and its management' by the Quebec Task Force: a critical evaluation. Spine 23(9): 1043–1049

Galasko G S B 1992 Back pain in children. In: Jayson M I V (ed) The lumbar spine and back pain, 4th edn. Churchill Livingstone, Edinburgh.

Gass E M 1995 The role of the physiotherapist in the management of chronic low back pain. In: Refshauge K, Gass E (eds) Musculoskeletal physiotherapy. Butterworth Heinemann, Oxford

Gill K P, Callaghan M J 1998 The measurement of lumbar proprioception in individuals with and without low back pain. Spine 23(3): 371–377

Grennan D M, Jayson M I V 1984 Rheumatoid arthritis. In: Wall P, Melzack R (eds) Textbook of pain. Churchill Livingstone, Edinburgh

Grieve G 1989 Common vertebral joint problems, 2nd edn. Churchill Livingstone, Edinburgh

Harding V 1998 Minimising chronicity after whiplash injury. In: Gifford L (ed) Topical issues in pain. Physiotherapy Pain Association yearbook 1998–1999. NOI Press, Falmouth, Adelaide

Herkowitz H 1995 Spine update: degenerative lumbar spondylolisthesis. Spine 20(9): 1084–1090

Hickey D S, Hukins D W L 1980 Relation between the structure of the annulus fibrosus and the function and failure of the intervertebral disc. Spine 5(2): 106–117

Hutton C W 1995 Osteoarthritis: clinical features and management. In: Butler R C, Jayson M I V (eds) Collected reports on the rheumatic diseases. Arthritis and Rheumatism Council for Research, Chesterfield

Keat A 1996 Reiter's syndrome and reactive arthritis. In: Butler R, Jayson M I V (eds) Collected reports on the rheumatic diseases. Arthritis and Rheumatism Council for Research, Chesterfield

Kirkaldy-Willis W H, McIvor G W D 1976 Lumbar spinal stenosis. Clinical Orthopedics 115: 2–3

Lipson S J 1988 Metaplastic proliferative cartilage as an alternative concept to herniated intervertebral disc. Spine 13(9): 105–160

Liston C B 1994 Low back pain: physical treatment in children and adolescents. In: Twomey L T, Taylor J R (eds) Physical therapy of the low back. Churchill Livingstone, Edinburgh

Markolf K L, Morris J M 1974 The structural components of the intervertebral disc. Journal of Bone and Joint Surgery 56-A(4): 675–687

McKenzie R 1981 The lumbar spine. Mechanical diagnosis and therapy. Spinal Publications, Waikanae, New Zealand

Mixter W J, Barr J S 1934 Rupture of the intervertebral disc with involvement of the spinal canal. New England Journal of Medicine 211: 210–215

Mooney M D, Robertson J 1976 The facet syndrome. Clinical Orthopaedics and Related Research 115: 149–156

Mourad L A 1991 Orthopedic disorders. Mosby Year Book, St Louis

Nathan H, Israel J 1962 Osteophytes of the vertebral column. Journal of Bone and Joint Surgery 44-A(2): 243–264

O'Sullivan P B, Twomey L T, Allison G T 1997 Evaluation of specific stabilising exercises in the treatment of chronic low back pain with radiological diagnosis of spondylolysis or spondylolisthesis. Spine 22(24): 2959–2967

Panjabi M M, White A A 1980 Basic biomechanics of the spine. Neurosurgery 7(1): 76–93

Panjabi M M, Cholewicki J, Nibu K et al 1998 Mechanisms of whiplash injury. Clinical Biomechanics 13: 239–249

Rai A 1995 Ankylosing spondylitis. In: Collected reports on the rheumatic diseases. Arthritis and Rheumatism Council for Research, Chesterfield

Rauschning W 1998 Lecture: patho-anatomical and clinical findings in spinal injuries and normal, functional and pathological anatomy of the spine. Swedish Medical Research Council, Stockholm

Schonstrom N 1994 Lumbar spinal stenosis. In: Twomey L T, Taylor J (eds) Physical therapy of the low back. Churchill Livingstone, Edinburgh

Sharma L, Yi-Chung Pai 1997 Impaired proprioception and osteoarthritis. Current Opinion in Rheumatology 9: 253–258

Sims K 1999 The development of hip osteoarthritis: implications for conservative management. Manual Therapy 4(3): 127–135

Spector T 1996 ARC research establishes a genetic basis for osteoarthritis. Arthritis Today 96

Spitzer W O et al 1995 Whiplash associated disorders: redefining whiplash and its management. Spine 20(85): 10s–73s

Taylor J R, Twomey L T 1986 Age changes in the lumbar zygapophyseal joints. Spine 11(7): 739–745

Taylor J R, Twomey L T 1994 The lumbar spine from infancy to old age. In: Twomey L T, Taylor J R (eds) Physical therapy of the low back. Churchill Livingstone, New York

Thacker M, Butler D 1997 Clinical problem solving. Physiotherapy Research 2: 201–211

Twomey L 1998 The sporting back. The Sporting Back Symposium, London

Twomey L T, Taylor J R 1987 Age changes in the lumbar vertebrae and the intervertebral discs. Clinical Orthopaedics and Related Research 221(224): 97

Twomey L T, Taylor J R 1991 Age related changes in the lumbar spine and spinal rehabilitation. Critical Reviews in Physical and Rehabilitation Medicine 2(3): 153–169

Twomey L T, Taylor J R 1993 The whiplash syndrome: pathology and physical treatment. Journal of Manual and Manipulative Therapy 1(1): 26–29

Twomey L T, Taylor J R, Oliver M J 1988 Sustained flexion loading, rapid extension loading of the lumbar spine, and the physical therapy of related injuries. Physiotherapy Practice 4: 129–137

Vernon-Roberts B 1992 Age-related and degenerative pathology of intervertebral discs and apophyseal joints. In: Jayson M I V (ed) The lumbar spine and back pain, 4th edn. Churchill Livingstone, Edinburgh

Walker D J 1995 Rheumatoid arthritis. In: Butler R C, Jayson M I V (eds) Collected reports on the rheumatic diseases. Arthritis and Rheumatism Council for Research, Chesterfield

Wiltse L, Newman P, MacNab I 1976 Classification of spondylolysis and spondylolisthesis. Clinical Orthopedics 117: 23–29

Wright V 1996 Psoriatic arthritis. In: Butler R C, Jayson M I V (eds) Collected reports on the rheumatic diseases. Arthritis and Rheumatism Council for Research, Chesterfield

Yasuma T, Ohno R, Yamauchi Y 1988 False-negative lumbar discograms. Journal of Bone and Joint Surgery 70A(9): 1279–1289

Yasuma T, Okamura T, Yamauchi Y 1990 Histological changes in aging lumbar intervertebral discs. Journal of Bone and Joint Surgery 72A(2): 220–229

Zipnick R, Gorek J, Kostiuk J P et al 1996 The aging spine. Spine 10(3)

FURTHER READING

Adams M 1996 Biomechanics of low back pain. Pain Reviews 3: 15–30

Butler R, Jayson M (eds) 1996 Collected reports on the rheumatic diseases. Arthritis and Rheumatism Council for Research, Chesterfield

Cyriax J 1982 Textbook of orthopaedic medicine: diagnosis of soft tissue lesions, 8th edn. Baillière Tindall, London

Grant R 1994 (ed) Physical therapy of the cervical and thoracic spine. Churchill Livingstone, Edinburgh

Grieve G P 1988 Common vertebral joint problems, 2nd edn. Churchill Livingstone, Edinburgh

O'Sullivan P B, Twomey L T, Allison G T 1997 Evaluation of specific stabilising exercise in the treatment of chronic low back pain with radiological diagnosis of spondylolysis or spondylolisthesis. Spine 22(24): 2959–2967

Stinson J T 1993 Spondylolysis and spondylolisthesis in the athlete. Clinics in Sports Medicine 2(3): 517–528

5

The muscles of the trunk

This chapter deals with muscle function, stabilizing mechanisms and injury. The initial summary of general muscle structure is intended as revision.

STRUCTURE OF MUSCLE TISSUE

There are three kinds of muscle tissue: skeletal, smooth and cardiac. Skeletal or striated muscles function under voluntary control and are concerned with body movement, contracting and relaxing on command; smooth or unstriated muscle tissues, those of the internal organs, work without conscious control; cardiac muscle, a mixture of the two, is involuntary but striated. In the context of this book, only skeletal muscle will be discussed.

Skeletal muscle is made up of individual muscle fibres. Each fibre is a single long cylindrical cell, enclosed by a membrane, the **sarcolemma**. The fibres are made up of **myofibrils** which are again divisible into individual filaments the centres of which are made up of contractile protein or **cytoplasm** (Ganong 1991, Mourad 1991). Muscle fibres are in bundles or **fasciculi**; each fibre is surrounded and separated from its neighbour in the fascicle by a connective tissue covering, the **endomysium**. Joining the many fasciculi together is more connective tissue, the **perimysium**, and the whole outer muscle covering is the **epimysium**. The three connective tissues provide pathways for nerves and blood vessels supplying the muscle cells. Collagen-producing fibroblasts play an important

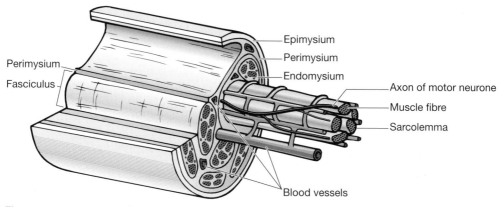

Figure 5.1 Muscle structure.

role in maintaining both the structure of a muscle and a suitable environment for muscle fibre function (Palastanga et al 1991, Jones & Round 1995) (Fig. 5.1).

MUSCLE TISSUE INNERVATION

Sensory receptors

Muscles contain free nerve endings and two specialized receptors.

The free nerve endings or **nociceptors** are scattered throughout the belly of the muscle and are responsible for mediating pain.

Muscle spindles are complex receptor organelles scattered throughout the muscle. They consist of highly specialized muscle fibres contained within a collagenous capsule filled with lymph and are designed to monitor change in length of the muscle and the rate of change. Because they are within the capsule of the spindle they are described as **intrafusal** fibres, as opposed to the **extrafusal** fibres which execute movement on contraction. Muscle spindles have both afferent and efferent nerve supply.

Golgi tendon organs are formed by multiple terminal branches of an axon weaving between the collagen fibres of a tendon; the region encompassed by these branches is surrounded by a fibrous capsule. Golgi tendon organs monitor the extent of muscle contraction and the force exerted by the muscle (Palastanga et al 1991).

The motor unit

Motor neurones form endings designed to deliver stimuli to extrafusal and intrafusal muscle fibres. The junction between motor neurone and muscle cell is known as the **motor endplate**. One motor neurone, through its axonal branches, supplies a number of fibres scattered throughout the muscle. The smallest amount of muscle that can contract in response to stimulation is not one single muscle fibre but all the fibres supplied by the motor neurone. Each single motor neurone and the fibres it supplies are a **motor unit**. The size of the action potential and the size of the twitch will be proportional to the number of fibres and type of fibres within the contracting unit (Jones & Round 1995).

The number of fibres in each unit varies from muscle to muscle and may be as few as 10 fibres per unit in the hand muscles and several thousand in the large quadriceps. The contractile properties of muscle fibres are determined by the nerve supplying the muscle. There are slow (**tonic**) motor units, innervated by small, slowly conducting motor nerves, and fast (**phasic**) motor units innervated by large, rapidly conducting motor nerves.

Motor recruitment

There is little response in skeletal muscles at rest; with minimal activity, a few motor units discharge, and with increasing effort more and

Table 5.1 Stabilizer and mobilizer characteristics of spinal muscles

Characteristic	Stabilizers	Mobilizers
Muscle type	Type 1	Type 2
Level	Deep	Superficial
Area of attachment	Monoarticular, segmental. Attached to every segment between origin and insertion	Biarticular, multisegmental. Do not attach segmentally at each level
Position	Medial tract	Lateral tract
Type of insertion	Muscle–osseous	Tendinous
Origin and insertion	Spinal vertebrae	Rib or trunk segments
Function and role	Work eccentrically. Static holding capacity. Stabilization, controlling excessive ROM or overstrain. Provide proprioceptive feedback	Work concentrically. Producing movement and power. Fast or large range movement

(adapted with permission from Comerford et al 1998)

Table 5.2 Motor unit function

Function	Slow motor units (tonic)	Fast motor units (phasic)
Fatiguability	Fatigue resistant	Fast to fatigue
Contraction force	Low	Moderate to high
Load threshold	Easily activated	Needs high stimulus
Recruitment	Activated first at low contraction	Increasingly recruited at higher contraction
Role	Fine control of postural and low load activity	Rapid or ballistic movement and high load activity

(adapted with permission from Comerford et al 1998)

more are brought into play. This process is called **recruitment of units**.

Functionally, muscles act predominantly as stabilizers or mobilizers although at certain times activity may demand a change of role (Goff 1972). Stabilizers and mobilizers are characterized in Table 5.1.

Physiologically, muscle fibres can be recruited tonically or phasically. Tonic fibre recruitment characteristics are slow-twitch fibres (type 1) which are slow to contract and slow to fatigue, with a strong sensory feedback. These are therefore used as stabilizers of movement and antigravity control. Phasic fibre recruitment characteristics are fast twitch fibres (type 2) which are fast to contract, fatiguing quickly, able to perform rapid, repetitive movements. These are used for mobilizing actions and rapid ballistic movements (Comerford et al 1998).

Ideally, stabilizing muscles should be used primarily with tonic fibre recruitment and mobilizing muscles with phasic recruitment. However, this distinction oversimplifies recruitment. The small slow (tonic) units are recruited first in most movements and the fast (phasic) units are generally recruited for more forceful activities. This is known as the Henneman Order Principle (Vander et al 1994). It has the advantage that the most frequently used units are the small, slow and fatigue-resistant fibres, providing fine control, while the large, fast and rapidly fatiguable units are only used for high-force contractions. The maximal contraction, speed, strength and fatiguability of each muscle depend on the proportions of the fibre types recruited (Ganong 1991, Jones & Round 1995, Comerford et al 1998) (Table 5.2).

All skeletal muscle fibres do not have the same mechanical and metabolic characteristics but all muscle fibres in a single motor unit are of the same fibre type. Most human muscles have slow and fast units interspersed with each other.

Stimulation

Muscle cells can be excited chemically, electrically and mechanically to produce an electrical discharge (**action potential**) and generation of force (**twitch**). The stimulus occurs at the motor endplate and the action potential is transmitted along the muscle fibre, initiating a contractile response (Ganong 1991, Mourad 1991).

A single action potential causes a brief muscle contraction or muscle twitch. Repeated stimulation before relaxation has occurred creates a **summation of contraction**. Rapid repeated stimuli elicit a **tetanic contraction**, causing complete tetanus when there is no relaxation at all (Ganong 1991, Jones & Round 1995).

Destruction of the nerve supply causes muscle atrophy; it also leads to excitability of the muscle with fine, irregular, non-visible **fibrillations** (contractions of individual fibres). These disappear when the nerve regenerates (Ganong 1991).

Normally, slow muscle fibres (type 1) used for minor adjustment of posture and position are required to be continuously active. Fast muscle fibres (type 2) have a pattern of activity where they are electrically silent for long periods and then discharge at short, high-frequency bursts. However, experiments indicate that it is the pattern of activity imposed on the muscle that regulates the fibre type. It has been found that fast fibres stimulated at low frequency for several hours a day change to slow fibres. Furthermore, it is not the frequency alone that is important but the total duration of the activity. Long periods of high-frequency stimulation are equally effective in changing the gene expression (Jones & Round 1995). This has significant clinical relevance with regard to the type of exercise chosen for muscle reeducation, affecting not only the type of contraction used but also the duration and speed of repeated contractions.

MUSCULAR ACTION

When stimulated, a muscle contracts so as to bring its two ends closer together. The strength of any contraction is determined by the number of motor units in action, the type of unit stimulated and the number of times per second that each unit is stimulated. Muscle cells either respond entirely to a stimulus or not at all. A stimulus strong enough to bring about a contraction is called a **liminal** stimulus; a less intense stimulus is **subliminal**. When a liminal stimulus is received, all fibres of a motor unit contract (Mourad 1991).

Types of muscle contraction

A muscle contraction can be isotonic or isometric. An **isotonic** contraction is one in which the muscle shortens and expands radially, moving its two ends closer together. An **isometric** contraction is one in which tension is developed but no change of length takes place, usually because of contracting against resistance.

Muscles contracting isotonically have an ability to work in opposite directions, working concentrically as they shorten, eccentrically as they lengthen or 'pay out'.

Each joint has controlling muscle groups, the prime movers or **agonists**, which move it in one direction, and an opposing group, the **antagonists**, which resist the agonists or move the joint the opposite way. **Synergists** are a group of muscles which work together under any load situation to generate force and movement. The normal coordinated contraction of synergists keeps a limb steady while the prime movers perform the action.

However, muscle balance and control are more complex than the simple interplay between muscle groups. Muscle length and muscle tension, motor control and recruitment, joint biomechanics and neural control are all involved (Mottram & Comerford 1998, Comerford et al 1998) (see below).

MUSCLES OF THE TRUNK

Stripped of its musculature, the vertebral column is wholly unstable. The muscles of the trunk provide support for the spine. They control movements of the whole vertebral column and stabilize vertebral posture during work or movement of the limbs (Troup 1979, Panjabi et al 1989). The muscles concerned with these activities are the muscles surrounding the vertebral column and the abdominal muscles.

Muscles of the vertebral column

Bogduk (1997) divides these into three functional groups.

1. **Psoas major** and **psoas minor**, which cover the anterolateral aspects of the lumbar spine.

The psoas muscles are attached to the lumbar vertebral bodies and discs at one end and the femur at the other. The principal action of psoas major is hip flexion. Psoas has a minimal movement role for spinal motion but provides a substantial axial compression to enhance segmental stability. Functionally, it eccentrically resists overrotation of the pelvis with respect to the trunk, for example in the swing phase of gait. It also contributes to abdominal bracing and increased intraabdominal pressure (IAP) for lifting (Bogduk 1997).

2. The **lateral intertransverse** muscles and **quadratus lumborum**, which connect and cover the front of the transverse processes. Working unilaterally, these muscles side flex the spine. Standing on one leg, quadratus lumborum prevents the pelvis dropping on the non-weight bearing side.

3. The lumbar back muscles, which lie behind and cover the posterior elements of the lumbar spine.

The lumbar back muscles

The muscles of the back are in roughly three layers, separated by and attached to the **thoraco-lumbar fascia** (see below). The deepest layer consists of short intersegmental muscles, the **lumbar interspinals** and **medial intertransverse**. The second layer consists of longer, polysegmental muscles travelling over several vertebrae, **lumbar multifidus** (Fig. 5.2) and the **erector spinae** muscles (Fig. 5.3). The most superficial layer are the longest and largest, polysegmental muscles, attached from the pelvis to the thoracic and cervical spine and the scapula (Fig. 5.4). By exerting an eccentric control, the erector spinae and multifidus are principally responsible for all movements that are gravity assisted.

Lumbar multifidus (LM). This is divided into a series of bands which originate from the lumbar spinous processes and laminae (Fig. 5.2). It acts as a powerful stabilizer of the vertebral column: the fascicles perform like extensible vertebral ligaments, adjusting their length to stabilize adjacent vertebrae, irrespective of the position of the vertebral column (Palastanga et al 1991). LM

is a rotator of the spine, but its major role as a stabilizer lies in *opposing* rotation, especially rotation in flexion. In resisting rotation it will oppose the independent contraction of the abdominal obliques (Bogduk 1997). Because of its polysegmental nature it can also exert an effect on any interposed vertebrae between its attachments, acting like bowstrings on the intervening vertebrae, maintaining the lumbar lordosis (Bogduk 1997).

The morphology is complicated by the pattern of innervation. All the fascicles attaching to the spinous process and lamina of one vertebra are innervated by the same nerve – the medial branch of the dorsal ramus that arises from below that one vertebra. As noxious stimulation of the lumbar facet joints evokes reflex activity in the paraspinal muscles, facet joint pain might be associated with abnormal activity in the relative LM fibres. Thus, this segmental innervation of LM may lay the ground for segmental dysfunction (Macintosh et al 1986).

LM has recently been the subject of considerable research. This is because of the role it plays in lumbar stabilization and the speed with which its activity and recruitment diminish during episodes of LBP (Macintosh et al 1986, Hides et al 1994, 1996, Richardson & Jull 1995a, Bogduk 1997, Sihoven et al 1997). Hides et al (1994), in examining the role of LM in spinal dysfunction, found a marked asymmetry in people with acute LBP, with decrease of LM cross-sectional area (CSA) ipsilateral to the symptoms and isolated to one vertebral level, the level of the symptoms. This suggested that the mechanism of loss for the CSA was not a generalized disuse atrophy or a generalized reflex inhibition, but that a selective spinal mechanism was in operation. The likely mechanism was an inhibition due to perceived pain which, via a long loop reflex, targeted the vertebral level of pathology to protect the damaged tissues. The rapid onset might indicate a metabolic effect inhibition.

In 1996 Hides et al followed this up with the discovery that LM does not spontaneously recover on remission of painful symptoms, so a lack of localized muscle support may be one

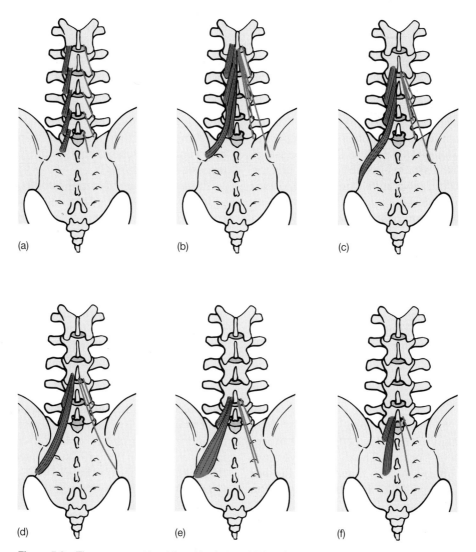

Figure 5.2 The component fascicles of lumbar multifidus. (a) The laminar fibres of multifidus. (b–f) The fascicles from the L1 to L5 spinous processes respectively. (Reproduced with permission from Bogduk and Twomey 1991.)

reason for recurrent LBP. Sihoven et al (1997) found that 75% of patients with radiating pain had electromyography (EMG) activities suggestive of nerve damage to LM. All this provides significant clinical support for the need to reeducate LM after any acute episode of pain.

The erector spinae (ES). This is a large, complex, powerful mass of muscle running alongside the length of the vertebral column (Fig. 5.3). It is composed of three columns, the iliocostalis, longissimus and spinalis muscles, relating to the lumbar, thoracic and cervical spines. Functioning bilaterally, it is the major extensor of the trunk but is also important in controlling flexion. Unilaterally it functions as a side flexor and rotator of the spine.

Muscles of the abdomen

Rectus abdominis (RAb) (Fig.5.5a)

The rectus abdominis muscle is the flat central muscle, attached to the pubic crest and

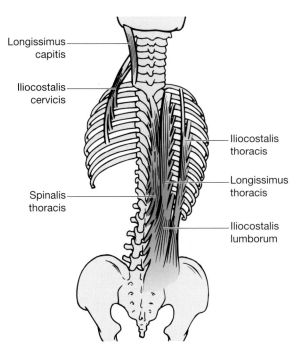

Figure 5.3   The erector spinae muscles. (Reproduced from Palastanga N et al 1989, with permission from Heinemann.)

ligaments of the pubis below and to the ribs and sternum above; its main action is flexion of the spine and rigidity of the abdominal wall, for example in abdominal bracing or increase in IAP.

External obliques

The external oblique muscles (EO) (Fig.5.5b) are the most superficial of the three sheets of muscle of the anterior abdominal wall, situated on the anterolateral aspect with the fibres running downwards and medially from the ribs towards the midline where they fuse with the linea alba.

Internal obliques

The internal oblique muscles (IO) (Fig.5.5b) lie deep to the external obliques. The fibres originate from the inguinal ligament, part of the iliac crest and from the thoracolumbar fascia. The fibres fan upwards to the lower four ribs, with the more anterior and lower fibres passing upwards

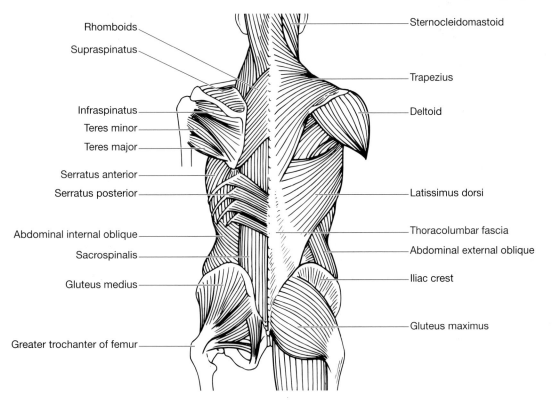

Figure 5.4   The larger muscles of the back.

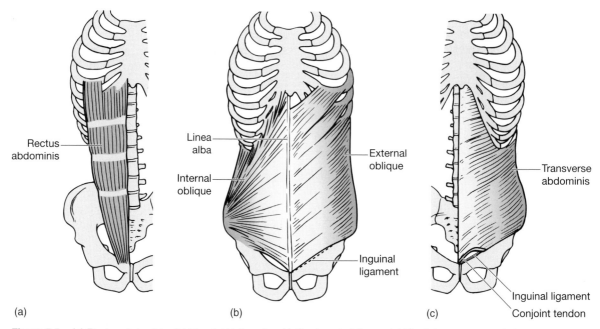

Figure 5.5 (a) Rectus abdominis. (b) The right internal and left external obliques. (c) The left transversus abdominis. (Reproduced from Palastanga N et al 1989, with permission from Heinemann.)

and medially to finally blend with the linea alba. Working together, the two oblique abdominals flex the lumbar spine, assist in respiration and support the abdominal contents; working independently, they rotate the trunk on the pelvis, for example moving a load from left to right.

Transversus abdominis

The transversus abdominis muscle (TA) (Fig. 5.5c) is the deepest of the three sheets of abdominal muscles. The fibres run horizontally around the abdomen, attaching via the thoracolumbar fascia to the transverse processes of each lumbar vertebra posteriorly, the lower six ribs, the iliac crest, the inguinal ligament and the linea alba anteriorly. It contracts with all trunk movements and is recruited prior to all other abdominal muscles with any sudden trunk perturbations. This is called an **anticipatory** contraction (Cresswell et al 1994, Hodges & Richardson 1996) (see 'Strategy for stabilization' below). As with LM, research has highlighted the role of TA in stabilization of the lumbar

spine and the possible link between dysfunction and LBP (Jull & Richardson 1994, Richardson & Jull 1995b, Hodges & Richardson 1996, Allison et al 1998) (see Chapter 9). For this reason, teaching the co-contraction of TA and LM, with low load and tonic recruitment, is an essential starting point in reeducation of spinal stability and should be almost routinely taught to everyone (see Chapter 17, Figs 17.1–17.5).

TA and the oblique abdominal muscles are used in dynamic abdominal bracing (used in 'back bracing') and in abdominal hollowing, both described in Chapter 17.

THORACOLUMBAR FASCIA

The thoracolumbar fascia consists of three layers of fascia effectively separating the three muscular layers of the lumbar spine. The layers of fascia are attached to the spinous processes, the transverse processes, the intertransverse ligaments and the ligamentous attachments of the muscles; the fascia reinforces the posterior ligamentous system through the orientation of its fibres (Kisner & Colby 1990, Sullivan 1994). In lumbar flexion, activity of the muscles attached to or surrounded by the fascia increases the tension of the fascia which in turn increases support and stabilization of the lumbar spine (Kisner & Colby 1990, Bogduk & Twomey 1991).

CONTROL OF MOVEMENT AND POSTURE

The unceasing interplay between muscle groups is the muscular mechanism of posture. The muscle system's stability function provides protection to articular structures by minimizing abnormal joint displacement, aiding stress absorption and prolonging cartilage life. For this reason injury could be more likely in the presence of poor muscular function (Panjabi 1992a).

The muscles required for lumbar stabilization are TA and the internal oblique abdominals, in co-contraction with LM and the erector spinae (Richardson et al 1992, Hides et al 1994, Richardson & Jull 1995a).

Classification of muscle function

Several systems of muscle function classification have been described. Comerford (Comerford et al 1998) reviews two of these systems.

1. A model based on muscles as stabilizers and mobilizers (see Table 5.1), mentioned previously.
2. A model using local and global muscle stability systems (Bergmark 1989) (Table 5.3).

Table 5.3 Local and global stability systems of the lumbar spine

Characteristic	Local	Global
Level	Deepest layer, originate and insert on lumbar spine	Superficial or outer layer, lacking segmental insertions
Control	Spinal curvature	Large torque producing
Function	Maintains mechanical stiffness of spine, controls intersegmental motion	Transfers load between thoracic cage and pelvis
Reaction response	Changes in posture and low intrinsic load	Changes in line of action and the degree of high load
Role	Increasing segmental stiffness, decreasing excessive motion, controlling low load	Movement production, control of high load

(abbreviated with permission from Comerford et al 1998)

The local muscle system is responsible for increasing segmental stiffness, decreasing intersegmental motion and maintaining control of low physiological load. The global muscle system is responsible for movement production and the control of high physiological load.

Stabilizers can be local or global (Table 5.4). The local stabilizers control stability segmentally. Global muscles have both stability and mobility roles. Global stabilizers control stability under all load situations, especially rotational forces. Global mobilizers are primarily designed for production of force and range of motion but

Table 5.4 Examples of stabilizer and mobilizer muscles

Local	Global	
Local stabilizer	Global stabilizer	Global mobilizer
For example:	For example:	For example:
Transversus abdominis	IO and EO abdominals	Rectus abdominis
Lumbar multifidus (deep fibres)	Spinalis	Iliocostalis
Middle and lower trapezius	Serratus anterior	Scalenae
Deep cervical flexors		
Vastus medialis obliquus	Gluteus maximus	Hamstrings

(abbreviated and adapted with permission from Comerford et al 1998) can contribute to stability under high load. In this book peripheral muscles can only be briefly mentioned. It is essential to attend movement dysfunction courses to learn the full skeletal concept.

Spinal stability

Spinal stability depends upon the combined function of the osseous, ligamentous, neural and muscular systems.

Panjabi (1992b) describes the spinal stabilizing system as consisting of three subsystems: the passive system, the active system and the control system (Fig.5.6).

A dysfunction of a component of any one of the subsystems may lead to one or more of the following.

- An immediate response from other subsystems to compensate.
- A long-term adaptation of one or more subsystems.
- An injury to one or more components of any subsystem.

Panjabi (1992a) also describes a 'neutral zone', a region of intervertebral motion around the neutral posture within which spinal motion is produced with minimal internal resistance. It may increase with injury to the spinal column or with weakness of muscles, which may in turn result in 'spinal instability' (stability dysfunction) and low back problems. It may decrease because of osteophyte formation, surgical fusion and muscle strengthening. The neutral zone is controlled by the stabilizing trunk muscles. Cholewicki & McGill (1996) propose that while the large muscles, such as ES and quadratus lumborum, provide the bulk of stiffness to the spinal column, the short segmental muscles are necessary to maintain stability; the spine will buckle if the activity of LM and ES is zero. Richardson & Jull (1995a) found that LM provides important antigravity control.

Quint et al (1998) state that the importance of neural control in stabilization of the spine cannot be overemphasized. The neural controller must not only select the appropriate muscles to stimulate but also decide on the appropriate activation level. Effective dynamic stability requires more than just adequate force generated by muscular tension. The force must be properly coordinated and an exact balance must exist between agonists and antagonists. This is optimized by the CNS to the point that the CNS initiates contraction of trunk muscles in advance of limb movement to ensure stability prior to the movement (Hodges & Richardson 1996, Gill & Callaghan 1998).

Strategy for stabilization

One strategy for stabilization is the early preprogrammed anticipatory recruitment of particular muscles. Another strategy is the regulation of muscle 'stiffness' achieved through cocontraction of agonist and antagonist on either side of a joint, using the tonic, slow-twitch motor units (Richardson & Jull 1995a). This biomechanical muscle stiffness is not the same as stiffness referring to the loss of ROM of a joint; it may be simplified as the passive or active tension that may resist a displacing force.

The early preprogrammed recruitment of trunk muscles (ES, EO and RAb) has been found in earlier investigations but Hodges & Richardson (1996) put forward a hypothesis which would combine the two strategies above: TA contracts before all other trunk muscles in anticipation of

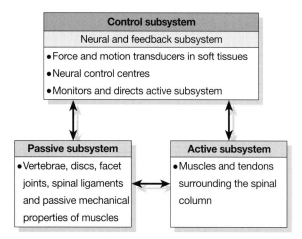

Control subsystem
Neural and feedback subsystem
• Force and motion transducers in soft tissues   • Neural control centres   • Monitors and directs active subsystem

Passive subsystem	Active subsystem
• Vertebrae, discs, facet joints, spinal ligaments and passive mechanical properties of muscles	• Muscles and tendons surrounding the spinal column

Figure 5.6 Spinal stabilizing system. (Adapted with permission from Panjabi 1992b.)

the initiation of the prime movers of a limb and the contraction of TA increases the stiffness of the lumbar spine, through raising the IAP and tensioning the thoracolumbar fascia. The stiffening would limit intersegmental translation and rotational forces and provide a more stable lever over which other trunk muscles can act. A delay in contraction of TA would reduce spinal stiffness at the time of initiation of the movement. Only 2° of segmental rotation is required to produce microtrauma of the structures of the lumbar spine (Hodges & Richardson 1996). The potential for this to occur as a result of delayed stiffness was significant.

Their findings were conclusive. TA was shown to contract before the other abdominals in anticipation of limb movement. In shoulder flexion TA contracted before the prime mover, anterior fibres of deltoid and the other abdominal muscles. Similarly, in shoulder abduction it contracted before middle deltoid and in extension both TA and RAb contracted before posterior deltoid. Unlike trunk loading, this anticipation cannot be reflexly mediated and must be preprogrammed by the CNS to precisely oppose the perturbing forces. In tests with LBP patients, none of the abdominal muscles was active before the shoulder prime movers while LM was the only muscle active significantly earlier. This indicates a significant deficit in the automatic motor command for control of disturbances to the spine in LBP which needs further investigation (Hodges & Richardson 1996).

Lumbopelvic stability

Under postural load specific ligament and muscle forces are necessary to stabilize the pelvis. Since load transfer from spine to pelvis passes through the sacroiliac (SI) joints, effective stabilization of these joints is essential. Stabilization can be increased by interlocking the ridges and grooves on the joint surface (form closure) or by compressive force structures like muscles, ligaments and fascia (force closure) (Pool-Goudzwaard et al 1998). Pool-Goudzwaard et al (1998) describe three muscle slings which contribute to force closure.

- A longitudinal sling consisting of LM, the deep layer of the thoracolumbar fascia and the sacrotuberous ligament.
- The posterior sling which can be energized by the coupled function of latissimus dorsi and gluteus maximus.
- The anterior sling which can be energized by the abdominal oblique muscles and by TA.

These mechanisms cannot be described in greater detail here, so further reading is essential.

CHANGES IN MUSCLE STRENGTH AND LENGTH

The strength of a muscle is directly related to its length. A postural adaptation in which a muscle either elongates or shortens will either relatively weaken or tighten the muscle.

Recruitment dysfunction

Adaptive responses in muscle, that is, changes in function and structure, take place as a result of recruitment dysfunction:

- when muscles that are predominantly stabilizers are recruited phasically and muscles that are mainly mobilizers are recruited tonically (Box 5.1)
- as a result of poor posture or a sedentary lifestyle. In any maintained poor posture stabilizing muscles 'give' and no longer control good vertebral alignment; the muscles which

---

Box 5.1 Recruitment dysfunction in activity

Recruitment dysfunction (substitution) occurs:
- *in walking*: lumbar rotation with pelvic roll/drop – instead of trunk stabilization and balanced hip flexion/extension (for example, the model's walk)
- *in walking*: strong upper thoracic rotation – instead of spinal stabilization with relaxed arm movement and good leg push-off (for example, the intensely muscular, thoracic rotation with flexed elbows)
- *in some repetitive arm activities*: inappropriate phasic shoulder girdle movement – instead of correct tonic thoracic/scapular stabilization with phasic shoulder and arm movement (Mottram 1997) (for example, in production line work, bowling in cricket, serving in tennis).

Box 5.2 Recruitment dysfunction in maintained postures

Alteration in muscle length/strength
1. With an increased dorsal kyphosis and protracted shoulders: long, weak posterior shoulder girdle muscles, especially lower trapezius; short tight pectoral region.
2. In the 'poking chin' posture – often associated with headaches: long, weak lower cervical extensors; long, weak upper cervical flexors.
3. With an increased lordosis: tight erector spinae, hip flexors and hamstrings; weak and long TA, oblique abdominals and gluteal muscles.

---

tend to weaken more easily are the muscles of the upper trunk and the oblique abdominals. The result is an adaptive change in length and strength of opposing muscle groups and an alteration of the ideal postural curves (Box 5.2) (Richardson et al 1992, Mottram 1997).

When overload, in the form of work or sport, is added to muscle imbalance, the spine can be vulnerable to injury (Sahrmann 1993, Comerford et al 1998).

Principles of exercise

Overdevelopment of one group of muscles by excessive exercise can lead to shortening and tightening of those muscles, with lengthening and weakening of their opposing group. Lengthened muscles must be shortened with exercise and shortened muscles must be stretched (Sahrmann 1993, Comerford et al 1998). Clinically, when maximum perceived effort is needed to perform a low load activity then it is likely that there is inefficient slow motor unit recruitment and dysfunction of the normal spindle response. Similarly, when less effort is needed to perform the same low load activity, it is likely that there is better facilitation of slow motor unit recruitment (Comerford et al 1998).

Dynamic postural control and normal low load functional movement are primarily a function of slow motor unit (tonic) recruitment. High load activity, strength or endurance training are functions using both slow (tonic) and fast (phasic) motor unit recruitment. However,

recruitment and hypertrophy in a muscle are very different processes: recruitment is modulated by the higher CNS and is powerfully influenced by the afferent proprioceptive system, whereas hypertrophy is a local adaptation to demand and is the result of overloading training (Comerford et al 1998).

Clinically this is significant in relation to the therapist's choice of exercise. For functional purposes recruitment of slow motor units will optimize postural holding/antigravity functions while recruitment of fast motor units will optimize rapid/ballistic movement and the production of force power. In the simplest terms, active flexion/extension movements of the spine will never optimize stabilization and sit-ups, unless performed in a specific manner, will never train the abdominal muscles to shorten, nor will they tighten and flatten the abdomen and thus stabilize the lumbar spine (Fleck & Schutt 1983). The curl-up, which has been used for abdominal muscle testing and strengthening (Kendall & McCreary 1983), favours rectus abdominis and, if performed at high speed, leads to *reduced* activity of the obliques and TA. In people who perform 100 sit-ups every day this often presents as a strong, tough abdomen with a low weak TA bulge below the umbilicus. However, if performed *slowly* over 50 times, the dynamic function does carry over to TA and the obliques' stabilizing function; once again, the speed of the activity is the important factor (Wohlfahrt et al 1993, Jones & Round 1995).

Dynamic stability and muscle balance depend on the specific action of individual muscles on or across a joint, the interaction between antagonists, the interaction between the relevant synergists and the effect of the combined actions of all the muscles working at one body segment, upon other segments up and down the kinetic chain (Comerford et al 1998).

Muscles can be strengthened and recruited in two ways.

- By slow, sustained, maintained contraction which shortens and strengthens weak long muscles and stretches shortened ones.
- By repetitive exercises.

Stabilization training (see Chapter 17)

Richardson & Jull (1995b) have given clear guidelines for stabilization training. Use low load or minimal intensity. RAb is best avoided in stabilization. TA and LM are the important local stabilizers. Oblique abdominals and interspinalis create global stability. Mobilizer muscles can assist stability under high load demands.

1. 'Abdominal drawing in' is the starting point, progressing to use in functional, upright, everyday positions.
2. Add trunk rotational control.
3. Add resisted isometric rotation.
4. Finally add load-graded limb movements.

Strengthening exercises

If repetitive strengthening exercises are used for a weak muscle group, it is important that when balance is achieved all groups are equally activated. It is permissible for the subject to 'feel' initially that they are working maximally during low load exercise so long as they do not fatigue or substitute by using trick movements. As stability improves, low load exercises should 'feel' easier (Comerford et al 1998).

Rissanen et al (1995) report that training with maximal or submaximal effort may reverse the atrophy of type 2 fibres in LM in patients with chronic LBP; this may well be a guideline for use in rehabilitation programmes.

High-force exercise can cause microdamage to muscle structure, especially when performed as strong eccentric contractions which are more stressful than concentric work.

MUSCULAR PAIN AND FATIGUE

Exercise and pain

Pain is experienced whenever, metabolically, a muscle is failing and is no longer in a steady state. The pain is caused by algesic substances being released from the active muscle. The precise level of pain in the tissues will be determined by the balance between the production of the noxious substance and its removal by the perfusing blood. Lactate is produced and accumulated by a working muscle but released potassium is a more likely candidate for the algesic substance (Jones & Round 1995).

There is a direct association between muscle pain and exercise, with two clearcut time factors (Mills et al 1989, Newham et al 1994, Jones & Round 1995).

Ischaemic muscle pain is pain which increases in intensity during exercise but stops as soon as movement ceases. It is caused by metabolic factors and appears to have non-lasting consequences. Intermittent claudication and angina pectoris are two clinical presentations of this condition but it can and does occur in any muscle denied its blood supply; for example, in a hand after carrying a heavy case or after maintaining any repetitive fast exercise.

Delayed-onset muscle pain (DOMS) is pain experienced about 8 hours after exercise, which may not reach peak intensity for 1–2 days. This is associated with high-force eccentric muscle activity and is of mechanical origin. Affected muscles also show weakness and damage which develop over days and can persist for weeks. The damage is reflected by tissue disruption, inflammation, degeneration and regeneration. Connective tissue damage may be the algesic source. Repetition of similar eccentric exercise rapidly brings about a reduction in pain and damage (Newham et al 1994). Although DOMS is most commonly associated with eccentric contractions it can also be induced by high-force isometric contractions if the muscle is exercised in an extended position, showing that muscle length seems to be more important than high-force work in eliciting pain (Jones & Round 1995).

There is no evidence that eccentric exercise is most effective for strength training. The loss of function and structure caused by unfamiliar high-force exercise of this kind is unlikely to be anything other then deleterious. Eccentric exercise, therefore, should be started at low force and only increased very gradually in order to avoid pain, damage and fatigue. Repeated training does give protection against damage (Newham et al 1994, Jones & Round 1995).

Myalgic pain

Tenderness, subsequently leading to severe pain, may develop in muscles, often associated with repetitive tasks. Areas, known as 'trigger points', can be identified from which the pain seems to radiate. Investigations have shown no tissue abnormalities in the area and the primary lesion may well be sensitization of the local sensory nerve (Jones & Round 1995).

Muscle spasm

Muscle spasm implies a reflex contraction of muscle surrounding an inflamed or injured structure (Mills et al 1989). Clinically this is frequently seen in global muscles. It is encountered in acute LBP as a dysfunction of motor recruitment resulting from the noxious input (pain) eliciting overactivity of the erector spinae, presenting as 'protective spasm' (Mottram & Comerford 1998). The muscles may be painful when this occurs but they are not necessarily part of the injury.

Muscle spasm can be a tonal disorder, taking the form of spasticity in neurological conditions (Thornton & Kilbride 1998).

Muscle cramp

Muscle cramp is an electrically active involuntary contraction. There are several causes, some chemical (from a decrease in body salts and potassium), some ischaemic, some neurological. Cramp occurs most frequently in the calf muscles and is a hazard for athletes (Mills et al 1989). There are usually some feelings of discomfort before the muscle goes fully into cramp. The pain of cramp is severe and distinctive and afterwards there is a feeling of tenderness. Cramps can usually be relieved by stretching the affected muscle or by stimulation of a sensory nerve in the skin. They are possibly prevented by a high sodium intake and quinine (Jones & Round 1995)

Muscle fatigue

Muscular fatigue is a loss of the ability to generate force but the term 'fatigue' requires elaboration. Briefly, long-lasting fatigue can be produced by repetitive high-force contractions and the changes can take 24–48 hours to recover. On the other hand, a maximum isometric contraction becomes intensely uncomfortable and unsustainable after about 30–45 seconds. Fast muscle fibres fatigue more quickly than slow fibres.

Things are further complicated by our sense of effort, when the motor input to the muscle seems to conflict with the proprioceptive feedback from the tissues (Jones & Round 1995).

DISORDERS OF MUSCLES

Muscles are intended for hard, tough work; however, muscle tissue and connective tissue can be damaged by trauma, disease and injury.

Trauma

Trauma may act to damage muscle via the nervous system: damage to upper motor neurones from head or spinal injuries (for example, in whiplash injuries) or to lower motor neurones (spinal or peripheral nerve lesions) or direct damage to the intramuscular nerve branches as they pass through the muscle (Herbert 1995, Stokes 1998).

Pathological diseases

These include pathologies such as neuropathies (for example, Guillain Barré), myopathies (such as the muscular dystrophies) and connective tissue diseases (such as RA) (Herbert 1995, Jones & Round 1995, Stokes 1998).

Local muscle injuries

Direct muscle injuries are of two types: in situ injuries and shearing injuries (Crisco et al 1994, Kalimo et al 1997).

In situ injury

In situ injury in its mild form is an exercise-induced injury, especially after eccentric loading, causing DOMS. Myofibrils are disrupted with possible sarcolemma damage, causing a brisk inflammatory reaction. With more excessive usage of untrained muscle, a severe in situ necrosis of myofibrils can occur. This can lead to a massive oedema and consequent compartment syndrome with severe ischaemia. In situ necrosis may also result from intramuscular injection of local anaesthetic.

Shearing injury

Shearing injury is the most common sports injury. It involves not only the myofibrils but also the connective tissue framework which can be torn. The myofibrils undergo segmental necrosis, the ruptured myofibrils contract and their ends are pulled apart; haemorrhage from the torn vessels fills the gap forming a haematoma which is later replaced by scar tissue. Functional recovery requires firm attachment of the myofibril stumps to the extracellular matrix by two chains of adhesion molecules and reestablishment of innervation. Two of the main shearing injuries are contusions and strains.

Contusion injuries. These, the result of a direct blow, are the most common traumatic muscle injuries, occurring frequently in contact sports. They can impair the ability of muscle to actively generate tension and can initiate pathological changes which alter the muscle's passive properties. Reinjury, muscle atrophy and contracture can occur with significant loss of time in training and competition (Crisco et al 1994).

Distraction strains and sprains. These can result from an excessive tensile force applied to an overstretched muscle, especially in jumping or sprinting. They occur near myotendinous junctions of superficial muscles, for example rectus femoris, semitendinosus and gastrocnemius.

Kalimo et al (1997) classify muscle injuries into three degrees:

1. *Mild*: tear of few muscle fibres, minor swelling, discomfort, minimal loss of strength and movement.
2. *Moderate*: greater damage with clear loss of strength.

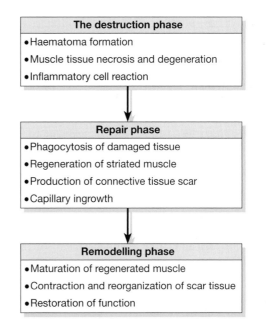

Figure 5.7   The process of repair in a muscle.

3. *Severe*: tear extending across the whole cross-section of muscle, resulting in total lack of function.

MUSCLE HEALING AND TREATMENT AFTER INJURY

Muscle healing

The process of repair in a muscle passes through three phases (Fig. 5.7) and treatment must coincide with this time schedule. Therapeutic management should be aimed at achieving the quickest and functionally most effective regeneration of the muscle.

Treatment

Muscle and ligamentous injuries should be carefully examined to estimate the degree of damage. A complete rupture should be referred for possible surgical repair. Ultrasound or MRI can be used for diagnosis. A short period of immobilization is needed to accelerate the formation of the granulation tissue. The length of immobilization or minimal loading is dependent upon the degree of the injury but should be as short as possible, with controlled activity started as soon as the swelling and haemorrhage have subsided. The aim should be to avoid muscle atrophy, loss of strength and extensibility which rapidly result from prolonged immobilization and, instead, to regain the former strength of the muscle with good orientation of the regenerating fibres, the resorption of connective tissue scarring and recapillarization of the damaged area (Kalimo et al 1997).

Days 1–3

The immediate treatment consists of RICE (rest, ice, compression and elevation), in order to minimize bleeding, prevent the formation of haematoma and interstitial oedema, shorten tissue ischaemia and accelerate regeneration. The rest period should be 1–3 days, depending on the degree of injury. Ice should be administered for 5 minutes only for the first 24 hours, increasing to 10–20 minutes later, at intervals of 30–60 minutes (Watson 1999). A maximal compression bandage should be used.

NSAIDs should be started early, providing there is no bleeding, but they are restricted only to early use as long-term NSAIDs may delay the repair phase. Glucocorticoids should not be used in treating muscle injury as they delay the elimination of haematoma and retard muscle regeneration (Mishra et al 1995, Kalimo et al 1997, Watson 1999).

High-frequency ultrasound has some beneficial effect in the initial stages in regeneration. If at the end of this time the contractile ability of the muscle is not improved, a large intramuscular haematoma or total rupture may be present.

Days 3–4 onwards

Minor ruptures and minor haematomas should be supported with elastic bandage and early mobilization started (Box 5.3). Stretching for scar tissue should be painless elongation, achieved gradually for periods of 15–20 seconds, proceeding up to a period of 1 minute. Final reeducation should be geared to the patient's normal activities and should be sports specific

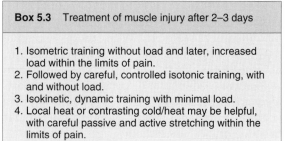

Box 5.3 Treatment of muscle injury after 2–3 days

1. Isometric training without load and later, increased load within the limits of pain.
2. Followed by careful, controlled isotonic training, with and without load.
3. Isokinetic, dynamic training with minimal load.
4. Local heat or contrasting cold/heat may be helpful, with careful passive and active stretching within the limits of pain.
5. Sport-specific training.

if they are involved in sporting activities (Magnusson et al 1995, Kalimo et al 1997).

If the muscle fails to improve, the possibility of an intramuscular (as opposed to an intermuscular) haematoma should be considered and followed by further clinical examination.

Early mobilization of muscular and ligamentous tissue is essential for good recovery. In the case of ligaments, movement enhances both the ligament substance and the insertion; alteration of the stress levels on a ligament can elicit changes in its biomechanical responses (Woo et al 1997). The healing of soft tissue depends upon aerobic metabolism which is enhanced by controlled activity rather than rest once the initial bleeding has ceased and swelling subsided. After recovery from any injury the soft tissue must be gradually stretched and strengthened to restore full function.

WEAKNESS OF MUSCLE

Muscular weakness can exhibit in two ways: an inability to achieve the required strength or an easy, rapid fatigue. The two should be differentiated. The former could be related to muscular denervation or loss of nerve supply, while the latter implies impaired blood supply (Mills et al 1989). Denervation can be the result of any neurological condition involving the CNS or peripheral nervous system.

As previously mentioned, it has been proven that the stresses and strains from muscular activity actually strengthen bone and that a lack of exercise leads to a decrease in strength and health generally, leaving the spine vulnerable to injury (Twomey & Taylor 1991).

Weakness is sometimes considered to be an inevitable part of ageing but there are several aspects to this apparent eventuality (Box 5.4).

Box 5.4   Ageing of muscles

There can be marked loss of muscle mass and decrease in strength after 50 years of age, sometimes reduced by 30% at the age of 90.
Possibly due to:
- Loss of motor units from disuse (Twomey and Taylor 1991) or from loss of motor neurones in the anterior horn (Jones and Round 1994). The loss can be substantially reversed with a programme of activity.
- Menopausal endocrine changes in women which cause a reduction in oestradiol levels, leading to muscle wasting. Men have testicular and adrenal testosterone available to convert into oestradiol. Hormone replacement can help to adjust this deficiency (Jones and Round 1994).
- Long-term corticosteroids which suppress the production of growth hormones and decrease the rate of muscle growth. Growth is restored if steroidal medication ceases.

Key points

1. Muscles are composed of slow and fast fibres.
2. Muscles can be recruited tonically or phasically.
3. Slow, tonic fibre recruitment should be used for reeducating spinal stabilization of the deep trunk muscles.
4. Recruitment reversal changes the characterization of muscles and may lead to dysfunction.
5. Dysfunction may lead to pain if provoked dynamically or statically.
6. Local muscle injury has a specific healing time and specific treatment schedule for regaining elasticity and strength.

REFERENCES

Allison G, Kendle K, Roll S et al 1998 The role of the diaphragm during abdominal hollowing exercises. Australian Physiotherapy 44(2): 95–102

Bergmark A 1989 Stability of the lumbar spine. A study in mechanical engineering. Acta Orthopaedica Scandinavica 230(60): 20–24

Bogduk N 1997 Clinical anatomy of the lumbar spine and sacrum. Churchill Livingstone, Edinburgh

Bogduk N, Twomey L 1991 Clinical anatomy of the lumbar spine, 2nd edn. Churchill Livingstone, Edinburgh

Cholewicki J, McGill S M 1996 Mechanical stability of the in vivo lumbar spine: implications for injury and chronic low back pain. Clinical Biomechanics 11(1): 1–15

Comerford M, Kinetic Control 1998 Dynamic balance of the human motor system. Course notes. Kinetic Control Ltd, Harrow

Cresswell A G, Oddsson L, Thorstensson A 1994 The influence of sudden perturbations on trunk muscle activity and intra-abdominal pressure while standing. Experimental Brain Research 98: 336–341

Crisco J J, Joki P, Heinen G T, Connell M D, Panjabi M M 1994 A muscle contusion injury model. Biomechanics, physiology and histology. American Journal of Sports Medicine 22(5): 702–710

Fleck S, Schutt R 1983 Types of strength training. Orthopedic Clinics of North America 14: 449–458

Ganong W F 1991 Review of medical physiology, 15th edn. Appleton Lange, Norwalk

Gill K P, Callaghan M J 1998 The measurement of lumbar proprioception in individuals with and without low back pain. Spine 23(3): 371–377

Goff B 1972 The application of recent advances in neurophysiology to Miss M. Rood's concept of neuromuscular facilitation. Physiotherapy 58(2): 409–415

Herbert R 1995 Adaptations of muscle and connective tissue. In: Refshauge K, Gass E (eds) Musculoskeletal physiotherapy. Butterworth Heinemann, Oxford

Hides J A, Stokes M J, Saide M, Jull G A, Coopers D H 1994 Evidence of lumbar multifidus wasting ipsilateral to symptoms in patients with acute/subacute low back pain. Spine 19(2): 165–172

Hides J A, Richardson C A, Jull G A 1996 Multifidus muscle recovery is not automatic after resolution of acute, first-episode low back pain. Spine 21(23): 2763–2769

Hodges P, Richardson C 1996 Inefficient muscular stabilisation of the lumbar spine associated with low back pain. A motor control evaluation of transversus abdominis. Spine 21: 2640–2650

Jones D A, Round J M 1995 Skeletal muscle in health and disease. A textbook of muscle physiology. Manchester University Press, Manchester

Jull G A, Richardson C A 1994 Rehabilitation of active stabilisation of the lumbar spine. In: Twomey L T, Taylor J R (eds) Physical therapy of the low back. Churchill Livingstone, Edinburgh

Kalimo H, Rantanen J, Jarvinen M 1997 Muscle injuries in sports. Baillière's Clinical Orthopaedics 2(1): 1–24

Kendall F, McCreary E 1983 Muscle testing and function, 3rd edn. Williams and Wilkins, Baltimore

Kisner C, Colby L 1990 Therapeutic exercise. Foundations and techniques, 2nd edn. F A Davis, Philadelphia

Macintosh J E, Valencia F, Bogduk N, Munro R R 1986 The morphology of the human lumbar multifidus. Clinical Biomechanics 1: 196–204

Magnusson S P, Simonsen E B, Aagard P 1995 Viscoelastic response to repeated static stretching in the human hamstring muscle. Scandinavian Journal of Medicine and Science in Sports 5: 342–347

Mills K R, Newham D J, Edwards R H T 1989 Muscle pain. In: Wall P D, Melzack R (eds) Textbook of pain, 2nd edn. Churchill Livingstone, Edinburgh

Mishra D K, Schmitz M C, Lieber R L 1995 Anti-inflammatory medication after muscle injury. A treatment resulting in short term improvement but subsequent loss of muscle function. Journal of Bone and Joint Surgery (Am) 77: 1510–1519

Mottram S L 1997 Dynamic stability of the scapula. Manual Therapy 2(3): 123–131

Mottram S, Comerford M 1998 Stability dysfunction and low back pain. Journal of Orthopedic Medicine 20(2): 13–18

Mourad L A 1991 Orthopedic disorders. Mosby Year Book St Louis

Newham D J, Edwards R H T, Mills K R 1994 Skeletal muscle pain. In: Wall P D, Melzack R (eds) Textbook of pain, 3rd edn. Churchill Livingstone, Edinburgh

Palastanga N, Field D, Soames R 1991 Anatomy and human movement. Heinemann Medical Books, Oxford

Panjabi M M 1992a The stabilizing system of the spine. Part II. Neutral zone and instability hypothesis. Journal of Spinal Disorders 5(4): 390–397

Panjabi M M 1992b The stabilizing system of the spine. Part I. Function, dysfunction, adaptation, and enhancement. Journal of Spinal Disorders 5(4): 383–389

Panjabi M M, Abumi K, Duranceau J, Oxland T 1989 Spinal stability and intersegmental muscle forces: a biomechanical model. Spine 14: 194–200

Pool-Goudzwaard A L, Vleeming A, Stoeckart R, Snijders C J, Mens J M A 1998 Insufficient lumbopelvic stability: a clinical, anatomical and biomechanical approach to 'a-specific' low back pain. Manual Therapy 3(1): 12–20

Quint U, Wilke H-J, Shirazi-Adi A, Parnianpour M, Loer F, Claes L E 1998 Importance of the intersegmental trunk muscles for the stability of the lumbar spine. Spine 23(18): 1937–1945

Richardson C A, Jull G A 1995a Muscle control – pain control. What exercises would you prescribe? Manual Therapy 1: 2–10

Richardson C, Jull G 1995b An historical perspective on the development of clinical techniques to evaluate and treat the active stabilising system of the lumbar spine. In: Sharpe M (ed) The lumbar spine. Australian Journal of Physiotherapy Monograph No. 1, Melbourne

Richardson C, Jull G, Toppenberg R, Comerford M 1992 Techniques for active lumbar stabilisation for spinal protection: a pilot study. Australian Physiotherapy 38(2): 105–112

Rissanen A, Kalimo H, Alaranta H 1995 Effect of intensive training on the isokinetic strength and structure of lumbar muscles in patients with chronic low back pain. Spine 20(3): 333–340

Sahrmann S A 1993 Diagnosis and treatment of movement system imbalances associated with musculoskeletal pain. Course notes, Washington University School of Medicine

Sihoven T, Lindberg K, Airaksinen O, Manninen H 1997 Movement disturbances of the lumbar spine and abnormal back muscle electromyographic findings in recurrent LBP. Spine 22: 289–295

Stokes M 1998 Neurological physiotherapy. Mosby Year Book, St Louis

Sullivan M S 1994 Lifting and back pain. In: Twomey L T, Taylor J R (eds) Physical therapy of the law back. Churchill Livingstone, Edinburgh

Thornton H, Kilbride C 1998 Physical management of abnormal tone and movement. In: Stokes M (ed) Neurological physiotherapy. Mosby Year Book, St Louis

Troup J D G 1979 Biomechanics of the vertebral column. Physiotherapy 65(8): 238–244

Twomey L T, Taylor J R 1991 Age related changes of the lumbar spine and spinal rehabilitation. Physical Rehabilitation and Medicine 2(3): 153–169

Vander A J, Sherman J H, Luciano D S 1994 Human Physiology, 2nd edn. McGraw Hill, New York

Watson T 1999 Tissue healing and repair. MACP Lecture, 24 June

Wohlfahrt D, Jull G, Richardson C 1993 The relationship between the dynamic and static function of abdominal muscles. Australian Physiotherapy 39(1): 9–13

Woo S L-Y, Chan S S, Yamaji T 1997 Biomechanics of knee ligament healing, repair and reconstruction. Journal of Biomechanics 30(5): 431–439

FURTHER READING

Chaitow L 1996 Muscle energy techniques. Churchill Livingstone, New York

Crosbie J, McConnell J (eds) 1993 Key issues in musculoskeletal physiotherapy. Butterworth Heinemann, Oxford

Daniels L, Worthington C 1986 Muscle testing: techniques of manual examination, 5th edn. W B Saunders, Philadelphia

Grisigona V 1991 Sports injuries. Butterworths, London

Jones D A, Round J M 1995 Skeletal muscle in health and disease. A textbook of muscle physiology. Manchester University Press, Manchester

Kendall F, McCreary E 1993 Muscle testing and function, 4th edn. Williams and Wilkins, Baltimore

Norris C M 1998 Sports injuries. Diagnosis and management. Butterworth Heinemann, Oxford

Richardson C, Jull G 1998 Therapeutic exercise for spinal segmental stabilisation in low back pain. Churchill Livingstone, Edinburgh

6

The nerve supply of the back

The human nervous system is the most highly developed and complicated in the animal kingdom, its structure and function being intricately bound together (Bowsher 1988). The system really needs to be considered as one as it is a continuous tract throughout the whole body. Butler (1991) describes it as being a continuum in three ways (Box 6.1).

However, for ease of description it is divided into the central nervous system, the peripheral nervous system and the autonomic nervous system.

THE CENTRAL NERVOUS SYSTEM

The central nervous system (CNS) consists of the **brain** and the **spinal cord**. Only an outline of their structure and function will be given here.

The brain, contained within the skull, is protected by the cranial bones and by three membranes known as the **meninges**: the **dura mater** on the outside, the **arachnoid mater** in the middle and the **pia mater** on the inside. It contains grey matter, consisting of cell bodies which receive, store and transform information, and

---

Box 6.1   The nervous system as a continuum
1. The connective tissues are continuous. 2. The neurones are connected electrically, so that an impulse generated at the foot is received in the brain. 3. The system is continuous chemically, the same neurotransmitters exist peripherally as centrally and there is a flow of cytoplasm inside axons.

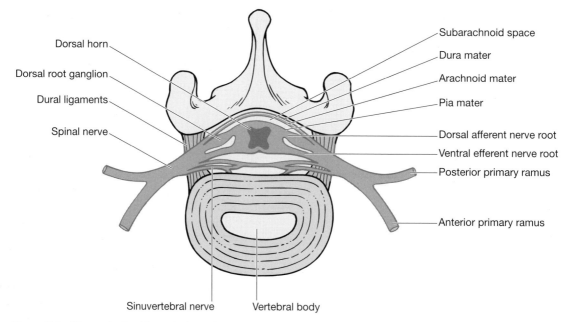

Figure 6.1 The contents of the spinal canal.

white matter, consisting of the nerve fibres which transmit information.

The spinal cord becomes continuous with the brain at the foramen magnum, the exit from the skull. The spinal cord consists of a central X-shaped core of grey matter around which the white matter is arranged (the ascending and descending pathways), all surrounded and protected by the same membranes as the brain. The dura mater of the spinal cord is a tough fibrous tube which is continuous with the cranial dura and descends down to the level of the sacrum. It is the toughest of the three sheaths and is separated from the wall of the canal by fatty pads and a plexus of veins. Between the arachnoid mater and the pia mater is the **subarachnoid space** containing cerebrospinal fluid (Johnston 1945, Palastanga et al 1998) (Fig. 6.1).

The spinal cord is suspended within the canal and is tethered to the bony structures by dural ligaments (Butler 1991). In the upright or extended posture, it hangs in a relaxed wavy line; on extreme flexion the cord elongates in the canal, moving forwards as it does so (Breig & Marions 1962, Breig & El-Nadim 1964, Troup

1986). From extreme spinal extension to complete flexion the spinal canal lengthens from 5 to 9 cm (Butler 1991). The changes in length and volume of the canal between flexion and extension, lateral flexion and rotation lead to major changes in the resting tension of the cord (Breig 1978). The ability of the cord to elongate within the canal on movement is highly relevant to the subject of spinal and neural mobility which will be discussed later in the text.

From the foramen magnum the spinal cord travels down through the canal for about 45 cm to the level of the first or second lumbar vertebra, where it tapers into a cone shape, forming the **conus medullaris**. From this point a delicate non-nervous filament, the **filum terminale**, descends to anchor the cord at the first coccygeal segment (Johnston 1945, Palastanga et al 1998).

A pair of nerve roots emerge from either side of the cord at appropriate levels of the cord's grey and white matter: an anterior and a posterior root. The anterior or ventral nerve root carries mainly efferent or motor nerve fibres; the posterior or dorsal nerve root carries mainly afferent or sensory fibres and transmits sensory fibres to the spinal cord. Above the level of the

IVF from which they will exit, the roots pierce through the dura mater, taking with them a continuation of the dura mater and arachnoid mater in the form of a dural sleeve, each root being covered by its own sleeve of pia mater which is continuous with the pia mater of the spinal cord. They pass down towards the relevant IVF in a soft tissue canal called the **radicular** or **intervertebral canal** (Bogduk & Twomey 1991).

The cervical nerve roots leave the cord level with their exit through the IVF. However, as the spinal cord is shorter than the spinal canal, the roots' emergence further down the cord no longer coincides exactly with their final exit; by the time the cord ends at the second lumbar vertebra, the lumbar and sacral nerve roots have already emerged from the cord and the mass of nerve roots, known as the **cauda equina**, descend in a cluster towards the sacrum, still enclosed in the dural sac (Johnston 1945, Palastanga et al 1998).

At the IVF the dorsal and ventral nerve roots unite to form a spinal nerve but prior to this, in the dorsal nerve root, there is a bulge containing the cell bodies of the sensory nerve fibres, the **dorsal root ganglion** (DRG) (Fig. 6.1). The dura mater becomes the **epineurium** or outer covering of the spinal nerve after they unite (Hewitt 1970).

The spinal nerve is quite short, only as long as the IVF, and contains motor and sensory nerve fibres and fibres from the autonomic nervous system. The spinal nerve immediately divides into two branches, the smaller posterior or dorsal ramus and the larger anterior or ventral ramus, which become the peripheral nerves of the body. Immediately after its formation the ventral ramus gives off the **sinuvertebral nerve** which is joined by a branch from the sympathetic nerve. The sinuvertebral nerve reenters the IVF, forming an ascending and descending branch which supplies the discs, vertebrae, ligaments, the blood vessels and the ventral and lateral aspects of the dura mater of the segment above and below its entry. Thus the dura mater, the dural sleeve of the nerve roots, the sheaths of the spinal nerves, the posterior longitudinal ligament, the annulus fibrosis, the blood vessels of the spinal canal and the periosteum of the vertebral bodies all become pain-sensitive structures within the spinal canal (Butler 1991).

THE PERIPHERAL NERVOUS SYSTEM

The peripheral nervous system (PNS) consists of 12 cranial nerves and 31 pairs of somatic nerves. The cranial nerves leave the brain inside the skull and travel directly to the eyes, ears, mouth, face and parts of the head.

The somatic nerves are a continuation of ventral and dorsal rami of the spinal nerves. The posterior primary rami supply the posterior muscles, the skin and structures of the facet joints. The ventral rami join together to form the cervical and brachial plexus, the nerves of the thoracic region and the lumbar and sacral plexus (Palastanga et al 1998). Although the particular area of skin supplied by a single nerve root (the **dermatomal supply**) (Fig. 6.2) is not identical in everyone, it is important during a neurological assessment to be aware of any sensory deficit and be able to link it with a motor deficiency which may be present (Table 6.1).

THE AUTONOMIC NERVOUS SYSTEM

The autonomic nervous system is made up of the **sympathetic** and **parasympathetic** nervous systems. They are antagonists in their effect: the sympathetic excites, with the 'fright, flight or fight' reaction, and the parasympathetic inhibits. The nerve fibres are distributed to the internal organs such as the various glands, viscera, blood vessels, muscles of the hairs and involuntary muscles of the body organs (Walton 1989, Bogduk 1991).

The sympathetic nervous system (SNS) forms a trunk which lies on either side of the anterior aspect of the vertebral column in two chains of fibres from C1 to the coccyx. The trunks are formed by preganglionic and postganglionic neurones of the SNS. The fibres of the SNS travel down through the spinal cord, exiting with the spinal nerve between T1 and L2. The efferent preganglionic fibres pass into the ventral rami

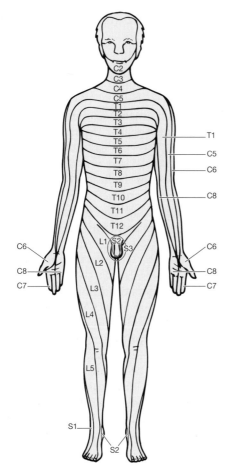 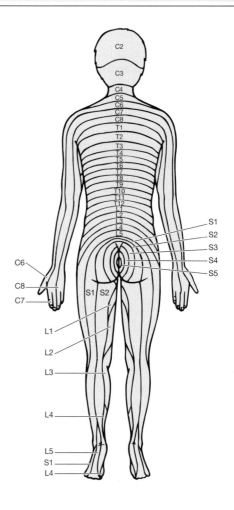

Figure 6.2 Map of the dermatomes.

and then enter the ganglia of the paravertebral sympathetic chain. There they synapse with the postganglionic fibres, which again rejoin the ventral rami of the spinal nerves. They continue to travel along with the somatic nerves, through the plexuses and into the individual peripheral nerves. Sympathetic postganglionic fibres also innervate sweat glands and blood vessels of the skin in a way that approximates the distribution of the somatic sensory nerves. The SNS is involved in changes in circulation, immune responses and endocrine function (Grieve 1988, Butler 1991, Ganong 1991, Bogduk 1991, Nayak & Shankar 1996). It has been found that the sympathetic chain can be affected by flexion/ extension movements of the vertebral column

and can be damaged by violent trauma as in whiplash injuries (Butler 1991).

The parasympathetic nervous system is distributed through cranial and sacral nerves. The cranial parasympathetic nerves supply the head, heart, lungs and upper part of the body and the sacral nerves branch to form the pelvic splanchnic nerves that supply the genitourinary organs and lower gastrointestinal tract. Although the parasympathetic nerves travel in the mixed peripheral nerves they are not part of the sympathetic chain (Johnston 1945, Ganong 1991, Bogduk 1991, Nayak and Shankar 1996).

The autonomic nervous system is greatly influenced by our emotions and vice versa. Excitement causes the heart to beat faster; anger

Table 6.1 Peripheral nerve functional tests

Nerve root	Main muscles	Resisted test movement	Reflex
C1	Rectus capitus ant. Longus capitus	Chin tuck in	
C2	Rectus cap.post. Maj. & min. obliques	Push chin up	
V cran.	Mastication	Jaw movement	
C3	Scalenes	Cervical lat. Flexion	
C4	Levator scapula Trapezius	Shldr. girdle elevation	
C5	Deltoid	Arm abduction	
C6	Biceps	Elbow flexion	Biceps jerk
C7	Triceps	Elbow ext.	Triceps jerk
C8	Thumb extensor Finger extensor	Thumb & finger extension	
T1	Intrinsic hand muscles	Finger adduction & abduction	
L2	Psoas-iliacus	Hip flexion	
L3	Quadriceps	Knee extension	Knee jerk
L4	Tibialis ant.	Foot dorsiflex.	Knee jerk
L5	Ext. hallucis long. Ext. digit. brev. Peronei Tib. post.	Big toe ext. Toe ext. Foot eversion Foot inv/PF	
S1	Gluteus max. Hamstrings Calf Peronei	Contract gluts. Knee flex. Heel raise Foot eversion	Ankle jerk
S2	Hamstrings Calf	Knee flex. Heel raise	
S3–4	Pelvic floor, bladder, genitals	Bladder control	

starts the adrenalin flowing, increasing energy for action; fear dries up the mouth. Butler (1992) has put forward the hypothesis that trauma to the sympathetic nervous system might possibly in turn create great emotional disturbance by chemical means.

NERVE STRUCTURE, NERVE ENDINGS AND IMPULSE TRANSMISSION

Nerve structure

The neurone or nerve fibre

The basic unit of the nervous system is the **neurone**. All neurones have three characteristic components: a **cell body**, **dendrites** and an **axon** (the nerve fibre).

The cell body contains the nucleus and apparatus necessary to sustain the metabolic activities of the cell. Cells are located in the grey matter of the brain and the spinal cord and in the dorsal root ganglia. The motor nerve fibres originate from the cell bodies of the ventral horn of the spinal cord and terminate at neuromuscular junctions; the sensory nerve fibres originate from the cell bodies of the dorsal root ganglia and terminate at sensory receptors or as free nerve endings in the tissues (Sunderland 1978, Lundborg 1988, Bogduk 1991).

Dendrites are short branching processes which radiate in various directions from the cell body. They receive information either through synapses with other nerves or from sensory nerve endings in the tissues and transmit it to the cell body (Bond 1984, Ganong 1991, Bogduk 1991).

The axon is a longitudinal, tubular extension of the cell membrane composed of a core of cell cytoplasm or **axoplasm** surrounded by a cell membrane, the **axolemma**. The axon or nerve fibre is the basic structure which carries the nerve impulses in the axolemma and also transports vital chemicals in the axoplasm along its entire length. The axoplasmic flow travels through the axonal transport system of the nerve fibre in both directions and three main flows have been identified (Box 6.2). The maintenance of this flow is vital, not only for the health of the nerve, which depends upon its relationship with the cell body, but also for the tissues it supplies, the

---

Box 6.2 The axonal transport system

Antegrade transport: from the cell body to the target tissue, carried at two speeds.
- Fast transport – functional materials, e.g. neurotransmitters and synthesizing enzymes for transmission at terminals.
- Slow transport – building materials for maintenance of the axon, e.g. microtubules, neurofilaments and proteins for the cell membranes.

Retrograde transport: from the target tissues to the cell body.
- Fast transport of 'recycled materials' and possibly 'trophic messages' about the state of the axon, the synapse and the environment around the synapse. Certain viruses can be carried in this way.

'target tissues'. The retrograde transport can be altered by physical constriction or loss of blood supply, inducing reactions in the nerve cell body, and the fast antegrade transport to the tissues can be slowed or blocked by deprivation of blood supply or the presence of toxic substances (Sunderland 1978, Lundborg 1988, Butler 1991, Melzack & Wall 1996, Ellaway 1998).

An adult has tens of thousands of axons to supply the foot alone and an axon can run all the way to the foot from the spinal cord without interruption – a distance of 1 metre (Melzack & Wall 1996).

So, in a neurone the axon forms the conducting element, the dendrites the receptive parts and the cell body the metabolic and genetic centre.

The peripheral nerve

Each peripheral nerve contains bundles of nerve fibres, sensory, motor and autonomic. There are two main types of fibres in peripheral nerves: **myelinated** and **non-myelinated**. All axons are surrounded by Schwann cells. In the case of the myelinated fibres, the Schwann cell produces the myelin, a laminated fat-protein insulating material, which forms multiple cuffs around the axon. At intervals of approximately 1 mm the myelin sheath is interrupted by small gaps, or **nodes of Ranvier**, which aid fast transport of

information as the action potential leaps from one node to the next. The non-myelinated axons lie singly or in groups, loosely enclosed in the cytoplasm of adjacent Schwann cells. The myelinated axons generally have a larger diameter than the unmyelinated axons (Butler 1991, Ellaway 1998).

The fibres in each bundle, both myelinated and unmyelinated, are protected by three sheaths of connective tissue: the **endoneurium** around the axons, the **perineurium** around each bundle or fascicle and the **epineurium** surrounding the whole nerve with its fascicular bundles (Fig. 6.3). The sheaths act as protective covers for the axons and contain blood vessels for the supply of nutrients.

The nerve sheaths themselves are innervated by the nervi nervorum (NN) and the blood vessels within the nerve sheath by the nervi vasorum, unmyelinated axons with 'free endings' in the layers of connective tissue (Willis 1997). The primary role of the NN is to guard the axons from physical injury by nociceptive signalling and to help regulate the neural environment through the release of neuropeptides that alter the blood–nerve barrier (Bove & Light 1997a,b). They are involved in any inflammatory process in their vicinity and may be the key element of nociception (see below).

Nerve fibres can be classified into types

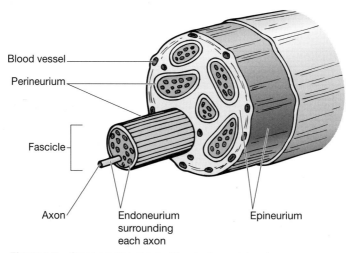

Figure 6.3 Cross-section of a multifascicular peripheral nerve.

Table 6.2 Nerve fibre types

Fibre type	Function	Speed in m/s
A: alpha	Proprioception, somatic motor	70–120
beta	Touch, pressure	30–70
gamma	Motor to muscle spindles	15–30
delta	Pain, temperature, touch	12–30
B	Preganglionic autonomic	3–15
C Dorsal root	Pain, reflex response	0.5–2
Sympathetic	Postganglionic sympathetic	0.7–2.3

A & B fibres are myelonated. C fibres are unmyelonated.
(Reproduced with permission from Ganong W F 1995
Review of medical physiology, 17th edn. Appleton and
Lange, Norwalk)

depending on their physiological characteristics, conduction velocity and diameter (Table 6.2) (Nayak & Shankar 1996). The sensory fibres are traditionally divided into three groups: the fast A-beta (large myelinated fibres) responding to non-noxious mechanical and thermal stimulation of touch, vibration, proprioception and heat; the slightly slower A-delta (smaller myelinated fibres) for noxious pinprick, pressure, strong temperature, chemical irritation (inflammation) and fast pain; and the slow C unmyelinated fibres responding most readily to noxious stimuli and carrying slow pain. About 60% of all afferents are in the C group (Melzack & Wall 1996).

Nerve endings

The nerve endings are in the tissues of the body, in the skin, muscles, ligaments, joint capsules and fat pads, organs of the abdomen, blood vessels and in the neural tissue sheaths (Butler 1991).

However, as previously mentioned, the inner portion of the disc and possibly the vertebral endplate are devoid of nerve supply, so two major load-bearing structures of the back can be damaged without eliciting pain. All other tissues of the motion segment receive a nerve supply and can communicate their responses to the brain.

Motor stimulation

Motor nerve endings deliver stimuli to muscles at the neuromuscular junction, the **motor endplate** (see p. 62). From the cell body the initial segment of the axolemma acts as a trigger zone and action potentials are generated at this site and conducted along the axon to the motor endplate.

Sensory stimulation

Sensory nerve endings and receptors in the tissues are complex and are of many different kinds. Receptors are structures, usually nerve endings, designed to respond to forms of energy (mechanical, chemical or thermal) and to convert a specific form of energy into electrical energy or a nerve impulse. **Mechanoreceptors** respond to change of position, supplying proprioceptive information; muscle tissue contains free nerve endings, Golgi tendon organs and muscle spindles (see Chapter 5) whilst **nociceptors**, or pain receptors, are associated with small myelinated and unmyelinated nerve fibres in the tissues. A-delta nociceptors respond to high-intensity mechanical and noxious thermal stimuli; C-fibre nociceptors in all tissues are activated by thermal, mechanical and chemical noxious stimuli. Because of their wide range of sensitivity, these are known as **C polymodal nociceptors** and are the free nerve endings of unmyelinated fibres where the nerve terminals themselves are the receptors. The C polymodal nociceptors are commonly silent unless activated by noxious stimulation. All stimulation results in the propagation of impulses along the afferent fibre towards the spinal cord (Bowsher 1997a, Ellaway 1998).

Impulse transmission

Nerve conduction

Nociception is the generation of nerve impulses by peripheral terminals of small-diameter sensory nerves to the spinal cord with the release of mediators in the dorsal horn (DH) (Rang et al 1994). Individual neurones convey information by conducting electrical action potentials along their cell membrane. These impulses are transmitted from one nerve to another at junctions or **synapses**. Synapses typically occur between the axon of one neurone and the dendrite of another but they can be between axons and cell bodies, axons and axons or even dendrites and dendrites (Bogduk 1991). So an axon has three direct functions: to encode, to conduct and to relay messages (Devor 1994). The transmission of impulses across a synapse occurs by either an electrical or a chemical process (Ellaway 1998).

Neurotransmitters

Transmission at most synaptic junctions is chemical and unidirectional, the impulse from the axon causing secretion of chemical neurotransmitters from the presynaptic membrane of the nerve terminal. This affects the postsynaptic terminal, increasing or decreasing the permeability of its membrane. The nature of the transmitter substance varies according to the function of the neurone and the nature of the receptor. The effect can be excitatory, causing depolarization of the postsynaptic membrane, raising the excitatory postsynaptic potential (EPSP) (Ellaway 1998) and generating an action potential, or inhibitory, altering the electric potential of the postsynaptic membrane, temporarily reducing its capacity to be stimulated (Bogduk 1991). This is known as **modulation** (see p. 104).

Neurotransmitters from the sympathetic nervous system, acetylcholine from the preganglionic neurones and noradrenalin from the postganglionic, act on adrenoceptors (adrenergic receptors) in the smooth muscle of blood vessels of the skin, the gut and the cardiac muscle (Thomson 1997).

Many different neurotransmitters and neuromodulators act on receptors in the body tissues, in the DRG and the DH. Primary afferent noxious stimulation of the DH and DRG results in the release of substance P, glutamate, calcitonin gene-related peptide and many others which, when carried in antegrade transport, act on the peripheral receptors and appear to 'prime' the receptor so that it remains ready for action. Likewise, in a phenomenon known as 'wind-up', prolonged activation of the DH neurones by C-fibre volleys (arriving at less than 3 seconds apart) causes them to respond with increasingly greater discharges (Bennett 1994). As result of

this the DH neurones become sensitive also to repeated A-beta stimuli, leading to central sensitization, that may lead to chronic pain states (Siddall & Cousins 1997) (see p. 107).

Summation is the excitatory effect of converging inputs at a synapse. There are two types of summation: **temporal** summation, when the effect is caused by frequent repeated impulses no more than 3 seconds apart, which leads to an increased intensity of burning pain (Bennett 1994), and **spatial** summation, when the aggregation of impulses from different neurones converges on the same postsynaptic membrane (Atkinson 1993).

The dorsal horn (DH)

The grey matter of the DH, the relay station of afferent transmission, can be divided into nine or 10 sections or **laminae** (Fig. 6.4). Lamina I is known as the **marginal zone**, lamina II the **substantia gelatinosa**, and laminae III, IV, V and VI are collectively known as the **nucleus proprius**. Laminae VII and VIII have no contact with the periphery, only from axons within the DH or descending from higher brain centres. Lamina IX is concerned with motor neurones in the anterior horn. Lamina X surrounds the central canal. Each lamina contains many different types of cells and all axons send branches to laminae deeper in the grey matter (Bowsher 1997b).

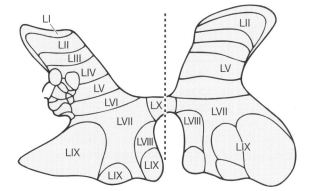

Figure 6.4 Laminae (I–X) in the grey matter of the dorsal horn of the adult human spinal cord – in the cervical region on the left and in the lumbar region on the right. (Reproduced from Bowsher 1997b, with permission from Butterworth Heinemann.)

Box 6.3   Neurones of the dorsal horn

Primary afferent nociceptors terminate on:
1. Nociceptive-specific (NS) projection neurones:
   - transmit rapidly to the brain via the spinothalamic tract
   - respond mainly to high-threshold, noxious afferents
   - are mainly in lamina I.
2. Wide dynamic range (WDR) projection neurones:
   - transmit to brain like NS neurones
   - respond to a range of stimuli both noxious, from A-delta and C fibres, and non-noxious, from A-beta fibres
   - are mainly in lamina V.
3. Excitatory and inhibitory interneurones communicating within the spinal cord itself:
   - respond to low threshold afferents and either enhance or diminish responsiveness to sensory input.

Table 6.3   The two main ascending CNS pathways

Tract	Projection	Perception of pain
Spinothalamic (STT) with branch to periaqueductal grey matter (PAG) in the brain stem	• Thalamus and then to somatosensory cerebral cortex	• Intensity, quality, location
Spinoreticular (SRT), sends to many regions	• Hypothalamus	• Autonomic response (raised blood pressure, irregular breathing)
	• Limbic system	• Emotional response
	• Frontal lobe of cerebral cortex	• Cognitive or meaningful response

Primary afferent nociceptors terminate mainly in laminae I, II and V: the unmyelinated polymodal C fibres end mainly in lamina II; A-delta high-threshold myelinated fibres terminate mainly in laminae I and V. They all terminate on three classes of neurones which either transmit to the brain or modulate the signals (Box 6.3) (Melzack & Wall 1996, Siddall & Cousins 1997, Johnson 1997, Bowsher 1997b). Messages which are transmitted to the brain cross the spinal cord and ascend in two main central tracts (Table 6.3) (Johnson 1997). The nociceptive system is complex; there is much debate over the role of differing levels of the CNS in the processing of pain and the role of the cerebral cortex is not definitive, so this simplified version must be viewed with caution (Johnson 1997).

The reflex arc

The reflex arc is a short-cut system in which the afferent input enters the dorsal horn in the usual way but instead of the message entering the ascending tracts, it is shot across to the ventral horn where motor impulses initiate immediate action. Proprioceptive information from muscles, tendons, joints and viscera, giving position and condition of deep structures, seldom reaches the brain. Most proprioception concerned with reflex activity is mediated through the spinal cord or

through the cerebellum from where posture and movement are controlled (Walton 1989).

THE BLOOD SUPPLY OF THE NERVOUS SYSTEM

Although the nervous system constitutes only 2% of body mass, it consumes 20% of available oxygen in the circulating blood. Nerve cells are especially sensitive to alteration in blood flow so an uninterrupted blood supply is imperative for the metabolic demands of normal neural function (Bowsher 1988, Butler 1991, Ganong 1991). The vertebral column has a rich supply of blood vessels supplied by the lumbar arteries and veins, giving off fine branches to all tissues (Dommisse & Grobler 1976, Crock & Yoshizawa 1976). They pass in and out of the IVF which becomes a veritable gateway for all structures entering or leaving the spinal canal. So the spinal cord, nerve roots and the peripheral nerves are well supplied with nutrients to the neural tissues.

DISORDERS AFFECTING THE TISSUES WITHIN THE SPINAL CANAL AND THE PERIPHERAL NERVES

Any disorder of the nervous system must involve at least one of the two relevant neural tissues:

impulse-conductive tissue and protective, supportive tissue (Butler 1991).

This book only considers disorders of the neural tissues within the spinal canal and the nerves related to spinal problems, not diseases or disorders of the central nervous system.

The most common neural disorders associated with vertebral problems are the mechanical and physiological consequences of stretch, friction and compression. These factors affect either the blood supply to the nervous system, the axonal transport system or the innervation of the connective tissue. The major factors in the resulting pathology are: intraneural oedema, neural ischaemia, traction injuries, friction fibrosis, inflammatory processes or infection. As nerve fibres are dependent upon an uninterrupted supply of blood for normal function, the vascular factors seem to be of greatest significance (Sunderland 1978, Lundborg 1988, Butler 1991).

An important factor to recognize is that injury at one part of the nervous system is likely to have clinical repercussions elsewhere along the system. Repercussions are more likely to appear at the vulnerable sites as well as at old injury sites and treatment at the local site will rarely suffice to best clear the signs and symptoms and prevent recurrences (Butler 1991).

Radiculopathy or nerve root pain

The central structures in the spinal canal need space and anything which jeopardizes this can lead to nerve root involvement or disturbance of the structures within the spinal canal. This space must be adequate during rest and during movement (see 'Spinal stenosis', p. 50) (Troup 1986).

Any abnormality which stretches or increases the resting tension of nerve roots can lead to ischaemia, severe pain, paraesthesia and anaesthesia. Nerve roots and neural tissue can be impinged upon or stretched by offending objects such as oedematous surrounding tissue, a bulging intervertebral disc, an osteophyte, a thickened ligamentum flavum or other bony impingement of the vertebral canal or IVF or restriction by scar tissue.

The impingement can lead to irritation or compression of the neural tissue but pain occurs only when mechanical irritation leads to ischaemia or inflammation (Troup 1986, Cailliet 1995).

The DRG is considered to be a major site of radicular pain and elicits probably the most disabling symptoms of all spinal pain. Mechanical compression of the DRG may also lead to intraneural oedema and a subsequent decrease in cell body blood supply, resulting in abnormal DRG activity and pain (Weinstein 1991).

Nerve irritation/inflammation

The nervi nervorum afferents respond to noxious mechanical, chemical and thermal stimulation; they also have receptors in adjacent muscles and tendons (Willis 1997). Thus nerve irritation can result from chemical irritation such as the inflammatory response from a nuclear extrusion or from the mechanical trauma of repeated injury, for example impingement of a disc or osteophyte.

Irritation of nerve tissue results in pain and sometimes in subjective feelings of paraesthesia and anaesthesia without actual loss of sensation. If the inflammation persists, intraneural tissues may be affected which is potentially damaging to the nerve fibre itself and can result in loss of conductivity (Lundborg 1988). Chronic neuritis or even minor nerve injuries can induce neuropathic pain syndromes (Greening & Lynn 1998) (see below and p. 105).

Nerve injury and neuropathy

Stretch and trauma

Nerves can be injured by stretch or by mechanical sources, both leading to inflammation (Box 6.4). Following injury when a nerve is cut across, the proximal stump seals off and forms a terminal swelling or 'endbulb'. Within a short time fine processes or axonal 'sprouts' emerge from the end and grow towards the 'target' tissue. Growth stops on arrival, spare sprouts are culled and peripheral receptor function is restored. If growth

---

> **Box 6.4** Injury to nerve sheaths
>
> 1. Stretch: initially the fascicles telescope but at the end of range damage through excessive shear leads to rupture of:
>   - epineurium
>   - perineurium
>   - axons
>   - blood vessels.
> 2. Mechanical sources: any trauma to a nerve is likely to damage NN axons, leading to:
>   - regrowth
>   - local healing
>   - ectopic impulses
>   - neuropathic and chronic pain syndromes.
> 3. Compression for 2 hours or more may lead to:
>   - external hyperaemia
>   - oedema
>   - demyelination.

---

is blocked, the sprouts turn back on themselves or form a tangled mass called a 'neuroma'. This can be the site for 'ectopic' or abnormal firing (Devor 1994).

Axons that have been demyelinated locally, but are otherwise in continuity, may also become hyperexcitable so that partial, incomplete nerve trauma can also lead to spontaneous, ectopic discharges (Devor 1994).

Compression

Compression can arise from steady external pressure, usually against underlying bony structures, or by entrapment within bony canals. Other causes include tumours, inflammatory masses, oedema and haemorrhage within confined spaces (whiplash injury) and the most common cause, spinal stenosis. Epineural oedema can result from quite mild compression or friction (Rydevik et al 1984).

Nerve compression can be acute or chronic.

• *Neuropraxia* is an acute block of conductivity due to ischaemia. This can result from a severe, abrupt, transient impingement or stretch of the nerve: for example, an acute prolapsed intervertebral disc (PID).

• *Entrapment neuropathy* or chronic compression occurs when a nerve is slowly or even intermittently compressed until the nerve fibres are destroyed and the nerve tissue is converted into fibrous tissue (Sunderland 1978, Nayak & Shankar 1996); for example, a posterior primary ramus entrapment from a stiff, thickened facet joint or a postoperative sciatic nerve entrapment with scar tissue.

Compression of neural tissue results in paraesthesia followed by loss of conductivity, resulting in loss of sensation and weakness. Ischaemia, a common component of nerve compression, can lead to irreversible damage (Breig & Marions 1962, Sunderland 1978, Bogduk & Twomey 1991).

Polyneuropathy

Polyneuropathies are divided into acquired and inherited types. Of the acquired neuropathies, the metabolic neuropathies make up the largest group (Nicklin 1998). Of these, **diabetic neuropathy** is the most commonly seen in the back pain clinic. It occurs with a 50% prevalence for patients with diabetes of 25 years duration. Demyelination is followed by axonal degeneration of the peripheral nerves. Symptoms often include pain and wasting of thigh muscles, paraesthesia in the feet with loss of vibration and position sense or loss of sensation and temperature sense, leading to foot ulcers. Presentation can also include cardiovascular, gastrointestinal and genitourinary involvement (Nayak & Shankar 1996).

Double crush syndrome

The double crush is a symptomatic lesion at two levels along the nerve. Mechanisms at fault are believed to be microcirculation loss, oedema caused by denervation, impairment of axonal flow and connective tissue abnormalities, for example tethering by scar tissue causing shear forces further along the nerve (Butler 1991). The most important of these appears to be the reduction in axon flow which can occur with light constriction.

If this occurs at a proximal site, the altered supply of nutrients down the nerve and the loss of information about the state of the target tissues to the cell body can cause sensitization of the target tissue interface (Butler 1991). 'Double crush' helps to explain the occurrence of combined entrapments of one nerve trunk at several levels, for example a cervical radiculopathy and a distal neuropathy (Raps & Rubin 1994, Baba et al 1998, Golovchinsky 1998). In this way an overt carpal tunnel entrapment of the median nerve could mask the coexistence of the prime lesion at the nerve root (Sunderland 1978, Lundborg 1988, Butler 1991).

The syndrome can also work in reverse when the initial injury is distal – for example, a severe Colles fracture with the next crush proximal, such as a median nerve entrapment at the elbow, followed by a root lesion (a triple crush) (Butler 1991). Situations like this tend to be even more likely when the patient has, some time previously, had a local vertebral problem. For this reason, therapists must be careful to direct treatment to the source of the problem and not ignore the spinal structures in any limb pain, for example tennis elbow, 'frozen shoulder', hip or knee pain (Wells 1997), or any traumatic limb injury which invariably involves vertebral structures.

Injury of non-neural tissue may also follow a neural lesion due to the interruption of axonal flow and the metabolic processes, for example injury to gastrocnemius muscle following a previous lumbar discogenic episode.

Extraspinal causes of sciatica

There can be causes of sciatic pain that do not originate in the lumbar spine. Up to one in five patients with an extraspinal cause of sciatica may have a radiologically abnormal lumbar disc which is not responsible for their symptoms (Dudeney et al 1998).

Cause can be related to:

- pathological conditions within the nerve as it courses from the neural foramina to the greater sciatic notch, e.g. diabetic radiculopathy, tumours of neural origin and

fibrosis or scarring of the sciatic nerve (Dudeney et al 1998)
- intrapelvic causes: tumours, haematoma in psoas muscle, endometriosis, tuboovarian abscess and aneurysms (e.g. abdominal aortic aneurysm) (Dudeney et al 1998)
- extrapelvic causes: gluteal artery aneurysms and pseudoaneurysms, tumours, gluteal abscess, piriformis muscle syndrome, avulsion fractures of ischial tuberosity and the migration of broken trochanteric wires after total hip arthroplasty (Dudeney et al 1998).
- entrapment of peripheral nerves in the lower limb masquerading as lumbar radiculopathy – femoral, saphenous, peroneal, tibial or sural nerves (Butler 1991, Dudeney et al 1998).

NEURAL DYNAMICS

During the movements of the body through flexion and extension the spinal cord is elongated and relaxed in the spinal canal, producing movement in the nerve roots (Breig 1978). In the course of normal everyday living, movement takes place in the neural environment, not only of the meninges and nerve roots within the spinal and radicular canals but also of the peripheral nerves within their mechanical interface tunnels throughout the body: bones, muscles, joints, fascia and fibro-osseous tunnels. The mechanical interface changes its dimensions as the body moves (for example, as muscles contract or the IVF alters in size); this in turn imposes forces on neural structures. During body movements the neural system slides and elongates within its interface while angulation, compression and cross-sectional

Table 6.4 Neurodynamic tests

Nerve tested	Test used
• Median nerve • Radial nerve • Ulnar nerve	• Upper limb tension test one (ULTT1) • Upper limb tension test two (ULTT2) • Upper limb tension test three (ULTT3)
• Femoral nerve • Sciatic nerve	• Prone knee bend (PKB) • Straight leg raise (SLR)

changes occur. Movement evokes physiological responses in the nerve, such as alterations in intraneural blood flow, impulse traffic and axonal transport (Lundborg 1988, Butler & Gifford 1989, Shacklock 1995).

Neurodynamic tests have been used for many years by therapists and medical practitioners to examine the response of neural tissue to applied stretch: the straight leg raise test (SLR), the prone knee bend test (PKB), the passive neck flexion test (PNF), the slump test (Maitland 1986) and the upper limb tension test (ULTT) (Elvey 1981, Butler 1991) (Table 6.4). More refined tests can attempt to direct stress towards specific peripheral nerves, for example the obturator nerve or sural nerve (Butler 1991).

These tests were previously referred to as examining adverse neural tension (ANT) or adverse mechanical tension (AMT). Elvey (1998) recently disputed the words 'mechanical' and 'tension' as they convey the wrong approach to the tests. He questions what tissues are restricting movement or eliciting pain and asks us to consider the possibility that resistance and symptoms may originate in structures protecting neural tissue. Support for this theory can be found in the work of Shacklock (1995), Wilson (1997), Katavich (1997), Elvey (1998) and Hall et al (1998). However, the validity of tension testing as a diagnostic test and informative tool in the process of clinical reasoning is not in doubt.

Disc protrusion, stenosis, spondylolisthesis, joint instability, scar tissue, high intramuscular pressure and overuse syndromes may cause musculo-skeletal dysfunction leading to mechanical stress on neural tissue. This stress may lead to damage or pathophysiology in neural tissue, resulting in pain and disability which is demonstrated by neural mechanosensitivity or pathodynamics (positive results of the tests) (Shacklock 1995, Greening et al 1999).

Hall et al (1998) have shown that increased muscle tone is one of the limiting factors in the SLR test. Wilson (1997) reports that muscles have the same protective function towards neural tissue as they have towards joints. This could demonstrate that the test is mainly mechanically limited by muscle contraction responding to demands from other tissues via the CNS, limitations that exist in referred somatic pain as well as in root pain (see Chapter 7). The tissues involved in an SLR are the hip and knee joints, the hamstring muscles, sacroiliac joints and lumbar spine, plus blood vessels, fascia, skin, connective tissue and the nerve itself (Wilson 1997).

Wilson (1997) also suggests that the pain may not be from adverse mechanical tension but from adverse sensitivity of receptor cells of the CNS to movement of neural tissue. Katavich (1997) examines the possibility that neural mobilization could decrease pain by activating the inhibitory systems and reducing muscle spasm. Mobilization of the nervous system, therefore, relies on influencing pain pathology via the mechanical treatment of neural tissue and the non-neural structures surrounding the nervous system, so these tests should be called neurodynamic tests (Shacklock 1995, Hall et al 1998).

When the tests are carried out, they should be considered as examination procedures and manoeuvres of tissues used to provoke or

---

Patient advice 6.1 Nerves

Patients need to know that nerves are not just telephone wires.
1. Nerves require a large blood supply.
2. Everyday movements provide this.
3. Demonstrate movements of the nerves that occur in daily living:
   - reaching up sideways to open a high cupboard door with wrist extended (median n.)
   - putting an arm backwards and sideways into a coat with wrist flexion (radial n.)
   - patting the side of your face with wrist extended (ulnar n.)
   - taking long strides in walking (sciatic n.)
   - knee flexion with hip extension in standing (femoral n., the least used in natural events!).
4. All static postures deny the neural tissues their blood supply.
5. Neural tissue deprived of blood leads to pain and pathology.
6. Movement is essential, therefore people in sedentary jobs *must* exercise.

stimulate a response; tension is not necessarily imparted or used.

Neurodynamic testing is a valuable tool when correlated with the full clinical presentation and restoration of normal range of movement should be one of the aims of treatment. When used clinically in the form of passive or active movements, great care must be taken not to overstretch or overwork the tissues as microtrauma can result (Patient advice 6.1).

Key points

1. All tissues, apart from the inner disc and VEP, are supplied with nerve endings and receptor organs.
2. Impulse transmission is electrical and chemical.
3. Nerve fibres transmit impulses at different speeds.
4. The DH receives, transmits, enhances or modulates impulses.
5. The degree of stimulation affects the CNS, causing summation and sensitization.
6. The nervous system can be severely damaged by a loss of blood supply.
7. The nervous system is a continuum and injury in one area can affect another.
8. Pathophysiology of the neural system can lead to pathodynamics, leading to limited neurodynamics.
9. Restoration of neural dynamics can be a guide towards full recovery.

REFERENCES

Atkinson J W 1993 Aspects of neuro-anatomy and physiology In: Tidswell M E (ed) Cash's textbook of neurology for physiotherapists, 4th edn. Mosby, London

Baba H, Maezawa Y, Uchida K et al 1998 Cervical myeloradiculopathy with entrapment neuropathy: a study based on the double crush concept. Spinal Cord 36: 399–404

Bennett G 1994 Neuropathic pain. In: Wall P D, Melzack R (eds) Textbook of pain, 3rd edn. Churchill Livingstone, Edinburgh

Bogduk N 1991 The nervous system. In: Palastanga N, Field D, Soames R (eds) Anatomy and human movement. Butterworth Heinemann, Oxford

Bogduk N, Twomey L T 1991 Clinical anatomy of the lumbar spine, 2nd edn. Churchill Livingstone, Edinburgh

Bond M R 1984 Pain. Its nature, analysis and treatment, 2nd edn. Churchill Livingstone, Edinburgh

Bove G M, Light A R 1997a The nervi nervorum. Missing link for neuropathic pain? Pain Forum 6(3): 181–190

Bove G M, Light A R 1997b The nerve of these nerves! Pain Forum 6(3): 199–201

Bowsher D 1988 Introduction to the anatomy and physiology of the nervous system, 5th edn. Blackwell Scientific Publications, Oxford

Bowsher D 1997a Nociceptors and peripheral nerve fibres. In: Wells P E, Frampton V, Bowsher D (eds) Pain management by physiotherapy. Butterworth Heinemann, Oxford

Bowsher D 1997b Central pain mechanisms. In: Wells P E, Frampton V, Bowsher D (eds) Pain management by physiotherapy. Butterworth Heinemann, Oxford

Breig A 1978 Adverse mechanical tension in the central nervous system. Almquist Wiksell International, Stockholm

Breig A, El-Nadim A F 1964 Biomechanics of the cervical spinal cord. Centre of Neurosurgery, UAR Armed Forces Hospital, Cairo, Egypt

Breig A, Marions O 1962 Biomechanics of the lumbo-sacral nerve roots. Acta Radiologica 1: 1141–1160

Butler D 1991 Mobilisation of the nervous system. Churchill Livingstone, Singapore

Butler D 1992 Lecture on Mobilisation of the Nervous System

Butler D, Gifford L 1989 The concept of adverse mechanical tension in the nervous system. Physiotherapy 75(11): 622–629

Cailliet R 1995 Low back pain syndrome. F A Davis, Philadelphia

Crock H V, Yoshizawa H 1976 The blood supply of the lumbar vertebral column. Clinical Orthopaedics and Related Research 115: 6–21

Devor M 1994 The pathophysiology of damaged peripheral nerves. In: Wall P D, Melzack R (eds) Textbook of pain. Churchill Livingstone, Edinburgh

Dommisse G F, Grobler L 1976 Arteries and veins of the lumbar nerve roots and cauda equina. Clinical Orthopaedics and Related Research 115: 22–29

Dudeney S, O'Farrell D, Bouchier-Hayes D, Byrne J 1998 Extraspinal causes of sciatica. Spine 23(4): 494–495

Ellaway P H 1998 Applied neuroanatomy and neuropathology. In: Stokes M (ed) Neurological physiotherapy. Mosby, St Louis

Elvey R L 1981 Brachial plexus tension tests and the patho-anatomical origin of arm pain. In: Idezack R M (ed) Aspects of manipulative therapy. Lincoln Institute of Health Sciences, Melbourne

Elvey R L 1998 OCPPP 45th Annual Conference. Course notes

Ganong W F 1991 Review of medical physiology, 15th edn. Appleton and Lange, Norwalk

Golovchinsky V 1998 Double crush syndrome in lower extremities. Electromyography and Clinical Neurophysiology 38: 115–120

Greening J, Lynn B 1998 Minor peripheral nerve injuries: an underestimated source of pain? Manual Therapy 3(4): 187–194

Greening J, Smart S, Leary R et al 1999. Reduced movement

of median nerve in carpal tunnel during wrist flexion in patients with non-specific arm pain. The Lancet 354(917): 217–218

Grieve G P 1988 Common vertebral joint problems, 2nd edn. Churchill Livingstone, Edinburgh

Hall T, Zussman M, Elvey R 1998 Adverse mechanical tension in the nervous system? Analysis of straight leg raise. Manual Therapy 3(3): 140–146

Hewitt W 1970 The intervertebral foramen. Moira Packenham-Walsh Foundation Lecture. Physiotherapy 332–335

Johnson M I 1997 The physiology of the sensory dimensions of clinical pain. Physiotherapy 83(10): 526–536

Johnston T B 1945 Gray's anatomy. Longman, Green, London

Katavich L 1997 Treatment of lumbar spinal pain with neural mobilisation. New Zealand Journal of Physiotherapy December: 23–26

Lundborg G 1988 Nerve injury and repair. Churchill Livingstone, Edinburgh

Maitland G 1986 Vertebral manipulation, 5th edn. Butterworths, London

Melzack R, Wall P 1996 The challenge of pain. Penguin Books, Harmondsworth

Nayak N N, Shankar K 1996 The peripheral nervous system. Physical Medicine and Rehabilitation 12(3): 387–412

Nicklin J 1998 Disorders of nerve II: Polyneuropathies. In: Stokes M (ed) Neurological physiotherapy. Mosby, St Louis

Palastanga N, Field D, Soames R 1998 Anatomy and human movement, 3rd edn. Heinemann Medical, Oxford

Rang H P, Bevan S, Dray A 1994 Nociceptive peripheral neurons: cellular properties. In: Wall P D, Melzack R (eds)

Textbook of pain. Churchill Livingstone, Edinburgh

Raps S P, Rubin M 1994 Proximal median neuropathy and cervical radiculopathy. Double crush revisited. Electromyography and Clinical Neurophysiology 34: 195–196

Rydevik B, Brown M D, Lundborg G 1984 Pathoanatomy and pathophysiology of nerve root compression. Spine 9: 7–15

Shacklock M 1995 Neurodynamics. Physiotherapy 81(1): 9–16

Siddall P J, Cousins M J 1997 Spine update. Spinal mechanisms. Spine 22(1): 98–104

Sunderland S 1978 Nerve and nerve injuries, 2nd edn. Churchill Livingstone, Edinburgh

Thomson J W 1997 Neuropharmacology of the pain pathway. In: Wells P E, Frampton V, Bowsher D (eds) Pain management by physiotherapy. Butterworth Heinemann, Oxford

Troup J D G 1986 Biomechanics of the lumbar spinal canal. Clinical Biomechanics 1(1): 31–43

Walton J 1989 Essentials of neurology, 6th edn. Churchill Livingstone, Edinburgh

Weinstein J 1991 Neurogenic and non-neurogenic pain and inflammatory mediators. Orthopaedic Clinics of North America 22(2): 235–246

Wells P 1997 Manipulative procedures. In: Wells P, Frampton V, Bowsher D (eds) Pain management by physiotherapy. Butterworth Heinemann, Oxford

Willis W D 1997 An alternative mechanism for neuropathic pain. Pain Forum 6(3): 193–195

Wilson E 1997 SLR. What are we testing? In Touch 4: 5–8

FURTHER READING

Butler D 1996 Mobilisation of the nervous system. Churchill Livingstone, Edinburgh

Elvey R L 1985 Brachial plexus tension tests and the pathoanatomical origin of arm pain. In: Glasgow E F, Twomey L T, Scull E R, Kleynhams A M, Idezak R M (eds) Aspects of manipulative therapy, 2nd edn. Churchill Livingstone, Melbourne, p. 116

Grieve G 1986 Modern manual therapy of the vertebral column. Churchill Livingstone, Edinburgh

Lundberg C 1988 Nerve injury and repair. Churchill Livingstone, Edinburgh

Palastanga N, Field D, Soames R 1998 Anatomy and human movement, 3rd edn. Butterworth Heinemann, Oxford

Petty N J, Moore A P 1998 Neuromuscular examination and

assessment. A handbook for physiotherapists. Churchill Livingstone, Edinburgh

Refshauge K, Gass E 1995 Musculoskeletal physiotherapy. Clinical science and practice. Butterworth Heinemann, Oxford

Stokes M 1998 Neurological physiotherapy. Mosby Year Book, St Louis

Sunderland S 1978 Nerve and nerve injuries, 2nd edn. Churchill Livingstone, Edinburgh

Walton Lord 1989 Essentials of neurology, 6th edn. Churchill Livingstone, Edinburgh

Wells P, Frampton V, Bowsher D 1997 Pain management by physiotherapy. Butterworth Heinemann, Oxford

7

Pain

THE MYSTERY OF PAIN

Pain is the most complicated area of human experience. Understanding it is a challenge to medicine, to the scientist, to the sufferer and to society (Melzack & Wall 1996). Although in recent years exciting new concepts regarding all aspects of the complex mechanisms of pain have been researched and explained, a certain mystery still remains.

Perhaps the enigma stems from the wide common usage of the word to describe all suffering from the mild sensations of a pinprick to the agony of bereavement to the relentless pain of an incurable disease. Hidden within this spectrum, there are associations with punishment, with martyrdom, with the intimation that stoicism leads to inner strength, that 'it must get worse before it gets better' and that pain is inflicted upon us and we are the victims of its aggression.

The origin of this attitude lies in the word itself. The term 'pain' is derived from the Greek *poine* (a tax) and the Latin *poena* (a punishment or penalty); the latter had both physical and mental implications in classical Latin. Thus the mind–body links in the word are present from its very earliest appearance in language and from the beginning our word 'pain' had an association with wrong doing (Fabrega & Tyma 1976).

The description of pain is rooted in historical and cultural factors. Religious and moral beliefs, age and gender all affect the individual's interpretation of and response to pain. Culture includes the distinctive features of a person's entire lifestyle and as such shapes psychological experience and social behaviour (Fabrega & Tyma 1976).

Another perplexing factor in our understanding of pain lies in the complicated relationship between injury and the degree of pain it elicits. Certain conditions defy straightforward physiological explanations of pain.

- *Congenital analgesia* is a condition in which there is an inability to feel pain, yet the nervous system is intact.
- *Episodic analgesia* is a condition in which there is a lack of feeling at the time of injury (Beecher 1959).
- Pain can be present in the absence of injury or long after injury has healed (Melzack & Wall 1996).

Thus injury may occur without pain and pain without injury. Fortunately, recent investigations are disclosing physiological links between the psyche/the CNS and the soma/physical pain which are beginning to explain the complicated mechanisms involved in pain perception. With new insight, perhaps all of us in the medical and therapeutic professions will be better equipped to understand the changing plasticity of the nervous system which, hopefully, will lead to more appropriate treatment of acute pain and the prevention of chronicity. Then, maybe, fewer patients will be 'accused' of being psychosomatic in their frustrated search for relief from ongoing problems.

DEFINITIONS OF PAIN

Pain is a symptom which humanity has tried to understand in terms of religion, philosophy and medicine from time immemorial (Fordham 1992). The constantly quoted definition of pain given by the International Association for the Study of Pain (1979) is probably the most apt as it encompasses the two aspects of physical and emotional sensation: pain is 'an unpleasant sensory and emotional experience associated with actual or potential tissue damage or described in terms of such damage'.

Pain is not a primary sensation – as are vision, hearing, touch, smell and thermal sensitivity – but an emotional disturbance resulting from the development of mechanical and/or chemical changes in body tissue of such nature and magnitude that they activate afferent systems that are normally quiescent. No matter how bizarre the clinical presentation, pain is always indicative of some degree of dysfunction (Wyke 1976).

'Pain is whatever the experiencing person says it is and it exists wherever he says it does' (McCaffery 1972). The fundamental point of reference for the medical profession's approach to pain is the patient's subjective experience of pain. In assessment, we *must* accept this important point and thoroughly examine dysfunction in every tissue system. At the same time, we need to move away from the dualistic thinking that pain is 'either in the tissues or a fault of the mind' (Thacker 1999) and integrate the complicated *mechanisms* of pain into our clinical thoughts.

THE PURPOSE OF PAIN

According to Sternbach (1989), pain is a warning sign; it enables the organism to sense impending tissue damage and thus avoid harm and prolong survival. Evidence supporting this evaluation comes from the studies of people with congenital insensitivity to pain who have died early in life because of a lack of the 'warning' of danger. Leriche (1939), cited in Melzack & Wall (1996), also points out that irregularities of pathology, for example cancer, can occur without pain. Although injury can occur without pain, pain usually, initially, signals tissue disorder.

Weinstein (1991) believes that basic nociceptor function is protective: nociceptors warn, sensitize and then contribute to the process of healing. However, the role of pain as a messenger changes depending upon its duration. In its briefest appearance it can be a helpful warning; in its longest display the very communication becomes a self-perpetuating reminder of what appears to be an insoluble situation, making pain appear to be the aggressor instead of the outcome of some form of assault (see 'Chronic pain', pp. 101, 107).

THE CONSCIOUS PERCEPTION OF PAIN

Emotional influences

Psychological evidence refutes the one-to-one relationship between stimulus and sensation. There are individual differences in each person's perception of pain and their response to it. The same injury can have different effects on different people and on the same person at different times (Melzack & Wall 1996). It is possible for a person to be in considerable pain but to hide it from others or, conversely, to complain a great deal about pain that appears minimal to other people. The mystery of undiagnosed pain with the fear of serious pathology can also be the cause of enormous suffering; people with diagnosed incurable disease can often cope better with their pain than those who do not know the cause. Uncertainty can promote the pattern of depression, disability and invalidism (Sternbach 1989). This is an important point for therapists to be aware of.

The conscious perception of pain is greatly influenced by the immediately prevailing emotional state. Diversion of attention reduces pain, albeit temporarily. Anxiety and preoccupation with it magnify the intensity. These observations are related to the strange phenomenon that allows the toleration of greater degrees of pain in moments of crisis. In an emergency, in war or sport for example, pain can be blocked off for hours to enable the person to continue with the essential activity. Soldiers who have had legs blown off have been known almost to ignore their plight until the next day, although they still reacted to the pain of an injection at the field hospital (Beecher 1959).

Verbal reports of personal pain frequently focus on emotional discomfort, describing pain in terms of personal misery, accompanied by evocative vocal and facial expressions (Craig 1994).

The most common concomitants of painful discomfort are anxiety, fear and depression, though other emotions may extend through to anger, aggression, subservience, sexual arousal and even laughter (Craig 1994). Fear, anxiety and depression are also capable of amplifying pain by provoking an autonomic nervous system visceral and skeletal activity which may in itself exacerbate pain (Craig 1994).

McCaffery (1972), Fordham (1992), French (1997), Treves (1999) and Gifford (1998a, 1999a,b,c) all give advice about helping patients to manage their pain (Patient advice 7.1).

Patient advice 7.1 The management of acute pain

1. Explain pain in a positive way: it is a symptom, not a disease; intense pain can come from quite benign disorders.
2. Relate this to 'their pain'.
3. Avoid use of words like 'crumbling spine', 'severe arthritis'.
4. Take care not to give wrong or worrying information. When describing a disc or facet joint, do so in interesting and very mechanical language.
5. Try to allay fear or anxiety: help them to choose the most appropriate way of coping with their pain without increasing pain avoidance.
6. Do not underestimate the timescale of healing, but give reassurance about recovery and early return to work.
7. Discuss the ergonomics of their work situation, including dynamic and static back care and posture.
8. Design a steady, progressive regime of activity/ exercise to restore full function.

Memory patterns

Emotionally traumatic life experiences, past experiences with pain and low-level abnormal inputs that produce self-sustaining neural activity can all become memory patterns which influence all other stimuli. Normally these mechanisms are inhibited by the central controlling system but when neural damage occurs, for example in a peripheral nerve lesion, the central inhibitory mechanisms are diminished, thus allowing spontaneous cell activity to occur even in the absence of noxious input, as for example in the case of phantom limb pain. Electrical stimulation of areas of the brain of a person who has had pain can reproduce the pain of previous experience whereas stimulation of someone who has never had pain elicits no reaction (McCaffery 1972, Weisenberg 1989, Gifford 1998b).

McCaffery (1972) quotes Pavlov (1927) who found that alarm and defence reactions could be initiated by any stimulus that had been previously associated with injuries, dangerous threat situations or frustrations. In this way sufferers of child abuse may have an unspoken hurt which remains part of every painful experience (Butler 1992).

Memories are hard to get rid of; therefore treatment that focuses on pain rather than function may not be helpful (Gifford 1999a).

Cultural, religious and social influences

McCaffery (1972) quotes Zborowski (1969): 'The fear of pain is said to rank only second to the fear of death'. However, in some cultures and religious sects pain is regarded as morally elevating or, when self-inflicted, as a means of expiating feelings of guilt attached to some supposed transgression (Wyke 1976). There are many initiation rites which involve pain-provoking rituals where the participants feel no pain at all (Melzack & Wall 1996). Stoicism is an attitude to pain which is reflected in certain cultural groups more than others and in certain family attitudes; age and gender often determine the acceptability of certain deviations from the norm within a group, with girls often allowed greater freedom to express pain than boys. These early experiences may influence our sensitivity to potentially painful stimuli and our pain behaviour throughout life (McCaffery 1972, French 1997).

Pain avoidance behaviour

Avoiding physical activity when pain is acute is rational and necessary to protect the tissues from further damage. However, pain avoidance in the extreme is one of the characteristics of chronic pain and it affects not only physical aspects but also social interaction, hobbies and work. There is little evidence that avoidance behaviour reduces chronic pain; symptoms may remain static while behaviour worsens. Avoidance behaviour may be an index of disability and an indication that the patient may have developed inappropriate coping strategies (French 1997, Waddell 1998, Gifford 1998a) (see 'The chronic pain state' below). This is where the therapist becomes a vitally important stimulus for the patient's understanding and possible rehabilitation.

DESCRIBING AND MEASURING PAIN

Describing and quantifying pain can appear to be confusing. The perception of pain and pain complaint are not necessarily synonymous.

Describing pain

Melzack & Wall (1996) point out the difficulties in scientifically measuring the language of pain. However, in a clinical situation, despite all the personality variations that may be present, it is astonishing how consistently people of one language and culture use the same adjectives to describe their pain, building up a recognizably meaningful picture. Within an English-speaking group, 'severe', 'stabbing', 'dull ache', 'burning', 'throbbing', 'crawling', 'shooting' and 'trickling' are some of the regular definitions. Some people manage to find uniquely evocative descriptions, but ones which are immediately recognizable to the listener.

In musculoskeletal conditions, the quality of pain as expressed by the patient can be an important guide to diagnosis (Melzack & Wall 1996). However, as the language, culture and religion of individuals greatly affect their attitude towards illness and the way in which they tolerate pain, the description of that pain may only be fully appreciated by people of the same group (Fabrega & Tyma 1976).

Measuring pain

'Pain thresholds' are used to explain people's different reactions when quantifying pain. The majority of people, regardless of background, have a uniform **pain sensation threshold** but the **pain tolerance threshold** is a greatly variable factor, being related to upbringing, past experience, expectations of bravery and cultural back-

---

Box 7.1   Pain thresholds

Pain sensation threshold is the least intensity level at which a sensation is first felt.

Pain tolerance threshold is the greatest intensity that a subject can bear.

Box 7.2   The role of nociceptors in the process of inflammation

1. Nociceptors evoke pain by signalling the presence of noxious physical or algesic chemicals in the tissues.
2. The barrage on afferents at the site leads to:
   - lowered response threshold
   - increased sensitivity to normal painful stimuli (primary hyperalgesia).
3. The nociceptors, responding to algesic stimuli, may release peptides and other neuromodulators that:
   - increase the excitability of neighbouring nociceptors in the surrounding area (secondary hyperalgesia).
4. This can in turn lead to an adaptive, protective mechanism which:
   - reduces stress on the injured parts
   - modulates the inflammatory process
   - promotes tissue repair.

---

ground (Box 7.1) (Hardy et al 1952, Zborowski 1952, Sternbach & Tursky 1965, Bowsher 1997a). The quality of pain plays an important role in tolerance threshold, the same person being able to tolerate one kind of pain, perhaps in one area, more than another.

Many methods have been devised to assess and measure pain. The three most commonly used are the Submaximal Effort Tourniquet Test and two pain assessment questionnaires: the McGill Pain Questionnaire and the Visual Analogue Scale (VAS) (Bowsher 1997a).

The Oswestry and Roland-Morris Functional Disability Scales are used to evaluate the correlation between functional disability and diagnosis (Leclaire et al 1997).

Other scales include Waddell's Non-organic Physical Signs in LBP, the Functional Capacity Evaluation and the Minnesota Multiphase Personality Inventory (Maruta et al 1997).

THE CLASSIFICATION OF PAIN

Pain from deep tissue damage differs from superficial damage and acute pain differs in its mechanisms and consequences from chronic pain, but pain can be divided timewise into three categories: transient pain, acute pain and chronic pain (Melzack & Wall 1996).

Transient pain

Transient pain is passing pain. A finger pinched in a door will elicit a sharp stab of pain for a short while and maybe a dull ache or throb afterwards, but if little or no damage has occurred the pain will gradually subside and there is no lasting anxiety (Melzack & Wall 1996).

Acute pain

Acute pain is pain which persists and the characteristics are the combination of tissue damage, pain and anxiety. The degree of anxiety and the result of injury will be influenced by factors such as personality and previous experience of injury (Melzack & Wall 1996).

Acute pain can be mechanical or inflammatory and the role of nociceptors in the process of inflammation has been described by Weinstein (1991) and Johnson (1997). Hyperalgesia, allodynia and spontaneous pain serve to protect the injured site and thus help the repair of damaged tissue (Box 7.2) (see 'Peripheral sensitization', p. 107).

As acute pain is associated with tissue damage, its duration is expected to be closely related to the healing of injury (Johnson 1997) (Fig. 7.1). The timescale of injury and healing described in Chapter 8 is an important guideline for treatment.

Chronic pain

The greatest challenges to pain relief are concerned with chronic pain. Defining chronic pain in itself presents a difficulty; perhaps each definition adds to the picture as a whole. It has been described as persistent or intermittent pain that lasts for more than 6 months (Fordham 1992). Melzack & Wall (1996) define it as pain

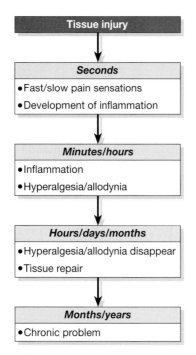

Figure 7.1 A summary of the time course of physiological events following an injury. (Reproduced with permission from Johnson 1997.)

that begins as acute pain but which lasts after healing has taken place; it often becomes a pain syndrome and a medical problem in its own right. Waddell (1998) points out that although the usual definition is simply 'pain that has continued for 3 months', 6–10% of adults may have persistent or recurrent pain which fulfils that criterion but they manage their pain, have little disability, deal with their symptoms and do not seek health care. The real problem is the 1–2% of adults with chronic, intractable, non-specific LBP and disability. They have been off work for years, have lost their jobs and use 80% of all health care, which fails to give lasting relief (Waddell 1998).

In terms of definition, the first difference between acute and chronic pain is its duration since both conditions may exhibit hyperalgesia, allodynia and spontaneous pain (Johnson 1997). The second difference is that chronic pain may not appear to show any clearly identifiable cause but instead is the result of multiple interacting causes (Melzack & Wall 1996).

As our techniques for examination become more sophisticated and our assessment and treatment more analytic on one hand and yet more functionally based on the other, maybe we can curtail the multiplicity of these interactions.

From the tissue-based viewpoint, Knight (1998), who is researching diagnostic and therapeutic techniques using laser endoscopy, is finding tissue pathology previously invisible on any scan or investigation, which could be the cause of chronic pain. There is also evidence that musculoskeletal dysfunction and lack of adequate trunk muscle stabilization may be a cause of ongoing spinal pain (see Chapter 5).

From the viewpoint of the apparently local injury but with far-reaching consequences, there is evidence that relatively minor nerve injuries, in which signs of changed nerve function are not initially apparent, may finally result in diffuse, painful, long-term symptoms with changed somatosensory thresholds (Devor 1994, Greening & Lynn 1998).

From the multifactorial viewpoint chronic pain conditions may in fact be due to a dysfunctional nociceptive system (Woolf 1994, Gifford 1999c). So, perhaps, the typical picture Waddell (1998) gives of a non-specific chronic pain state with 'persistent pain out of all proportion to physical findings' may have this complicated, reorganized synaptic circuitry of the PNS and CNS systems (see 'The chronic pain state' below).

The question which still remains unanswered is: how many of these chronic pain sufferers may be the result of poor diagnosis, poor treatment with unresolved neural and musculoskeletal dysfunction, central sensitization of their acute pain, poor education and poor self-management?

Whatever the reason for its existence, whilst acute pain may promote survival (by its warning mechanisms), chronic pain is usually destructive physically, psychologically and socially. Emotional and behavioural disturbances can result in the patient feeling victimized, desperately seeking someone who can solve their problem (Craig 1994).

However, it is important to remember that many people live and work with ongoing pain without exhibiting marked dysfunction or disability; it is only the 1–2% of chronic pain sufferers who present a social and financial problem.

Psychogenic pain

When psychological factors appear to play a predominant role in a person's pain, the pain used to be labelled as 'psychogenic'. Hysteria and hypochondriasis are grouped in this class. Hysteria is described as the translation of mental conflict into a somatic disturbance which has no acceptable organic basis and hypochondriasis is the unrealistic fear of disease (Adams et al 1994). People are presumed to be in pain because they need or want it but Melzack & Wall (1996) believe that chronic pain is usually the *cause* rather than the *result* of neurotic symptoms. Present-day understanding of pain mechanisms discloses a multicomplex and multilevel problem, recognizing three dimensions of pain that are largely responsible for an individual's behaviour pattern (Box 7.3) (Johnson 1997, Gifford 1998b); each dimension is integrally connected with the others.

In many cases of litigation, for example in whiplash injuries, patients are accused of prolonging their symptoms and told that their complaints of pain and trappings of disability only persist until legal proceedings have ceased (Treves 1999). Treves (1999) reports that Shapiro & Roth (1993) find no evidence that settlement of claims leads to resolution of symptomatology. Posttraumatic stress often causes negative labelling of psychosomatic pain, but a more complex, multifactorial understanding is necessary.

THE PHYSIOLOGY OF PAIN

There are three physiological responses of nociceptive neurones (Rang et al 1994).

1. Normal excitation by noxious stimuli (chemical, thermal mechanical).
2. Spontaneous activity associated with neuronal damage (neuropathic pain).
3. Pathological sensitization (increased response to low-intensity stimuli) – peripheral and central sensitization

Normal or nociceptive excitation

Afferent nerves are sensitive to a wide variety of noxious stimuli – thermal, mechanical and chemical. When a painful stimulus is applied to the body there is usually a double pain sensation: 'first' or 'fast' pain followed by 'second' or 'slow' pain (Box 7.4) (Price 1996, Johnson 1997, Bowsher 1997a).

Chemical excitation is from endogenous algesic (pain-producing) substances released by damaged cells. A detailed description of the complicated physiology of nociception is given in *Textbook of pain* (Wall & Melzack 1994), Bowsher (1997a,b,c,d), Weinstein (1991), Siddall & Cousins (1997) and Johnson (1997).

Non-neurogenic pain mediators

At the onset of tissue damage non-neurogenic pain mediators are released from damaged tissue, evoking an inflammatory reaction. Among others, these include potassium and hydrogen ions, bradykinin, serotonin, histamine and prostaglandins. The interactions among these chemicals affect local nociceptor responses and stimulate the action potential transmission of 'fast' pain (high-threshold A-delta fibres) and 'slow' pain (C-polymodal fibres). C-polymodal nociceptors are especially sensitive to these

---

Box 7.3 The three dimensions of pain

- *Sensory* dimensions: the location, intensity, quality and behaviour of pain
- *Affective* dimensions: the emotional reaction to pain
- *Cognitive* dimensions: the thoughts associated with pain

Box 7.4 The two sensations of pain

1. *First or fast* pain: immediate, sharp, well-localized sensation, usually ceases as soon as the stimulus is removed. Carried by A-delta fibres.
2. *Second or slow* pain: a dull, poorly localized, sometimes throbbing, lasting ache; continues for some time after removal of the stimulus. Carried by C fibres.

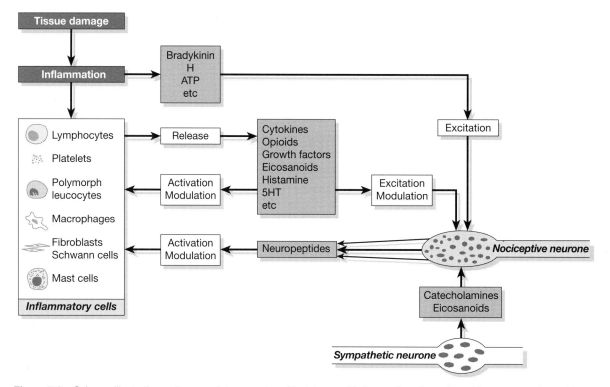

Figure 7.2 Scheme illustrating various mediators produced by injury and inflammation. A number of factors are released from damaged tissue, from immune cells and other blood cells. These can act directly on nociceptors or can stimulate the production and release of other mediators from immune cells and sympathetic neurones. (Reproduced with permission from Rang et al 1994.)

pain-producing chemicals. Rang et al (1994) give a clear scheme to illustrate this immediate response (Fig. 7.2).

Neurogenic pain mediators

The action potentials stimulate the production of neurogenic pain mediators in the form of neuropeptides from the cell bodies of primary afferents within the DRG. These neuropeptides, for example substance P, are then delivered by axonal transport to both the central (the DH) and peripheral processes of neurones. Substance P released from the peripheral ends of nociceptive afferents then enhances the inflammatory process (Weinstein 1991).

The action potentials into the CNS activate nociceptive-specific or wide dynamic range cells in the DH where the information is processed and transmitted to the brain (see Chapter 6).

It is important to remember that nerve fibres are not simply inert conductors of information but can themselves be damaged. Nerve sheaths are dynamically involved with movement and are susceptible to trauma, deformation and the chemical consequences of injury, with the nervi nervorum also signalling pain (Bove & Light 1997a,b).

Nociceptive activity occurs both at the periphery and in the CNS. However, pain only becomes pain when it is perceived as such by the brain and at any level of transmission, pain can be modulated.

The modulation of pain

Modulation means that information from a receptor can be changed, either enhanced, diminished or even suppressed, at the periphery or in the CNS (Bowsher 1997b).

Peripheral modulation. Peripheral modulation or **adaptation** takes place when the receptors themselves cease to respond to stimulation. This occurs daily when skin receptors cease to respond to ongoing contact with our clothes, because the contact no longer requires a response.

Adaptation also occurs at the periphery with the use of aspirin, which raises the response threshold of peripheral nociceptors, and also with morphine injection which can act at the peripheral end of afferent neurones (Bowsher 1997c). Local anaesthetics act by stabilizing the membranes of nerve cells, blocking the generation of impulses so that the nerve remains in its resting state (Melzack & Wall 1996). Drugs can be used to affect pain at a wide range of sites along the nociceptive pathways, acting either against the pathological processes producing pain at the periphery or by modulation of the response at the cerebral level.

Central modulation. In 1965 Melzack & Wall proposed a new theory based on modulation, **the gate control theory**, which revolutionized the concepts of pain. Prior to this there were two theories of pain.

• The *specificity theory* proposed that pain is a sensory phenomenon in its own right with special receptors, special routes of transmission through the CNS and special centres for registration, appreciation and interpretation in the brain (Hayward 1981, Bond 1984).
• The *pattern theory* stemmed from a group of theories formed as a reaction against the specificity theory. An intensity theory emerged which says that specific receptors for pain do not exist and that pain arises as a result of stimulation by any means, so long as the intensity of that stimulation passes a certain threshold (Bond 1984).

The gate control theory incorporates elements of both these theories but also takes into account the role played by emotion in the experience of pain and attitude towards it. The theory proposed an imaginary gate in the spinal cord which regulates the onward transmission of noxious input from the DH to the brain. Normally this gate is opened by the small-diameter afferent fibres (A-delta and C-poly-modal) en route to the brain. However, the gate can be closed by descending inhibitory pathways from the brain (including previously learned responses) or by other incoming powerful afferent stimulation from large A-beta nerves (e.g. from the mechanoreceptors in muscles and joints). Increased activity in either of these two pain-suppressing systems would initiate the release of inhibitory neurotransmitters from interneurones in the DH which would 'switch off' activity in the central nociceptive transmission cells (the WDR and NS cells). Sensory input is, therefore, subjected to the modulating influence of the gate *before* it evokes pain perception and response (Melzack 1982, Johnson 1997).

Descending projections arise from the hypothalamus, periaqueductal grey matter (PAG) and nucleus raphe magnus to form descending inhibitory pathways which terminate at spinal level to modulate incoming nociceptive signals. A variety of neurotransmitters, manufactured in the grey matter of the brain and present in the DH, have been implicated in descending inhibition. These include endorphins (endogenous morphine-like substances), enkephalins and dynorphins (all opioid peptides) as well as other neurotransmitters such as serotonin and noradrenalin (Fields & Basbaum 1984, Porter 1986, Melzack & Wall 1996, Siddall & Cousins 1997).

Thus noxious afferent stimulus can be modified by our prelearned attitudes, by descending chemical inhibition from the brain and by change of chemistry in the DH. All this influences the choice of modalities used in clinical therapy (Box 7.5) (Bowsher 1997c, Gifford 1998b).

Neuropathic or neurogenic pain

Neurogenic pain differs from all other pains. It is often seen clinically in combination with nociceptive pain but its origins are different. It is not caused by activation of either peripheral nociceptors or nociceptors within the nerve tissue but by damage or malfunction of the peripheral and central nervous systems. It results in a change of baseline somatosensory sensitivity (Box 7.6) (Devor 1994, Johnson 1997).

Box 7.5   Modalities that influence modulation

- Any counterirritant applied to the area of pain – this is what 'rubbing it better' has always done!
- High-frequency, low-intensity stimulation: transcutaneous electrical nerve stimulation (TENS) or vibration, A-beta stimulation.
- Low-frequency, high-intensity stimulation: acupuncture, A-delta stimulation (Alltree 1997).
- Chemical or pharmacological modulation (opioids).
- Mobilizing techniques in physiotherapy: mid-range, repetitive movements which stimulate the gate closing, A-beta stimulation.
- The attention to pain, the value put on pain and the concern shown about pain: central modulation (Gifford 1998a).

Box 7.6   Somatosensory changes in neurogenic pain

1. Aberrant inputs to central nociceptive cells (peripheral sensitization)
2. Ectopic impulse generation
3. Hyperactive central nociceptive cells (central sensitization)
4. Loss of A-beta inhibition
5. Sympathetic hyperactivity

Neurogenic pain can result from quite minor peripheral nerve damage, immediately after injury or after a delay of weeks or months. Recent research implicates the nervi nervorum in the role they may play in neurogenic vasodilation leading to local inflammation, hypersensitivity and spontaneous discharge (Willis 1997, Bove & Light 1997a,b, Sorkin et al 1997). Examples of neurogenic pain occur in any neural inflammation or in conditions such as causalgia, complex regional pain syndrome (reflex sympathetic dystrophy), partial avulsion of nerve roots (for example in whiplash), postherpetic neuralgia and trigeminal neuralgia (Bowsher 1997d, Greening & Lynn 1998, Gifford 1999a).

Neurogenic pain is characterized by typical excruciating, burning, unbearable pain in the area served by the damaged nerve. Sensitivity can spread to the surrounding areas removed from the damaged nerve and the skin can become so sensitive that pain can be triggered by small movements or even vibration produced by loud noises (Melzack & Wall 1996). A heightened sensitivity to noradrenalin stimulation may develop and normal levels of sympathetic nervous system activity may provoke C fibre firing. Therapeutically it is important to realize that quite minor manipulation of a peripheral nerve can trigger sensitivity to noradrenalin, resulting in increased pain (Greening & Lynn 1998).

The area can be hot, discoloured, swollen and sweating and patients often feel the need to wrap wet towels around the limb for relief (Melzack & Wall 1996, Bowsher 1997d). The consequences of minor nerve injury may be far reaching. Injury to peripheral nerves may take time to generate a response, remaining silent for the first day or two (for example in whiplash injury) then slowly increasing their activity over the following weeks (Gifford 1999a). Pathophysiologic changes in injured nerves constitute a principal cause of post-injury chronic pain (Devor 1994).

Neurogenic pain is virtually unresponsive to opioid analgesics (narcotics) but local anaesthetic applied distal to the injury can relieve it for long periods. Medically, the best treatment appears to be the tricyclic drugs amitriptyline or despramine. TENS and high-frequency vibration may be helpful and some forms of manual therapy, for example mobilizing surrounding neural tissue interfaces to relieve compressive effects, minimizing C fibre input activity and restoring neural function (Bowsher 1997d, Greening & Lynn 1998).

Other abnormal sensations associated with neuropathic pain are hypoaesthesia (loss of sensation), hyperalgesia (increased response to a normally painful stimulus), allodynia (pain due to a stimulus which is not normally painful) and hyperpathia (pain that continues to increase after cessation of stimulus) (Bennett 1994, Greening & Lynn 1998).

Sensitization of the nociceptive system

There is increasing recognition that the concept of pain within the nervous system is no longer a 'hard wire' system but that after prolonged, noxious stimulation, long-term changes occur. This 'plasticity' of the system alters the body's response to further peripheral stimuli. The mechanisms that sensitize the nociceptive system following tissue damage operate in both the periphery and the CNS. Both peripheral and central sensitization initially encourage protection, avoiding further injury, and are therefore adaptable and protective but they can both become maladaptive and unhelpful (Devor 1994, Gifford 1999b).

The acute pain state

Peripheral sensitization. Cell damage leads to the accumulation of algesic substances which generates action potentials to the CNS, triggering an antidromic reaction sending substance P down the nerve to the periphery; this in turn enhances the inflammatory reaction. Further chemical reaction sensitizes C-polymodal and to a lesser extent A-delta nociceptors, lowering their threshold of activation, increasing their sensitivity to a given stimulus and increasing the number of nociceptors firing, with increased barrage of input to the CNS. An inflammatory soup of chemicals in the area leads to primary and secondary hyperalgesia and allodynia and is the normal, inflammatory process of acute pain described in Box 7.2 which is both protective and adaptive (Siddall & Cousins 1997). As normal healing takes place the hyperexcitability reduces and the tissues return to normal function.

Chronic constrictive injuries (CCI), where nerves are subject to mechanical compression or mechanical torsion (for example, carpal tunnel), may also result in peripheral sensitization of nociceptors with the lowering of thresholds (Greening & Lynn 1998). In CCI, ischaemia of myelinated fibres (A-beta fibres) results in demyelination which can lead to both the loss of A-beta normal input and the production of ectopic impulses (discharge without specific stimulation). Ectopic impulses can also occur at the site of a neuroma, formed by damaged axons at the site of trauma. In this way sensitization of non-noxious A-beta afferents occurs, causing them to respond as if they were noxious afferents (Siddall & Cousins 1997, Greening & Lynn 1998).

Central sensitization. Afferent input generated by tissue damage will increase the excitability of neurones in the spinal cord, 'sensitizing' neurones in the DH and spinothalamic tract (Woolf 1994). The combined effect of the nociceptive barrage changes the sensitivity of the WDR and NS cells in the DH, reducing their threshold to all stimulation and increasing their response to incoming information from normally non-noxious stimuli (A-beta fibres) (Price 1996, Johnson 1997, Bowsher 1997d). There is also an expansion of the receptive field in the DH. The key is the initial C-fibre evoked central hyperexcitability, 'wind-up' or temporal summation of pain (Woolf 1994, Price 1996) (Box 7.7).

In the presence of central changes when A-beta fibres evoke painful symptoms, their inhibitory influence is lost and the central nociceptive output to higher centres is increased (Bowsher 1997d, Siddall & Cousins 1997, Johnson 1997, Greening & Lynn 1998). With abnormal sensitivity and loss of inhibition, when even normal touch and movement result in a 'pain-type' discharge pattern, the onset of pain behaviour is quite understandable (Greening & Lynn 1998).

The chronic pain state

Nociceptive, neuropathic, psychological, cultural, religious and environmental factors contribute to the experience of pain and chronic pain must be seen in its entire context.

Under normal circumstances the acute pain state and the increased sensitivity associated with it should resolve and the nociceptive

---

Box 7.7 Cell changes in the dorsal horn

- Reduction in threshold; non-noxious stimuli become painful (allodynia).
- Amplification response to afferent input with exaggerated pain (hyperalgesia).
- Expansion in the receptive field with sensitivity in uninjured areas.

system should return to normal functioning. However, after long-term changes, when the 'plasticity' of the nervous system is altered, the pain can become a chronic pain state with continuing nociceptive dysfunction. This is becoming a more and more likely source of ongoing pain and is currently an area of intense research (Johnson 1997).

Neuropathic pain is particularly persistent, possibly because a loss of inhibition from injured axons (A-beta fibres) helps to maintain sensitization. The pathophysiology connected with neurogenic pain is complex, difficult to diagnose and difficult to manage. Sensory conduction tests are often normal but somatosensory function tests, for example vibration tests, are often abnormal (Greening & Lynn 1998).

The nociceptive system operates in a number of modes (Woolf 1994) (Box 7.8). Modes 1,2 and 3 reproduce plasticity of the system while in mode 4 cells of the DRG die, axons of the DH degenerate or atrophy and contacts between synapses become modified and changed in their response. The regeneration of injured neurone endings in the DH causes regrowth into new sites, resulting in alteration of the DH circuitry (Woolf 1994). Controversy exists over the extent to which changes within the CNS become self-perpetuating or require ongoing noxious peripheral input to maintain them.

Patients with 'non-specific' chronic pain and unexplained limb pains may have undiagnosed continuing tissue dysfunction. Conditions such as non-specific arm pain, whiplash and non-specific back pain may present with positive symptoms usually associated with nerve injury, for example paraesthesia, hyperalgesia, allodynia, spontaneous pain and loss of function, but with normal reflexes, muscle power and sensation (Greening & Lynn 1998, Gifford 1998b).

The loss of the chemicals that modulate pain may also play a role in chronic low back pain. Normally enkephalins and endorphins in the cerebrospinal fluid play an important role in the suppression of pain. Their quantity is maintained and increased by activation of large muscle groups. It has been found that chronic back pain sufferers have a diminished amount of these endorphins in their cerebrospinal fluid (Nachemson 1985). Pain avoidance leads to lack of movement, so could this also be a significant factor? Certainly, activity is a vital part of all rehabilitation.

Waddell & Main (1998), describing the 'biopsychosocial' model, believe that chronic pain and disability become disassociated from the original physical problem and that continued attempts to treat tissue damage actually reinforce pain and perpetuate the problem. Pain and disability are fundamentally different. Pain is symptomatic whereas disability is a diminished or restricted capacity for everyday activity and is easier to evaluate than pain. Concentrating on the 'disease model' or the neurophysiology of pain is not the answer.

Gifford (1998a, 1999a,b) incorporates neurophysiological involvement and all elements of pain mechanisms into what he calls the mature organism model (MOM) (Fig. 7.3), taking every aspect of the human pain problem into consideration. In patients, clinicians should concentrate on pain mechanisms and restoration of function rather than focusing on local tissue dysfunction and give the message that 'hurt' does not necessarily 'harm' (Gifford 1998b).

Cohen et al (1992) present their own version of a chronic pain paradigm which identifies three levels of contributing factors: nociceptive, neurogenic and psychogenic. This is a clear, simple expression of the important factors (Box 7.9).

Researchers dealing with the problems of chronic pain are hoping that a picture may emerge whereby the potential causative factors of chronic low back pain (CLBP) may be

---

Box 7.8 The four modes of the sensory motor system

1. *Control mode*: normal somatosensory function
2. *Suppressed mode*: transmission suppressed by inhibitory mechanisms, e.g. descending inhibitory mechanisms, TENS, analgesics, acupuncture, etc.
3. *Sensitized mode*: excitability increased (allodynia and hyperalgesia)
4. *Reorganized mode*: potentially irreversible reorganization of synaptic circuitry

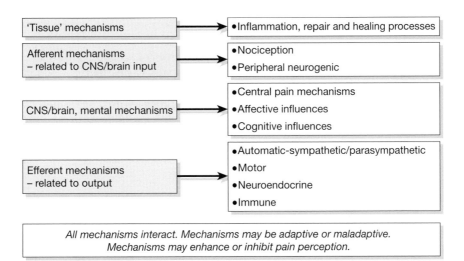

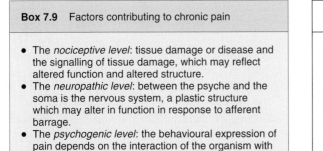

All mechanisms interact. Mechanisms may be adaptive or maladaptive.
Mechanisms may enhance or inhibit pain perception.

Figure 7.3   Pathobiological mechanisms related to pain perception and physical and mental/psychological dysfunction. (Reproduced with permission from Gifford 1999a.)

Box 7.9   Factors contributing to chronic pain

- The *nociceptive level*: tissue damage or disease and the signalling of tissue damage, which may reflect altered function and altered structure.
- The *neuropathic level*: between the psyche and the soma is the nervous system, a plastic structure which may alter in function in response to afferent barrage.
- The *psychogenic level*: the behavioural expression of pain depends on the interaction of the organism with past experiences, culture and environment.

Patient advice 7.2   Treatment for chronic pain

It is *essential* for therapists to understand the mechanisms of pain and the predisposing factors which may lead to chronicity.

It is *unhelpful* for therapists to misunderstand those mechanisms and assume 'psychological' causes for the source of pain.

- Avoid words like 'tension' – they are unhelpful and offer no positive actions or understanding.
- Mobilize/exercise joint or tissue dysfunction.
- Explain pain and discuss the way to cope with it and continue normal living.
- Then focus on function and the mechanisms of pain, rather than local pain.
- Discuss and explain the essential need to move.
- Encourage helpful physical awareness without fear of movement.
- Explain the important role patients play in their own recovery.
- Discuss ergonomic adaptations or improvements at work.
- Suggest appropriate activities with graded progressions to fit the patient's ability.

---

identified more clearly and prevented at an earlier stage. The new cry is for further research in the systematic data collection of predictors of chronic back pain and disability.

Twomey & Taylor (1987) hypothesize that if acute pain were always fully resolved, chronic pain would be minimized (See 'Treatment of acute pain', Chapter 10). With new clinical approaches to neural and muscular involvement in acute pain, with the awareness of the need to regain full function wherever possible, with the realization that all acute pain sufferers need to be educated to understand pain and to be unafraid of its manifestations, maybe we will be able to decrease the number of non-specific chronic back pain sufferers (Patient advice 7.2).

THE NATURE OF BACK PAIN
Transient back pain

Transient pain can be the twinge of the overstretch from a maintained posture or from a slightly awkward movement. It is a passing pain but one which should not be ignored as it serves as a warning to avoid repetition by using back care or exercising out of it in the right way (see Chapter 17).

Acute back pain

Acute back pain can either build up from daily, sustained posture (long standing, long sitting, long stooping) or repeated movements (digging, shelf stacking) or it can occur suddenly following a traumatic event (lifting, falling). Tissue damage may have taken place, no matter how small, and the situation requires attention: first to heal the damage and reduce the pain, then to restore full function to the whole area. The chances for successful rehabilitation are reduced in patients whose pain persists for more than 6 months. Even after 3 months of persistent pain, the attitude of the person may be altered, introducing anxiety, pain avoidance behaviour and all the mechanisms of chronic pain (Nachemson 1985) (see Chapter 16).

Chronic back pain

Waddell (1998) describes the features of chronic back pain as: persistent pain which may be out of all proportion to physical damage; progressive inactivity and disability; disturbed mood; unhelpful beliefs; increasing requests for medical help; treatment failure and side-effects; additional social and family stress; anger and hostility.

This classifies the 1–2% of chronic back pain sufferers with disability and should not be applied to patients attending clinics with intermittent ongoing episodes of pain who manage to cope for the greater part of their lives (see 'Treatment of chronic low back pain' in Chapter 10).

THE PHYSIOLOGY OF BACK PAIN

Pain can arise from any pathological process that stimulates nociceptors in any pain-sensitive structures of the back (Bogduk & Twomey 1991); this means any tissue connected to or around the motion segment that has a nerve supply, including the innervated neural connective tissue itself (Bove & Light 1997a,b).

Back pain varies in type depending upon its cause. It can originate from a mechanical or chemical disturbance of tissue or a combination of both (Wyke 1976, McKenzie 1981). Pain can be experienced either locally, at the site of injury, or it can be referred into more distant areas.

Mechanical pain

Pain is produced by the application of mechanical forces as soon as the mechanical deformation of innervated structures is sufficient to irritate nociceptors or free nerve endings (McKenzie 1981).

Pain can occur with or without tissue damage. With an absence of damage, the pain is from stretched or briefly ischaemic tissues, followed by relief as soon as the stress is removed. The pain can be caused by postural stress, musculoskeletal dysfunction, shortened scar tissue or disc protrusion (McKenzie 1981).

The nerve root, together with any pain-sensitive structure within the vertebral canals or the IVF, can be stretched, bent or tethered at any point. Compression of the nerve root evokes paraesthesia and anaesthesia but not pain. However, if a nerve is compromised in any way for a long period, oedema can result which would lead to a chemical disturbance in the nerve tissue (Bogduk & Twomey 1991).

Chemical pain

Chemical or inflammatory pain is produced by chemical changes in the tissues which irritate nociceptors or local nerve endings. It is caused by damage in trauma, infection, disease or ischaemia with resulting inflammation.

Mechanical and chemical pain are both present in all trauma, strains, sprains, soft tissue lesions and disc lesions where there is extrusion of matter or wherever there is an inflammatory reaction (Box 7.10).

TYPES OF BACK PAIN

While the source of pain may be mechanical or chemical, the sensation of pain can be experienced either locally or referred into other areas.

Local pain

Local pain arises from the somatic or skeletal tissues. It is a localized mechanical or chemical disturbance of any of the pain-sensitive structures of the motion segments, including the muscles which are attached to or pass over them. The structures can be affected individually or in a combined way. The pain is experienced at the site of the injury, the patient often being able to pinpoint the exact spot. The character of the pain depends upon its mechanical or chemical origin (see above).

Referred pain

Referred pain is pain perceived in a region topographically displaced from the area that is the source of the pain. Not all pain in the back is necessarily due to disorders of the lumbar spine. Lumbar pain may originate in visceral or vascular disease and this possibility must be assessed carefully on examination. Referred pain from the spine experienced in the limbs or trunk can be either **somatic** or **radicular** in origin but as with all pain there must be a mechanical or chemical irritant (Bogduk 1986, Bogduk & Twomey 1991).

Experiments in the past suggested that all referred pain followed a specific pattern into areas of the body but it has been found that referral from deep structures is not consistent from person to person (Hockaday & Whitty 1967).

Somatic referred pain

Somatic referred pain is the mislocation of pain. Two mechanisms are known.

- The existence of bifurcated axons in sensory nerves. This means that sensory units which have one branch supplying skin and another branch coming from some other subcutaneous structure have only one cell body in a DRG and a single proximal axon travelling to the DH, so that messages from both areas are received at one source.
- Convergence of separate peripheral sensory units onto the same cell in the spinal cord. The mechanism appears to be that afferent impulses from affected vertebral structures activate neurones in the CNS which also receive impulses from afferents in the limbs or other areas and the perception of these messages becomes confused (Bowsher 1997c).

Somatic referred pain can originate in any of the spinal structures, especially the disc or the facet joints. The pain is deep, vague and aching. The distance of referral is usually relative to the intensity of spinal stimulus. This relationship becomes very evident during the recovery of referred pain of this nature: as the condition improves, the pain centralizes, withdrawing towards the vertebral source of pain (Mooney & Robertson 1976, McKenzie 1981). It is important to explain this process to patients to avoid them becoming extremely concerned when, possibly for the first time, they have a severe LBP on disappearance of their leg pain.

Radicular referred pain

Radicular referred pain originates from mechanical stimulation or traction of clinically damaged nerve roots or involvement of the DRG itself. The pain is of a shooting, lancing type, often all the way down the limb in a specific line of dermatomal distribution (Bogduk & Twomey 1991).

Compression of an undamaged nerve elicits paraesthesia and anaesthesia only. However, as it is impossible to say when a sound compressed nerve root may become damaged, any nerve deformation can eventually give rise to pain of a radicular nature together with altered sensation, weakness of muscle, paraesthesia and possibly anaesthesia (Bogduk & Twomey 1991).

Pain is becoming less and less of a mystery as research investigates its mechanisms but the involved interconnections still present many fascinating unsolved problems.

The approach of clinicians, therapists, nurses and carers is summarized by Porter (1986), who says that we need to listen, observe, record and learn from patients' experiences in order to unravel the mystery of pain, and by Maitland (1986) who says, simply, we must listen, we must search and we must believe (see Chapter 10).

Key points

1. Pain is initially a warning of possible tissue damage.
2. Transient and acute pain are a time-progression of tissue injury.
3. In acute pain, chemical changes in the tissues promote peripheral and central nervous system changes which normally resolve in a recognized timescale.
4. Chronic pain and disability may have many components:
   - poor initial treatment in the acute stage
   - undiagnosed tissue pathology
   - musculoskeletal joint and muscle dysfunction
   - damage to nerve tissue and/or altered neural dynamics
   - a maladaptive, dysfunctional nociceptive system
   - worry and desperation in the search for a solution.
5. Both acute and chronic pain are influenced by:
   - emotional, cultural and religious attitudes to pain
   - behavioural, environmental and social factors.

REFERENCES

Adams N, Ravey J, Bell J 1994 Review of personality characteristics in chronic back pain patients. Physiotherapy 80(8): 511–519

Alltree J 1997 Acupuncture. In: Wells P, Frampton V, Bowsher D (eds) Pain management by physiotherapy. Butterworth Heinemann, Oxford

Beecher H K 1959 The measurement of subjective responses. Oxford University Press, Oxford

Bennett G F 1994 Neuropathic pain. In: Wall P D, Melzack R (eds) Textbook of pain. Churchill Livingstone, Edinburgh

Bogduk N 1986 The anatomy and pathophysiology of whiplash. Clinical Biomechanics 1: 92–101

Bogduk N, Twomey L T 1991 Clinical anatomy of the lumbar spine, 2nd edn. Churchill Livingstone, Edinburgh

Bond M R 1984 Pain: its nature, analysis and treatment, 2nd edn. Churchill Livingstone, Edinburgh

Bove G M, Light A R 1997a The nervi nervorum. Missing link for neuropathic pain? Pain Forum 6(3): 181–190

Bove G M, Light A R 1997b The nerve of these nerves! Pain Forum 6(3): 199–201

Bowsher D 1997a Acute and chronic pain and assessment. In: Wells P, Frampton V, Bowsher D (eds) Pain management by physiotherapy. Butterworth Heinemann, Oxford

Bowsher D 1997b Nociceptors and peripheral nerve fibres. In: Wells P, Frampton V, Bowsher D (eds) Pain management by physiotherapy. Butterworth Heinemann, Oxford

Bowsher D 1997c Modulation of nociceptive input. In: Wells P, Frampton V, Bowsher D (eds) Pain management by physiotherapy. Butterworth Heinemann, Oxford

Bowsher D 1997d Central pain mechanisms. In: Wells P, Frampton V, Bowsher D (eds) Pain management by physiotherapy. Butterworth Heinemann, Oxford

Butler D 1992 Mobilisation of the nervous system. Course notes

Cohen M L, Arroyo J F, Champion G D, Browne C D 1992 In search of the pathogenesis of refractory cervicobrachial pain syndromes. Medical Journal of Australia 156: 432–436

Craig K D 1994 Emotional aspects of pain. In: Wall P D, Melzack R (eds) Textbook of pain. Churchill Livingstone, Edinburgh

Devor M 1994 The pathophysiology of damaged peripheral nerves. In: Wall P D, Melzack R (eds) Textbook of pain. Churchill Livingstone, Edinburgh

Fabrega H, Tyma S 1976 Language and cultural influences in the description of pain. British Journal of Medical Psychology 49: 349–371

Fields H L, Basbaum A I 1984 Endogenous pain control mechanisms. In: Wall P D, Melzack R (eds) Textbook of pain. Churchill Livingstone, Edinburgh

Fordham M 1992 Pain. In: Wilson-Barnett J, Batehup L (eds) Patient problems. Scutari Press, London

French S 1997 The psychology and sociology of pain. In: Wells P, Frampton V, Bowsher, D (eds) Pain management by physiotherapy. Butterworth Heinemann, Oxford

Gifford L 1998a Pain, the tissues and the nervous system: a conceptual model. Physiotherapy 84(1): 27–36

Gifford L 1998b Personal communication

Gifford L 1999a Tissue and input related mechanisms. In: Gifford L (ed) Topical issues in pain. Physiotherapy Pain Association Yearbook 1998–1999. NOI Press, Falmouth, Adelaide

Gifford, L 1999b The 'central' mechanisms. In: Gifford L (ed) Topical issues in pain. Physiotherapy Pain Association Yearbook 1998–1999. NOI Press, Falmouth, Adelaide

Gifford, L 1999c The mature organism model. In: Gifford L (ed) Topical issues in pain. Physiotherapy Pain Association Yearbook 1998–1999. NOI Press, Falmouth, Adelaide

Greening J, Lynn B 1998 Minor peripheral nerve injuries: an underestimated source of pain? Manual Therapy 3(4): 187–194

Hardy J D, Wolff H G, Goodell H 1952 Pain sensations and reactions. Williams and Wilkins, Baltimore

Hayward J 1981 Information – a prescription against pain. Royal College of Nursing, London

Hockaday J M, Whitty C W M 1967 Patterns of referred pain in the normal subject. Brain 90(3): 481–495

International Association for the Study of Pain Subcommittee on Taxonomy 1979 Pain terms: a list with definitions and notes on usage. Pain 6: 249–252

Johnson M I 1997 The physiology of the sensory dimensions of clinical pain. Physiotherapy 83(10): 526–536

Knight M 1998 The bio-psycho social model – the dumping ground for the diagnostically destitute. Second National Symposium. The Changing Face of Back Pain Management, Chester

Leclaire R, Blier F, Fortin L, Proulx R 1997 A cross-sectional study comparing the Oswestry and Roland-Morris functional disability scales in two populations of patients with low back pain of different levels of severity. Spine 22(1): 68–71

Leriche R 1939 The surgery of pain. Williams and Wilkins, Baltimore

McCaffery M 1972 Nursing management of the patient with pain. J B Lippincott, Philadelphia

McKenzie R 1981 The lumbar spine and mechanical diagnosis. Spinal Publications, Waikanae, New Zealand

Maitland G D 1986 Vertebral manipulation, 5th edn. Butterworths, London

Maruta S, Goldman S, Chan C W, Ilstrup D M, Kunselman A R, Colligan R C 1997 Waddell's nonorganic signs and Minnesota Multiphasic Personality Inventory profiles in patients with chronic low back pain. Spine 22(1): 72–75

Melzack R 1982 Recent concepts of pain. Journal of Medicine 13(3): 147–160

Melzack R, Wall P 1965 Pain mechanisms: a new theory. Science. 150(3699): 971–979

Melzack R, Wall P 1996 The challenge of pain. Penguin, Harmondsworth

Mooney V, Robertson J 1976 The facet syndrome. Clinical Orthopaedics and Related Research 115: 149–156

Nachemson A 1985 Recent advances in the treatment of low back pain. International Orthopaedics (SICOT) 9: 1–10

Pavlov I P 1927 Conditioned reflexes. Oxford University Press, Oxford

Porter R W 1986 Management of back pain. Churchill Livingstone, Edinburgh

Price D D 1996 Selective activation of A-delta and C nociceptive afferents by different parameters of nociceptive heat stimulation: a tool for analysis of central mechanisms of pain. Pain 68: 1–3

Rang H P, Bevan S, Dray A 1994 Nociceptive peripheral neurons: cellular properties. In: Wall P D, Melzack R (eds) Textbook of pain. Churchill Livingstone, Edinburgh

Shapiro A P, Roth R S 1993 The effect of litigation on recovery from whiplash. Spine 7(3): 531–556

Siddall P J, Cousins M J 1997 Spine update. Spinal pain mechanisms. Spine 22(1): 98–104

Sorkin L S, Wagner R, Myers R R 1997 Role of the nervi nervorum in neuropathic pain. Pain Forum 6(3): 191–192

Sternbach R A 1989 Acute versus chronic pain. In: Wall P D, Melzack R (eds) Textbook of pain, 2nd edn. Churchill Livingstone, Edinburgh

Sternbach R A, Tursky B 1965 Ethnic differences among housewives in psychophysical and skin potential responses to electric shock. Psychophysiology 1(3)

Thacker M 1999 Whiplash – is there a lesion? In: Gifford L (ed) Topical issues in pain. Physiotherapy Pain Association Year Book 1998–1999. NOI Press, Falmouth, Adelaide

Treves K 1999 Understanding people with chronic pain following whiplash: a psychological perspective. In: Gifford L (ed) Topical issues in pain. Physiotherapy Pain Association Year Book 1998–1999. NOI Press, Falmouth, Adelaide

Twomey L T, Taylor J R 1987 Innervation, pain patterns, and mechanisms of pain production. In: Twomey L T, Taylor J R (eds) Physical therapy of the low back. Churchill Livingstone, Edinburgh

Waddell G (ed) 1998 The back pain revolution. Churchill Livingstone, Edinburgh

Waddell G, Main C J 1998 A new clinical model of low back pain and disability. In: Waddell G (ed) The back pain revolution. Churchill Livingstone, Edinburgh

Wall P D, Melzack R 1994 Textbook of pain. Churchill Livingstone Edinburgh

Weinstein J 1991 Neurogenic and nonneurogenic pain and inflammatory mediators. Orthopedic Clinics of North America 22(2): 235–246

Weisenberg M 1989 Cognitive aspects of pain. In: Wall P D, Melzack R (eds) Textbook of pain, 2nd edn. Churchill Livingstone, Edinburgh

Willis W D 1997 An alternative mechanism for neuropathic pain. Pain Forum 6(3): 193–195

Woolf C J 1994 The dorsal horn: state-dependent sensory processing and the generation of pain. In: Wall P D, Melzack R (eds) Textbook of pain. Churchill Lvingstone, Edinburgh

Wyke B 1976 Neurological aspects of low back pain. In: Jayson M I V (ed) The lumbar spine and back pain. Pitman Publishing, London

Zborowski M 1952 Cultural components in response to pain. Journal of Sociological Issues 8: 16

Zborowski M 1969 People in pain. Jossey-Bass, San Francisco

FURTHER READING

Baldry P E 1993 Acupuncture, trigger points and musculoskeletal pain. Churchill Livingstone, Edinburgh

Diamond A W, Coniam S W 1997 Management of chronic pain. Oxford University Press, Oxford

Gifford L (ed) 1999 Topical issues in pain. Physiotherapy Pain Association Yearbook 1998–1999 NOI Press, Falmouth, Adelaide

Greening J, Lynn B 1998 Minor peripheral nerve injuries: an underestimated source of pain? Manual Therapy 3(4)

Melzack R, Wall P 1996 The challenge of pain. Penguin Books, Harmondsworth

Merskey H, Bogduk N 1994 Classification of chronic pain. IASP Press, Seattle

Shipton E A 1999 Pain, acute and chronic. Edward Arnold, London

Waddell G 1999 The back pain revolution. Churchill Livingstone, Edinburgh

Wall P 1999 Pain. The science of suffering. Weidenfield and Nicolson, London

Wall P D, Melzack R 1999 (eds) Textbook of pain. Churchill Livingstone, Edinburgh

Wells P, Frampton V, Bowsher D 1997 Pain management in physiotherapy. Butterworth Heinemann, Oxford

8

Injury

THE PROCESS OF INJURY AND HEALING

It is important for therapists to remember the timescale involved in the process of injury and healing. The process described occurs in any soft tissue trauma and takes place in three stages: injury, inflammation and repair (Table 8.1) (Evans 1980, Oakes 1982). The concept of the 'collagen timescale' described by Evans (1980) is particularly relevant because good functional recovery is governed by the time constraints of normal physiological healing and does not necessarily relate to the level of pain (Fitzgerald 1997).

Injury

During the course of any soft tissue injury, a sprain, bruise or crush, the local network of blood vessels is damaged; some tissues are deprived of blood supply and the cells die. Fibrous tissue in the area may also be structurally damaged and

Table 8.1   Injured tissue: the timescale of healing

Time	Processes occurring
First 3–5 days	Inflammatory exudate still increasing, depending on the severity of the injury
After 3–5 days	Repair starts: exudate removed, collagen laid down, scar tissue replacing exudate
1–3 weeks	Gradual repair taking place
3 weeks–6 months	Scar tissue formed and starts to shorten

so within a few minutes of injury the area contains a collection of dead and dying cells.

A series of chemical changes then take place. The dying cells break down and release chemicals which affect other nearby cells and capillaries, causing the blood vessels to become more permeable. Any bleeding into the area releases dead red blood cells, dead platelets and plasma. The platelets in turn release thrombin, an enzyme, which turns one of the plasma proteins (fibrinogen) into fibrin. Fibrin forms a network of fibres, enmeshing the debris of dead cells into a blood clot. So, the area begins to feel sore, stiff and achy and the next phase, inflammation, has started (Evans 1980).

Inflammation

The four signs of inflammation are calor (heat), rubor (redness), dolor (pain) and tumor (swelling).

Heat and redness

Immediately after injury, there is a brief vaso-constriction in the area followed by dilation of the blood vessels as a result of chemical action and the axon reflex of arterioles (Thomson et al 1991). The area is flooded with blood and becomes pink and warm. Change of colour may never be noticeable in the back due to the quantity of muscle bulk between the injury and the skin but heat is palpable.

Pain

Chemicals released into the tissue start the physiological processes of pain described in Chapter 7.

Swelling

Swelling occurs immediately only if there has been substantial bleeding; otherwise it takes a few hours to manifest. Four hours after injury, white cells begin to migrate through the vessel walls into the damaged area to start their job of scavenging and devouring the debris. The area now contains a mass of inflammatory exudate,

the pressure of which further irritates nerve endings, enhancing the pain. The inflammatory exudate may still be increasing for 3–5 days depending upon the severity of the injury or the amount of reinjury inflicted (Evans 1980).

Repair

Finally, on the third to fifth day the process of repair begins, a process that lasts approximately 6 weeks. Nearby cells begin to divide and multiply. Whilst the exudate is gradually being removed by the white cells, new capillaries bud and grow in from the perimeter of the debris, bringing fresh oxygen. Fibroblast cells start to lay down fibrils of collagen in the exudate which grow to become bundles of collagen or fibrous tissue and healing takes place. The larger the quantity of exudate, the greater the amount of fibrous tissue. In other words, the quantity of scar tissue depends upon the amount of swelling.

Healed tissue is never exactly the same as it was before; although it is replaced, the new structure and properties are not identical with the original. Scar tissue has the property of gradually shortening when it is fully formed, a process which occurs from the third week to the sixth month after injury (Evans 1980, Torrance 1986).

From this timescale clear guidelines emerge for the treatment of injury (Patient advice 8.1) (see Chapter 18). It is important for patients to

---

Patient advice 8.1   Self-treatment of injury

- Explain injury to the patient in positive terms, stressing the deleterious effect of immobilization and the advantageous effect of gentle movements.
- Reduce inflammation with ice and antiinflammatory treatment to avoid the formation of extensive scar tissue.
- If severe, bed rest for only 2–3 days.
- Respect the injury for at least 3–5 days and avoid provocation, for example active sports, for 3–6 weeks, depending on severity.
- Return to work as soon as possible, taking back care into consideration.
- Gradually restore normal movement and normal activities, ensuring return to full range of movement finally.

understand this. People are often desperate if pain lasts longer than 2 weeks. They either feel there is some serious pathology behind their pain and become extremely concerned about it or they feel they are being oversensitive and dig the garden to prove there is nothing wrong, possibly reinjuring the tissue. Both reactions are deleterious in relation to the healing process.

Healing cannot be accelerated but correct handling can avoid delay caused by repeated injury and correct understanding can avoid anxiety.

Ignoring the injury period by allowing repeated damage and increased exudate to develop not only lengthens the time of healing but inevitably leads to increased scar formation and loss of previous movement range.

REFERENCES

Evans P 1980 The healing process at cellular level. Physiotherapy 66(8): 256–259

Fitzgerald D 1997 Physiotherapy in the management of pain in sport. In: Wells P E, Frampton V, Bowsher D (eds) Pain management by physiotherapy. Butterworth Heinemann, Oxford

Oakes B W 1982 Acute soft injuries: nature and management. Australian Family Physician 10(Suppl): 3–16

Thomson A, Skinner A, Piercy J 1991 Causes of disease: inflammation. In: Tidy's physiotherapy, 12th edn. Butterworth Heinemann, Oxford

Torrance C 1986 The physiology of wound healing. Nursing 5: 162–168

9

The causes of back pain

THE CLINICAL PICTURE

The search for the cause of back pain would be simple if the fault could be attributed to a specific structure but there is rarely one source of pain. Painful conditions of the back can arise from a disturbance of any pain-sensitive structure of the motion segment (Spitzer et al 1987, Bogduk 1994, Adams 1996).

Since the 1970s, research has led to greater understanding of the relationship between the intricacies of pain and the role played by the nervous system. Similarly, the link between the mechanics of joint movement and musculoskeletal dysfunction has been clarified.

Most disorders of the vertebral column enumerated in earlier chapters can be present without pain or can be a part of the pain picture of a patient seeking treatment. Degenerative changes or musculoskeletal dysfunction can be present for years, remaining asymptomatic, and then from trauma, overuse or new use, pain may result.

One of the most revealing overall discoveries has been that *structural change in itself need not give pain* (McKenzie 1981). An MRI may show a disc protrusion but the person may never have had pain; similarly, a person may have marked osteoarthritis changes but no symptoms. Clinically we are seeing situations where X-rays may show osteophytes at certain levels of the spine, disc narrowing at others, spinal abnormalities (such as spondylolisthesis) and bony disorders (osteoporosis) and yet on examination the pain may be coming from quite another source, possibly from a more healthy-looking motion segment under stress because it is taking greater strain. Pain arises only when the function of an 'at-risk' tissue is compromised and altered, for whatever reason. To minimize this overstrain, good posture and controlled trunk motion are essential.

The maintenance of posture and the performance of good trunk motion are the results of coordinated load sharing between the passive and active systems and the stabilizing mechanisms of the trunk are controlled by the neural system (Panjabi 1992). A dysfunction of the musculoskeletal system may result in excessive load sharing of the passive system that can cause abnormal motion and greater strains on certain structures, accompanied by increased pain and discomfort (Quint et al 1998). Waddell (1998) describes dysfunction as a yet 'untapped mine of knowledge'. He believes there is a need to look more closely at the soft tissues and their physiology, at physical dysfunction and the effects of disuse, a need to consider more complex, dynamic patterns of movement which lead to a change in the balance of movement.

In conclusion, there is no one cause of neuromusculoskeletal back pain but the potential for it lies in **predisposing** (indirect) and **precipitating** (direct) factors (McKenzie 1981) (Box 9.1). Dysfunction plays a role in both these factors, possibly being an integral part of the first and either a contributing factor or consequence of the second.

Box 9.1 The causes of LBP

1. Dysfunction – which can be part of both 2 and 3.
2. Predisposing factors:
   - postural stress – dynamic, sustained and adolescent
   - work-related stress – both physical and emotional
   - disuse and loss of mobility
   - obesity
   - debilitating conditions.
3. Precipitating factors:
   - new use
   - misuse
   - overuse
   - abuse or trauma.

DYSFUNCTION

The functional pathology of the neuromuscular system has been studied by clinicians and researchers during the past years. They are providing more and more evidence that changes in muscular function play an important role in the pathogenesis of many painful conditions of the musculoskeletal system and constitute an integral part of postural defects in general.

Panjabi (1992) postulated that dysfunction of the spinal stabilizing systems may lead to injury and LBP. Cholewicki & McGill (1996) found that the stability of the lumbar spine is diminished during periods of low muscular activity, making it vulnerable to injury in the presence of sudden unexpected loading. The spine will buckle if the activity of the lumbar multifidus (LM) and the erector spinae is zero, even when the forces in large muscles are substantial. This could explain the occurrence of spinal injury during activities requiring low muscular force. Cholewicki & McGill (1996) put forward a hypothesis that there is greater risk of injury when decreased demand requires less muscular effort; for example, a person could work all day on a demanding job and then 'put his back out' stooping to pick up a pencil from the floor in the evening. Buckling behaviour can be limited to a single level from inappropriate activation of muscles.

In all joints a state of movement balance should exist when the path of the instantaneous centre of rotation (PICR) during active movement is consistent with the standard kinesiology for the joint (Sahrmann 1993). All joints have force couples acting about all three axes of movement. The forces have strength and direction and a change in the strength of one force alters the PICR of the joint. Remembering that only 2° of intersegmental rotation is required to produce microtrauma in the lumbar spine (Hodges & Richardson 1996), it is not surprising that changes in the PICR cause microtrauma that may lead to pain and possibly to pathology (Sahrmann 1993).

Mimura et al (1994) have shown that the ROM of axial rotation increases and lateral flexion decreases with disc degeneration. As the IVD and facet joint sources of pain are well documented

Table 9.1 Dysfunction (reproduced with permission from Comerford et al 1998)

Area of occurrence	Dysfunction	Result
Locally	Faulty recruitment and motor control of deep segmental stability system	Poor control of the neutral joint position
Globally	An imbalance between monoarticular stabilizers and biarticular mobilizers	Abnormal overpull or underpull around the joint

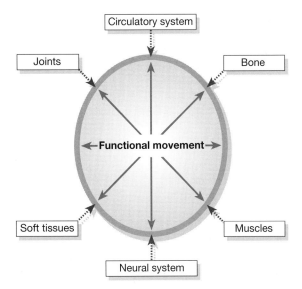

Figure 9.1 The boundaries of functional movement. (Reproduced with permission from Kettle 1999.)

and segmental instability is a recognized source of LBP (Bogduk 1994, Adams 1996, Siddall & Cousins 1997) this decreased ROM, for example, could be a potential troublespot.

Dysfunction can occur locally or globally (Sahrmann 1993, Comerford et al 1998) (Table 9.1). The body tends to take the path of least resistance and with daily activity that path offers less and less resistance, becoming a site of greatest relative flexibility, while other paths increase in stiffness. For example, in flexion the lumbar spine may be more flexible relative to the hips due to lengthened erector spinae and short hamstrings, or the thoracic spine may be more flexible relative to the lumbar spine due to tightened erector spinae, short hip flexors and possibly short hamstrings. Thus inappropriate movement occurs at the site of greatest relative flexibility, putting these segments at risk of abnormal strain and stress during full movements, for example stooping to pick up something or being pressed down in a rugby scrum (Comerford et al 1998).

Clinically patients are presenting with pain related to dysfunction every day. The question seems to be: which comes first, the pain or the dysfunction? As dysfunction can exist without pain (possibly because the tissues have never been compromised or put under repetitive/ sustained/sudden stress) and pain can exist without *known* prior dysfunction (for example, when pain is initiated by trauma), the link appears to be impossible to prove scientifically. When pain and dysfunction are linked but the dysfunction remains untreated, the pain may resolve but the dysfunction may persist, possibly predisposing to chronic pain (Hodges & Richardson 1996, Hides et al 1996, Comerford et al 1998): an important point for therapists.

In many people subclinical dysfunction exists within self-imposed boundaries where limitation of movement within boundaries maintains the asymptomatic state (Fig. 9.1). As long as the patient lives within these boundaries there is no pain. However, the boundaries can be encroached upon by trauma (whiplash), abuse or overuse, age changes, local dysfunction or muscle imbalance and the subclinical patient becomes symptomatic (Fig. 9.2). Physiotherapy re-establishes the boundaries and restores function, so increasing the patient's three-dimensional area of functional movement (Kettle 1999).

The movement system is made up of articular, myofascial, neural and connective tissue systems (Fig. 9.3). Good function requires the integrated and coordinated interaction of these systems and all four systems need to be assessed in their relation to each other (Mottram & Comerford 1998).

Clinical situations in which movement dysfunction plays a major role in contributing to the pathology include: postural pain, pain of

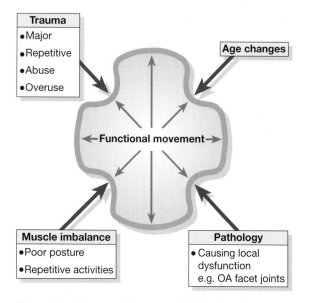

Figure 9.2 The assault on musculoskeletal function with encroachment on the boundaries. (Reproduced with permission from Kettle 1999.)

insidious onset, static loading or holding pain, pain from overuse (low-force repetitive strain or high-force/impact repetitive strain), recurrent patterns of pain and chronic pain (Cholewicki & McGill 1996, Comerford et al 1998).

PREDISPOSING FACTORS

Postural stress

Posture is a composite of the positions of all the joints of the body at any given moment and static postural alignment is best described in terms of the positions of the various joints and body segments. Posture may also be described in terms of muscle balance (Kendall et al 1993).

The variety of different postures is profuse, some with increased and some with decreased curves. However, allowing for slight variation in skeletal type, there is a basic standard which involves a minimal amount of stress and strain and is conducive to maximal efficiency of body function (Kendall et al 1993) (see Chapter 11).

Although there is a considerable amount of literature stating that there is no proven link between posture and LBP (Dieck et al 1985, Raine & Twomey 1994, Gass & Refshauge 1995, Refshauge et al 1995), there is now an equal wealth of evidence connecting dysfunction to a lack of muscular stabilization in patients with back pain (Pheasant 1991, HSE 1992, Griegel-Morris et al 1992, Adams 1996, Mottram 1997, Kember 1998). Twomey and Taylor (1994b) thought that poor posture was a prelude to LBP.

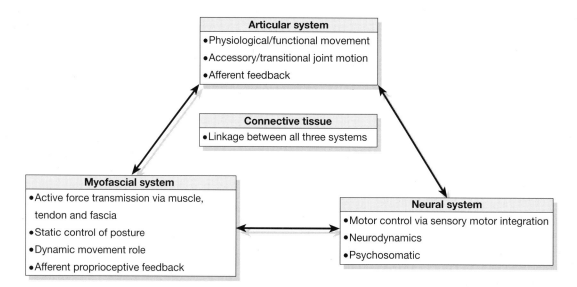

Figure 9.3 The movement system of the spine. (Reproduced with permission from Comerford et al 1998.)

Box 9.2 Dysfunction linked to habitual and sustained postures

---

Habitual movements
- Normal movements done correctly, too many times, e.g. repetitive strain from stooping in gardening
- Repetitive movement performed in an inappropriate posture, e.g. sitting slumped while typing in sustained wrist flexion resulting in carpal tunnel pathology (Comerford et al 1998) or playing an instrument with incorrect posture resulting in hand or arm pain (Kember 1998)
- Abnormal movement, e.g. shoulder injury from loss of scapular/thoracic stabilization (Mottram 1997)

Sustained postures
- Any sustained position, in standing upright, stooping or sitting, e.g. LBP in nurses or headaches, neck/arm pain or LBP in office workers

---

The vertebral column posture is ideally dynamic rather than static as the tissues adapt to prolonged static loading by further creep of the column (Twomey & Taylor 1994a). However, both habitual movements and sustained postures play a major role in the development of dysfunction (Box 9.2). Faulty movement can *induce* pathology, not just be a result of it (Sahrmann 1993). Repetitive movement patterns can lead to overactivity in some muscles and lack of activity in others, while lack of general support can come from the overall weakness associated with a sedentary lifestyle (Richardson et al 1992). A sedentary lifestyle can also predispose to the development of lumbar disc disorders, especially if the spine is maintained in flexion for most of the working time (Bullock & Bullock-Saxton 1994).

Dynamic postures

Repetitive extension. This occurs mainly in sport: in tennis (serving), in cricket (fast bowling), in gymnastics and in the high jump; also in building work, in tasks such as painting a ceiling.

The greatest danger lies in sudden, forced extension which can fracture the pars interarticularis and damage the interspinous ligament (Twomey & Taylor 1994b).

Repetitive flexion. This is a frequent daily insult. It is often performed with some rotation,

often with a weight in the hands, rarely resuming the upright and so never restoring the lordosis. It occurs in occupations such as building work or road work, gardening, nursing, housework, jobs involving the care of young children, industrial packaging, sheep shearing and shelf stacking in supermarkets.

This places stress on all structures of the articular triad. The interspinous ligaments suffer first, then the facet joints and finally the discs (Adams 1996). When rotation is added to flexion, the facet joints are less able to protect the discs and so they become increasingly vulnerable. Lifting during repetitive bending creates an added vulnerability to sudden stress or trauma (Twomey & Taylor 1994b). Change can occur either by accumulated fatigue or in a single incident, for example a stumble or a fall (Adams 1996) (Patient advice 9.1).

Sustained postures

All sustained posture is abusive, even in a good position or even involving light work. In any maintained position the spinal curves change, joints sag into their end of range, hanging the body weight onto stretched soft tissue. The stress may not be sufficiently great to cause pain until the cumulative effect builds up.

Pain can occur in any sustained upright posture (walking slowly round an exhibition) or during activities in the stoop/slouch (as in vacuuming or driving) or when moving out of the sustained position (changing from sitting to standing).

Occupations involving sustained standing or prolonged sitting have been proven to have a high incidence of LBP (Bullock & Bullock-Saxton 1994, Adams 1996). Static posture is particularly provocative especially when asymmetric and awkward, for example, working with machinery which requires a distorted body posture maintained for hours without respite (Boyling 1992).

Lack of movement causes the synovial fluid to be inactive, the circulation to slow down, waste products to accumulate in the muscles, blood supply to the neural tissue to decrease and the neuromuscular input to be minimal. Pathological changes may take place in the muscles, connective

Patient advice 9.1 Repeated stooping

- Try to avoid stoop: stand with one foot in front of the other, keep the back stabilized and bend the knees.
- Take care with reaching forwards in stoop.
- Avoid moving a weight outside the area formed by both feet.
- Beware of twisting in a stooping position.
- Move the legs rather than reach or twist.
- Observe lifting techniques.
- Constantly stand up and arch the back, restoring the lordosis (Fig. 9.4).

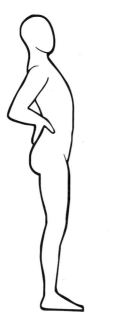

Figure 9.4 The routine back arch after sitting or stooping.

tissue of tendons, joint capsules and joint ligaments and muscle imbalance may develop (Bullock & Bullock-Saxton 1994, Adams 1996). Static postures actually initiate age change and degeneration (Twomey & Taylor 1994a). Activity usually eases the pain.

Sustained extension. This occurs mainly in prolonged standing. Fatigue in the stabilizing muscles causes an increase in the lumbar lordosis, shifting the axis of movement further posteriorly.

The result is compression concentrated on the posterior annulus fibrosus with an impairment of the supply of metabolites; loss of disc fluid and height; reduction in the volume of the

spinal canal; and increased loading on the facet joint surfaces. The spinous processes approximate each other, actually impacting in a condition in the elderly known as 'kissing spines' (Taylor & Twomey 1994, Adams 1996). The compressed innervated posterior annulus fibrosus could be a major cause of LBP as the lordosis increases (Adams 1996) (Patient advice 9.2).

Patient advice 9.2 Sustained standing

- Pain in sustained standing is normal; movement is necessary to relieve it.
- Correct posture frequently, pulling in the lower abdomen.
- *Move*: transfer weight from one leg to the other, rock the pelvis, sit for a few minutes, if possible put one foot up on a step or stool, keep changing position.
- Flatten low back against a wall for a few seconds to eliminate the stressed lordosis.
- Be careful of shopping centres because slow walking is a sustained posture.
- At home, try Figs 9.5 and 9.6 as possible relieving positions.

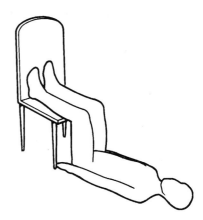

Figure 9.5 Recovery position for an aching back.

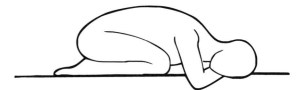

Figure 9.6 Recovery position for pain in standing.

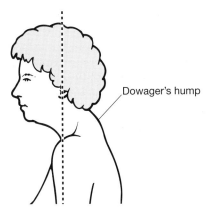

Figure 9.7 Forward head posture with cervico-thoracic kyphosis ('dowager's hump').

Sustained flexion. Maintained stoop in standing and prolonged slouch-sitting have a similar effect on the lumbar spine. Stoop-standing can involve outstretched arms with added weight stress on the back as hands manipulate objects away from the body. Slouch-sitting involves not only thoracic and lumbar spine flexion but also the weight of the arms, head and thorax is thrust into the tissues of the upper and lower back. There is increased flexion at the C7/T1 junction, the 'dowager hump' posture, and in order to correct eye position the upper cervical joints are forced into extension, with the forward head posture (Fig. 9.7).

Sustained flexion occurs in occupations such as nursing, certain industries, research, dentistry, museum conservation work, all sedentary office occupations and driving. Computer workers function with static vertebral postures (often maintained with tension around the shoulder area), a frequently awkward head position and hands that are held fixed on the keyboard, the fingers alone moving (see Chapter 15).

This results in stretch of interspinous ligaments; facet joints slide and lock; anterior compression of the disc forces intradiscal pressure posteriorly towards the stretched posterior annular wall (Adams 1996). Creep causes loss of fluid in all soft tissues; after change of activity it takes many hours for fluid to be reabsorbed and the shape of the tissues to be reestablished. When the amount of creep involved is considerable,

---

Patient advice 9.3   Prolonged stoop and prolonged sitting

The spine in stooping is the same as in sitting slouched.

In sitting
- The pelvis is tilted back and lumbar spine flattened: support the lumbar spine.
- Shift position and correct posture frequently.
- Crossed legs may adversely affect leg circulation, but it rests the abdominal oblique muscles (Snijders et al 1995) and adds a change of position.
- Avoid crossing legs with sciatic pain.
- Office workers: shoulder pain is not from 'tension', it is from poor posture. Analyse the work-related posture, frequently correct it and try to reduce arm pain by correcting poking chin posture.
- Use 'pause exercises'.
- Avoid remaining still for long.
- Exercise into stiffness but take care with exercise into pain.
- Correct posture in driving.
- Try Figure 9.5 for recovery from LBP.

In stoop
- Try to avoid stoop: raise the work surfaces or lower the seat.
- Arch out of stoop every 5 minutes (Fig. 9.4).

---

then recovery back to the original starting posture (**hysteresis**) is extremely slow (Twomey & Taylor 1994b). The recovery takes longer with ageing, hence the time it takes for elderly backs to recover after stooping.

Daily sustained slouch-sitting with shoulder protraction may result in shortening and tightening of anterior soft tissues and lengthening and weakening of the posterior elements. This may lead to dysfunction around the shoulder girdle, with inadequate scapula stabilization, headaches, and neck and arm pain (see 'Postural correction', p. 152).

Adolescent postures and pain

LBP now appears to be a relatively common complaint in adolescence and considerable clinical attention has been paid to the subject; 17–18% of adolescents questioned in Finland (Taimela et al 1997) and 38.5% of Flemish adolescents had LBP at the time of investigation (Staes et al 1995). Cowieson & Nicholls (1997) in the UK report a 'sizeable problem that may have implications for the prevalence of back pain in the adult population'. Taimela et al (1997) found a familial predisposition for juvenile disc herniation and non-specific LBP, but there were also risk factors of physical inactivity, sports injuries and heavy physical loading.

Obesity in children and adolescents is also an increasing problem which needs to be addressed by dietary control as well as the use of exercise – supervised aerobics, extra gym classes, walking, jogging and cycling (CSP 1995, Epstein et al 1996).

Duggleby & Kumar (1997) found that there was a potential link between the adolescent growth spurt and the increased prevalence of LBP. During the growth spurts in human development, the first between the ages of 6 and 8 and the second between 12 and 14, the rate of bone growth supersedes the growth rate of soft tissue. Muscles and soft tissue lag behind the bone length by about 6–8 months. This leads to tightness of tissues, especially those of the lower limbs, with considerable neuromuscular involvement (Butler 1991). Headaches, knee problems, calf pains and poor posture can result, with shortened hamstrings and calf muscles.

With less school gymnastic activity, unless a child attends dance classes, yoga classes or stretches regularly and correctly before all sport, these muscles remain shortened. Tight hamstrings limit pelvic anterior rotation during forward flexion. This can lead to stress on the lumbar spine in flexion activities or stress on the thoracic spine as it 'gives' to compensate for limited pelvic rotation; LBP or thoracic pain may result. There is also a correlation between recurrent hamstring injuries and LBP and between LBP and a limited SLR in adolescents (Mierau et al 1989, Muckle 1990).

Adolescents who outgrow their peer group or who try to hide early breast development may adopt a thoracic kyphosis, usually accompanied by a poking chin. Since the sympathetic trunk in the cervical spine is placed towards the anterior part of the vertebral bodies, sustained upper cervical extension of a poking chin posture may place undue tension on the sympathetic trunk; possible symptoms might be nausea, vague thoracic pains and headaches (Butler 1991). These symptoms, of course, need not only be associated with the adolescent poking chin.

Organized, competitive sports provide many predisposing factors for adolescent back pain which range from the activities themselves to physical factors related to the participants to external factors such as the surface played on, the equipment or apparatus (Liston 1994). When bones are growing faster than muscles, strong repetitive activities can provide increased pressure on bone apophyses and lead to injury; the vertebral epiphyses and apophyses of the vertebral ring may be disrupted or distorted from overloading, which may disrupt growth (Liston 1994, Reynolds 1997). Back injuries can be the result of contact, impact or stress injury.

Studies also show that there is a link between foot abnormalities and LBP and that the malalignment may precipitate LBP symptoms (Campbell 1995).

In addition, in the UK and in Ireland research has investigated the possible connection between adolescent back pain and the present need for school children to carry heavy bags (Casey & Dockerell 1996, NBPA 1997). Heavy bag carrying may encourage a muscle imbalance which could predispose to a postural scoliosis (see p. 21).

In view of all these possible causative factors of back pain in children and adolescents, Cowieson & Nicholls (1997), Vicas-Kunse (1991) and Twomey & Taylor (1994a) suggest that vigorous prophylactic back education is warranted for young school children which should be continued throughout their primary and secondary education (Box 9.3). Because the immature spine is at greater risk of injury it is critical for

---

Box 9.3 Advice in schools

Primary and secondary school children should be taught:
1. simple biomechanics with postural and physical awareness
2. the need to start good habits: sitting, standing, lifting, pulling, pushing, carrying
3. regular stretching and strengthening exercises

coaches and athletic trainers to have a thorough understanding of the growing spine (Reynolds 1997), added to which great care should be taken to provide adequate training for correct sporting techniques with strong muscles to control movement. Postural irregularities which develop in childhood may result in more serious dysfunctions later in life.

However, in a clinical situation, back pain in children and adolescents could also be indicative of serious underlying pathology, for example infective discitis and osteomyelitis; spondylolysis and spondylolisthesis; IVD herniation; Scheuermann's disease; or the results of trauma (Liston 1994). Further investigations must be made if these are suspected.

Work-related stress

Physical stress: from both force and vibration

Force. In industrial occupations there is often too great a force required to perform a job with too little time to relax in order to recuperate. There should also be adequate training for any occupation which involves the use of force (Boyling 1992).

Vibration. This stimulates the release of neuropeptides from the DRG which mediates a progressive degeneration of the functional motion segment (Weinstein 1991). Cyclic loading inflicted upon the body by any tools, by the use of hands or by materials can cause unnatural stresses, especially around the neck and shoulders: for example, the use of pneumatic drills, constant hammering or enforced heavy-glove wearing (Boyling 1992, Pope & Hansson 1992).

All driving, especially of heavy vehicles such as tractors, can provide a vibration stress which may cause creep, leading to mechanical fatigue which can affect the axial loading of the discs (Anderson 1987, Twomey & Taylor 1994a, Klaber Moffett et al 1995).

Emotional stress: work frequency, duration and pressure

In all occupations there should be a change of rhythm between activity and pause or rest. The body and mind need to 'recover' from sustained postures or prolonged concentration. Problems arise that are related to the level of skill and confidence of the performer, the performer's age in relation to the magnitude of the task and, not least, the financial element whereby pressure is added by the call for increased productivity (Boyling 1992). Stress from the demand for greater activity, greater performance, with greater competition, is a problem in the whole working population.

Disuse and loss of mobility

A decrease in the range of movement of a joint potentially reduces its response to sudden demand. Loss of mobility may result from disuse or poor recovery from injury.

Disuse

Prolonged inactivity leads to muscle atrophy, loss of strength and adaptive shortening of soft tissue. Inactivity hinders cartilage and soft tissue nutrition whereas movement stimulates the activity of synovial fluid within joints and accelerates ongoing regeneration in all tissues. Thus a sedentary lifestyle leads to poor muscle tone, lack of aerobic fitness, poor posture and a predisposition to osteoporosis (Salter et al 1975, Williams & Sperryn 1979, Evans 1980, Taylor & Twomey 1994).

Mobility of the hips and knees plays a fundamental role in back care. If adequate knee flexion in weight bearing is impossible, the protective techniques of knee flexion to avoid stoop can never be mastered and stooping will be inevitable when lifting or retrieving something from the floor, low cupboard or low drawer. Weakness and immobility of the hips and knees advance insidiously with age unless a concerted effort is made to counteract them. Exercising is one way but conscious attention to daily habits plays a vital and even more important role (Patient advice 9.4).

As the health of joints is dependent on low stress movements maintaining the transfer of nutrients across the joint surfaces and as

---

Patient advice 9.4   Knee mobility

Stress the need to use every opportunity to use the legs.
- Keep knees mobile and strong.
- Avoid relying on arms by leaning on worktops to reach into a low cupboard.
- Do not avoid squatting because the knees 'feel weak'.
- Half-squat with feet apart and one foot in front of the other.
- If it feels difficult to rise from half-squat at first, go on repeating it at every opportunity and it will get easier.

---

osteoarthritis changes begin in areas where collagen is not often stressed by movement (Twomey & Taylor 1994a) and possibly in joints with reduced proprioception, maintaining full knee ROM in everyday activities has a good chance of warding off degeneration.

Poor recovery from episodes of back pain

In episodes of LBP poor recovery, inadequate treatment, lack of reeducation and continuing dysfunction may lead to loss of mobility. Restoration of full function is an essential part of recovery with the possibility of providing protection against recurrence and chronicity.

Obesity

Scientific evidence that being overweight is related to LBP is scanty and not well documented. However, chronic LBP and symptoms of disc herniation appear to be more prevalent in instances where the fat distribution results in a large abdomen (Han et al 1998). The weight of a large abdomen pulls the lumbar spine into an increased lordosis, possibly evoking the usual stresses of maintained extension; creep will increase and overload on the spine may accelerate wear and tear (Twomey & Taylor 1994b). A prolonged burden of excess weight may also cause LBP through increased load compression on IVDs or indirectly through altered gait, evoking further spinal stresses (Han et al 1998).

Loss of mobility is a covert companion to obesity. No matter how apparently mobile an obese person's joints remain, tissue bulk obstructs full movement of any joint, whether the back, the hips or the knees, with the result that these joints can never be put through their full range. Added to which there is an increased weight-bearing burden on the knees.

Obesity imposes a vast claim on medical facilities generally (Han et al 1998) and it has been identified as a risk factor for coronary heart disease (HEA 1997). Dieting is a complicated problem for many because it is so tied up with inner needs and desires and professional help should be sought if self-imposed restraint is impossible. A weight problem is best discussed with a doctor before entering into any dietary regime. Physical activity or a walking exercise programme can lead to positive changes in the level of fitness of obese women, aged 60 and over, including weight loss, a decrease in percentage of body fat, waist to hip ratio and body mass index and an increase in cardiovascular fitness (Dallas 1997, HEA 1997).

Debilitating conditions

Joint pain is frequently a symptom of a viral condition, for example influenza, though there is little research on the subject. Care should be taken of the back during the period of recuperation in order to avoid any possible risk of injury. LBP presentation in clinics is often associated with an episode of a minor systemic illness.

PRECIPITATING FACTORS

Precipitating factors are the direct and sudden causes of back pain which can provoke a previously pain-free back or trigger pain in a back which has a previous history of trouble. Either of these might have an undisclosed dysfunctional element. They can be summarized as abnormal stress on a normal back; normal stress on an abnormal back; and normal stress on an unprepared normal back (Bullock & Bullock-Saxton 1994).

Injury can range from a minor 'sprain type' facet joint or soft tissue injury, to a disc lesion or to the more extensive bony and soft tissue damage of trauma.

New use

Any previously unperformed and unpractised activity can be structurally provocative (abnormal stress on normal back) and so can a familiar movement, not performed for some time and now beyond the capabilities of structures involved (normal on unprepared normal). Examples of these are: taking on a lifting job after a previously sedentary occupation; digging a new garden after years of living in a flat; playing a strenuous game of squash for the first time in middle age.

Misuse

Awkward movements

Accustomed movement performed in an awkward way can cause injury ranging from a disc protrusion to a 'locked' facet joint; for example, rotation in flexion, especially when holding a weight (Twomey & Taylor 1994b) (normal on unprepared normal).

No matter how light the object, an incorrect move can precipitate a problem when stability is diminished (Cholewicki & McGill 1996). Bending quickly to pick up a toy on the carpet, reaching sideways and twisting to turn out the light and stretching upwards into a cupboard are all normal movements which cause injury only when performed without adequate stabilization and control.

Awkward objects

Manual handling is a hazard at all times, no matter how small the load, but if the load is awkward, the potential for injury is greater (abnormal on normal); human beings are particularly awkward to handle as they are mobile, floppy and unpredictable. It is therefore important to assess all objects and plan the move before attempting any action. It is essential to have special training for all manual handling work (see Chapter 14).

Overuse

Non-stressful activity repeated over a long period of time or stressful activity repeated too many times will finally fatigue structures beyond their ability to adapt to demands, and tissue injury results accompanied by severe pain (McKenzie 1981) (abnormal on normal). This can be initiated by low force repetitive strain or high force/ impact repetitive strain (Comerford et al 1998). Whereas the former tends to be an occupational group stress, the latter with added extension and possibly rotation occurs in many sports injuries.

Abuse or trauma

Back injury can occur in any accident, violent movement or fall (abnormal on either). Depending upon the severity of the trauma (e.g. road traffic accident), injury can include tissue bruising, damage to facet joint cartilage, ligamentous rupture, muscular strain, bony fracture, end-plate fracture or IVD damage. Whiplash is one of the most common traumatic presentations but even coughing and sneezing can precipitate injury.

The term 'sprain' in relation to the vertebral column is open to dispute. Research to date finds no evidence of the pathology of sprain occurring in the back (Bogduk & Twomey 1991). It is, however, a useful term for a clinical picture involving a series of signs and symptoms that cannot be accurately ascribed to any particular tissue of the back but which closely resemble the signs and symptoms evoked by a peripheral joint sprain such as a sprained ankle, something experienced by most people (Bogduk & Twomey 1991).

Sprain-type injuries can involve multiple joints, as in accidents, or a single joint if injury occurs whilst performing a minor movement.

RISK SITUATIONS

Certain unusual risk situations frequently present as causative factors in clinical practice.

Lifting after sitting for long periods

Lifting is a risk factor at any time but lifting after a period of long sitting is an infrequently recognized precipitating factor for LBP (Twomey & Taylor 1994a) (normal on unprepared normal). The most common presentation is as a pre- or post-holiday accident. At the end of a long journey, after sitting still for hours in a flat-back posture, the passenger reaches to lift heavy suitcases from the boot of the car or off the airport luggage carousel, possibly using a flexion/rotation/lateral flexion combined movement. The result can be immediate pain or pain later that day or on waking the next morning.

The avoidance technique is relatively simple and will be stressed in Section 2 of this book: it is essential to restore the lordosis by arching the back immediately on rising from sitting (see Fig. 9.4). This does two things: it reestablishes the tissues for recovery from creep and it initiates 'back awareness'.

Slouching after vigorous exercise

Slouching when grossly fatigued is a clinical encounter which to my knowledge has not been researched, but which appears too frequently in clinic to be ignored (normal on unprepared normal). After a hard day's work, possibly followed by a game of squash or heavy activity in the garden, ending with a hot bath, the most provocative position appears to be total relaxation for several hours in a large arm chair. The fatigued tissues are put under stress but give no warning until rising from the chair or rising from bed the next morning. After strenuous activity, lying supine or prone for 10–15 minutes as in Figure 9.5 or Figure 9.8 may be more recuperative.

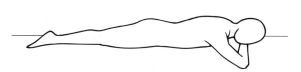

Figure 9.8   Recovery position for sustained flexion.

Reaching up or stretching

Reaching up or stretching suddenly in an off-balanced position provides the abusive combined movements of rotation, lateral flexion and extension (abnormal on normal).

Smoking

There is evidence of a link between smoking and LBP. Smoking may affect the nutrition of the disc (Battie et al 1991, Klaber Moffett et al 1995) or the link may be that smoking decreases the fibrinolytic activity (healing process) and thus may contribute to chronic pain (Meade et al 1979).

BACK PAIN IN PREGNANCY

Surprisingly little research has been undertaken to determine the cause of LBP in pregnancy. Postural change, particularly the increase in lordosis, has been cited as the cause, but the pathophysiological mechanism of the pain production has not been reported (Bullock et al 1987, Franklin & Conner-Kerr 1998). As LBP starts very early in pregnancy it is thought that changes in posture do not play a significant role, in spite of the increase in anterior pelvic tilt (Bullock et al 1987, Franklin & Conner-Kerr 1998). The sacroiliac area has been described as the most common area of pain, with or without symphysis pubis pain (Franklin & Conner-Kerr 1998).

Progesterone and relaxin, two of the pregnancy hormones, induce changes in collagen which result in a softening and relaxing effect on the spinal ligaments, especially those around the sacroiliac joints and symphysis pubis, which can widen by 3–4 mm (Polden & Mantle 1990, Franklin & Conner-Kerr 1998). Women with severe pelvic girdle pain in pregnancy have been found to have significantly higher serum levels of relaxin than those who are pain free. Pregnancy may also be a risk factor for post-partum disc prolapse if there has been a preexisting condition (Russell & Reynolds 1997).

Increased abdominal bulk, fluid retention and postural change add extra strain at the very moment of vulnerability. There is frequently an increased thoracic kyphosis, often enhanced by the increase in breast size as well as an increased lordosis in the early stages of pregnancy (Bullock et al 1987, Sandler 1996). Alteration of posture around the upper thoracic and lower cervical spine may lead to thoracic outlet syndrome which should not be confused with carpal tunnel syndrome caused by local oedema (Sandler 1996).

Idiopathic osteoporosis in pregnancy may be more common than the current literature suggests, so it is something therapists need to be aware of (Dunne 1994, Khastgir & Studd 1994, Rizzoli & Bonjour 1996) (see 'Osteoporosis', p. 17).

Patients can present with LBP, sometimes referring into the buttock and leg, thoracic spine pain, symphysis pubis pain and sacroiliac pain, often increased in side lying.

Treatment and prevention

Treatment

Assess. Look at spinal dysfunction, hip and sacroiliac joints. If the pain is acute, advise mainly rest and positional changes. Later, possibly consider gentle mobilization in side lying (Polden & Mantle 1990). The thoracic spine may play a very relevant role in the overall pain and perhaps physiotherapists should direct more attention to it (Bullock et al 1987). A pelvic support or trochanteric belt can be helpful. Give postural and positional advice, especially relieving positions (Box 9.4).

Prevention

Give all the usual advice about postural care in standing, with added work on TA and oblique abdominals. In sitting, recommend plenty of lumbar support. Advise against wearing high heels because of their indirect effect on the lumbar spine.

Baby preparation. Discuss preparation for the new baby: the height of cots, prams, places for changing mats, etc., and encourage planning all

---

> **Box 9.4**   Relieving positions in pregnancy
>
> - Lying supine: a small towel folded under the waist to support the lumbar spine
> - Side lying: a pillow between the legs
> - See Figs 9.5 and 9.6 for pain relief positions
> - Turning over: from the crook lying position, press both knees together to avoid sacroiliac stress
> - Sitting astride a chair the wrong way round, leaning forwards onto the back of the chair
> - Getting out of bed: teach method in Chapter 16 (p. 204)

---

this beforehand. However, stress the need for baby safety whilst caring for the back; for example, explain that even tiny babies can fall off high, unprotected surfaces.

Carrying the baby. Keep the baby close, carrying the baby in front or behind in a baby carrier. Baby carriers are good but they should not be used for long periods; the front carriers put a strain on the thoracic spine and the back ones, though less stressful, can stress the lumbar spine. This can be avoided by altering the position of the carrier and compensating with postural adaptation.

Epidural anaesthesia

The spectre of a link between epidural local anaesthetics in childbirth and CLBP has emerged but the survey data do not prove causation (McQuay 1994). Epidural haematomas are rare but when they do appear they resemble lumbar disc herniation (Watanabe et al 1997); post-epidural symptoms can include headache, migraine, neck pain, paraesthesia and visual disturbances (Russell & Reynolds 1997).

Many factors related to various conditions may be associated with higher risk of LBP, for example stressed positions in difficult labours and preexisting LBP (Russell 1995). In the clinic a number of patients who have had epidural analgesia present with LBP and it is easy to feel there is a strong link between the two. As thousands of epidurals are given each year with no apparent negative result, further research is very necessary.

REFERENCES

Adams M A 1996 Biomechanics of Low back pain. Pain Reviews 3: 15–30

Anderson J A D 1987 Back pain and occupation. In: Jayson M I V (ed) The lumbar spine and back pain, 3rd edn. Churchill Livingstone, Edinburgh

Battie M C, Videman T, Gill T et al 1991 Smoking and lumbar intervertebral disc degeneration: an MRI study of identical twins. Spine 16: 1015–1021

Bogduk N 1994 Innervation pain patterns, and mechanisms of pain production. In: Twomey L T, Taylor J R (eds) Physical therapy of the low back, 2nd edn. Churchill Livingstone, Edinburgh

Bogduk N, Twomey L T 1991 Clinical anatomy of the lumbar spine. Churchill Livingstone, Edinburgh

Boyling J 1992 Repetitive strain injury. Personal communication

Bullock M I, Bullock-Saxton J E 1994 Low back pain in the work place: an ergonomic approach to control. In: Twomey L T, Taylor J R (eds) Physical therapy of the low back. Churchill Livingstone, Edinburgh

Bullock J E, Jull G A, Bullock M I 1987 The relationship of low back pain to postural changes during pregnancy. Australian Journal of Physiotherapy 33(1): 10–17

Butler D 1991 Mobilisation of the nervous system. Churchill Livingstone, Edinburgh

Campbell R H 1995 Chronic low back pain and mechanical foot abnormalities. Musculoskeletal Management 1(1): 21–25

Casey G, Dockerell S 1996 A pilot study of the weight of schoolbags carried by 10-year old children. Physiotherapy Ireland 17(2): 17–21

Chartered Society of Physiotherapy (CSP) 1995 Press release. Physiotherapists concerned about unfit, fat, flabby young people. Chartered Society of Physiotherapy, London

Cholewicki J, McGill S 1996 Mechanical stability of the in vivo lumbar spine: implications for injury and chronic low back pain. Clinical Biomechanics 11: 1–15

Comerford M, Kinetic Control Ltd 1998 Dynamic stability and muscle balance of the lumbar spine and trunk. Kinetic Control course notes

Cowieson F M, Nicholls J A 1997 Non-specific back pain in children: a hidden problem? British Journal of Therapeutics and Rehabilitation 4(3): 129–132

Dallas M I 1997 Exercise walking for obesity management in older adult women. Issues on Aging 20(2): 8–11

Dieck G S, Kelsey J K, Goel V K et al 1985 An epidemiological study of the relationship between postural asymmetry in the teen years and subsequent back and neck pain. Spine 10(10): 872–877

Duggleby T, Kumar S 1997 Epidemiology of juvenile low back pain: a review. Disability and Rehabilitation 19(12): 505–512

Dunne F 1994 Idiopathic osteoporosis occurring in pregnancy. Journal of the Association of Chartered Physiotherapists in Gynaecology 75: 18–20

Epstein L H, Coleman K J, Myers M D 1996 Exercise in treating obesity in children and adolescents. Medicine and Science in Sports and Exercise 28(4): 428–435

Evans P 1980 The healing process at cellular level. Physiotherapy 66(8): 256–259

Franklin M E, Conner-Kerr T 1998 An analysis of posture and back pain in the first and third trimesters of pregnancy. Journal of Orthopaedic and Sports Physical Therapy 28(3): 133–138

Gass E M, Refshauge K M 1995 Theoretical basis underlying clinical decisions. In: Refshauge K, Gass E (eds) Musculoskeletal physiotherapy: clinical science and practice. Butterworth Heinemann, Oxford

Griegel-Morris P, Larson K, Mueller-Klaus K, Oatis C A 1992 Incidence of common postural abnormalities in the cervical, shoulder, and thoracic regions and their association with pain in two age groups of healthy subjects. Physical Therapy 72(6): 425–430

Han T S, Schouten J S A G, Leon M E J, Seidell J 1998 The prevalence of LBP and associations with body fatness, fat distribution and height. International Journal of Obesity 21: 600–607

Health Education Authority (HEA) 1997 Young people and physical activity. HEA, London.

Health and Safety Executive (HSE) 1992 Manual handling operations regulations. Guidelines on regulations. HMSO, London

Hides J, Richardson C, Jull G 1996 Multifidus recovery is not automatic after resolution of acute, first episodic low back pain. Spine 21: 2763–2769

Hodges P W, Richardson C A 1996 Inefficient muscular stabilisation of the lumbar spine associated with low back pain. Spine 21(22): 2640–2650

Kember J 1998 The physical therapist's contribution: neck and shoulders. In: Winspur I, Wynn Parry C B (eds) The musician's hand: a clinical guide. Martin Dunitz, London

Kendall F P, McCreary E K, Provance P G 1993 Muscle testing and function, 3rd edn. Williams and Wilkins, Baltimore

Kettle D 1999 Personal communication

Khastgir G, Studd J 1994 Pregnancy-associated osteoporosis. British Journal of Obstetrics and Gynaecology 101: 836–838

Klaber Moffett J K, Richardson G, Sheldon T A, Maynard A 1995 Back pain: its management and cost to society. University of York Centre for Health Economics, York

Liston C 1994 Low back pain: physical treatment in children and adolescents. In: Twomey L T, Taylor J R (eds) Physical therapy of the low back. Churchill Livingstone, Edinburgh

McKenzie R 1981 The lumbar spine: mechanical diagnosis and therapy. Spinal Publications, Waikanae, New Zealand

McQuay J H J 1994 Epidural anaesthesia. In: Wall P, Melzack R (eds) Textbook of pain. Churchill Livingstone, Edinburgh

Meade W, Chakrabarti R, Haines A et al 1979 Characteristics affecting fibrinolytic activity and plasma fibrinogen concentrations. British Medical Journal 1: 153–156

Mierau D, Cassidy J D, Yong-Hing K 1989 Low-back pain and straight leg raising in children and adolescents. Spine 14(5): 526–528

Mimura M, Panjabi M, Oxland T R, Crisco J J, Yamamoto I, Vasavada A 1994 Disc degeneration affects the multidirectional flexibility of the lumbar spine. Spine 19(12): 1371–1380

Mottram S 1997 Dynamic stability of the scapula. Manual Therapy 2(3): 123–131

Mottram S, Comerford M 1998 Stability dysfunction and low back pain. Journal of Orthopaedic Medicine 20(2): 13–18

Muckle D S 1990 Recurrent hamstring injuries as an expression of lumbar stress syndromes. Journal of Orthopaedic Rheumatology 3: 75–82

National Back Pain Association (NBPA) 1997 School bag survey '97 – findings and recommendations. Health Regulation Authority NBPA, Teddington

Panjabi M M 1992 The stabilizing system of the spine. Part I. Function, dysfunction, adaptation, and enhancement. Journal of Spinal Disorders 5(4): 383–389

Pheasant S 1991 Ergonomics, work and health, Macmillan, London

Polden M, Mantle J 1990 Physiotherapy in obstetrics and gynaecology. Butterworth Heinemann, Oxford

Pope M H, Hansson T H 1992 Vibration of the spine and low back pain. Clinical Orthopaedics 279: 49–59

Quint U, Wilke H-J, Shiraz-Adl A, Parnianpour M, Loer F, Claes L 1998 Importance of the intersegmental trunk muscles for the stability of the lumbar spine. A biomechanical study in vitro. Spine 23(18): 1937–1945

Raine S, Twomey L 1994 Posture of the head, shoulders and thoracic spine in comfortable erect standing. Australian Physiotherapy 40(1): 25–32

Refshauge K, Bolst L, Goodsell M 1995 The relationship between cervicothoracic posture and the presence of pain. Journal of Manual and Manipulative Therapy 3(1): 21–24

Reynolds N L 1997 Back injuries in the young athlete. Orthopedic Physical Therapy Clinics of North America 6: 491–503

Richardson C, Jull G, Toppenberg R, Comerford M 1992 Techniques for active stabilisation for spinal protection: a pilot study. Australian Physiotherapy 38(2): 105–112

Rizzoli R, Bonjour J P 1996 Pregnancy-associated osteoporosis. Lancet 347: 1274–1275

Russell R 1995 Epidural analgesia and back pain. Current Anaesthesia and Critical Care 6: 212–217

Russell R, Reynolds F 1997 Back pain, pregnancy and childbirth. British Medical Journal 314: 1062–1063

Sahrmann S A 1993 Diagnosis and treatment of movement system imbalances associated with musculoskeletal pain. Washington University School of Medicine, course notes

Salter R B, Simmonds D F, Malcolm B W 1975 Effects of continuous passive motion on the healing of articular cartilage defects. Journal of Bone and Joint Surgery 57A(4): 570

Sandler S E 1996 The management of low back pain in pregnancy. Manual Therapy 1(4): 178–185

Siddall P J, Cousins M J 1997 Spine update. Spinal mechanisms. Spine 22(1): 98–104

Snijders C J, Slagter A H E, van Strik R et al 1995 Why leg crossing? The influence of common postures on abdominal activity. Spine 20: 1989–1993

Spitzer W O, LeBlanc F E, Dupuis M et al 1987 scientific approach to the assessment and management of activity related spinal disorders. A monograph for clinicians. Report of the Quebec Task Force on spinal disorders. Spine 12: 75

Staes F, Vervaet L, Stappaerts K, Evaraert D 1995 Low back pain in Flemish adolescents: a preliminary study. Musculoskeletal Management 1(2): 93–98

Taimela S, Kujala U M, Salminen J J, Viljananen T 1997 The prevalence of low back pain among children and adolescents. A nation-wide, cohort-based questionnaire survey in Finland. Spine 22(10): 1132–1136

Taylor J R, Twomey L T 1994 The lumbar spine from infancy to old age. In: Twomey L T, Taylor J R (eds) Physical therapy of the low back. Churchill Livingstone, Edinburgh

Twomey L T, Taylor J R 1994a Back and joint pain: a rationale for treatment with manual therapy. In: Twomey L T, Taylor J R (eds) Physical therapy of the low back. Churchill Livingstone, Edinburgh

Twomey L T, Taylor J 1994b Lumbar posture, movement and mechanics. In: Twomey L T, Taylor J R (eds) Physical therapy of the low back. Churchill Livingstone Edinburgh

Vicas-Kunse P 1991 Educating our children: the pilot school program. Spine 5(3): 497–501

Waddell G 1998 The pain revolution. Churchill Livingstone, Edinburgh

Watanabe N, Ogura T, Kimori K et al 1997 Epidural hematoma of the lumbar spine, simulating extruded lumbar disk herniation: clinical, discographic, and enhanced magnetic resonance imaging features. Spine 22(1): 105–109

Weinstein J 1991 Neurogenic and non-neurogenic pain and inflammatory mediators. Orthopedic Clinics of North America 22(2): 235–246

Williams J G P, Sperryn P N 1979 Sports medicine. Edward Arnold, London

FURTHER READING

C S P 1998 Symphysis pubis dysfunction. Association of Chartered Physiotherapists in Women's Health, London

Grieve G P 1994 Counterfeit clinical presentations. Manipulative Physiotherapist 26: 17–19

Grisigano V 1991 Sports injuries. Butterworths, London

Liston C B 1994 Low back pain: physical treatment in children and adolescents. In: Twomey L T, Taylor J R (eds) Physical therapy of the low back. Churchill Livingstone, Edinburgh

Magee D J 1997 Orthopaedic physical assessment, 3rd edn. W B Saunders, London

Polden M, Mantle M J 1990 Physiotherapy in Obstetrics and Gynaecology. Butterworth Heinemann, Oxford

Reynolds N L 1997 Back injuries in the young athlete. The young athlete, part 1. Orthopedic Physical Therapy Clinics of North America 6(4): 491–503

Back care

SECTION CONTENTS

10

Treatment and prevention of low back pain

THE DIAGNOSTIC TRIAGE

Up until recently little consensus existed with regard to the most effective management and treatment of acute LBP, resulting in a wide variation in fundamental approach. The Quebec Task Force (Spitzer et al 1987) were the first to lay down guidelines for the management of back pain in primary care, followed in the US in 1994 by the Agency for Health Care Policy and Research (AHCPR) and in the UK by the Clinical Standards Advisory Group (CSAG 1994) and the Royal College of General Practitioners (RCGP 1996, with review in 1999). The CSAG guidelines consist of a diagnostic triage which should be the basis of primary care back pain management and treatment (Box 10.1). The early management of pain determines the final outcome, therefore

---

Box 10.1   The CSAG Diagnostic Triage (reproduced with permission from CSAG 1994)

- *Simple back ache*: onset age 20–55; lumbosacral region, buttocks and thighs; mechanical in nature; varies with activity and time; patient well; prognosis good
- *Nerve root pain*: Limb pain more severe than vertebral; paraesthesia or anaesthesia; reduced tension tests; motor and sensory changes; prognosis reasonable
- *Serious pathology or 'red flags'*: age of onset <20 or >55; violent trauma; constant progressive pain; thoracic pain; PMH carcinoma; systemic steroids; drug abuse, HIV; patient systemically unwell; weight loss; widespread neurology; cauda equina syndrome

---

Box 10.2 Early management for acute simple back pain

- Prescribe simple analgesics or NSAIDs.
- Advise rest only if essential: 1–3 days maximum.
- Encourage normal movement within the limits of pain.
- Arrange physical therapy if symptoms last more than a few days.
- Educate in relation to pain.

Box 10.3 The value of X-rays

X-rays are only of value to discount:
- fractures in trauma
- osteoporosis, especially after prolonged steroidal use
- spondylolisthesis or other bony anomalies
- tumour or infection, in combination with blood tests.

Box 10.4 CSAG 'red flags', inflammatory disorders and cauda equina symptoms (reproduced from CSAG 1994)

Further investigations if no improvement in less than 6 weeks:
- the 'red flag' warnings of Box 10.1
- Inflammatory disorders – morning stiffness, persistent limited spinal movement in all directions, peripheral joint involvement; iritis, skin rashes, colitis, urethral discharge, family history.

Immediate investigations, cauda equina symptoms:
- difficulty with micturition
- loss of anal sphincter tone or control
- saddle anaesthesia
- widespread or progressive motor weakness in legs or gait disturbance.

---

accurate diagnostic triage is fundamental to appropriate referral and management.

The RCGP guidelines stress that bed rest is not recommended for simple acute pain and that continuation of normal activities within the limits of pain should be encouraged (Box 10.2) (see Chapter 16 on coping with acute pain). X-rays are of limited value and should only be used to discount certain pathologies or deformities, as they show no soft tissue lesions (Box 10.3).

The success of treating acute LBP depends on early advice and education in relation to pain. (CSAG 1994, Malmivaara et al 1995, Turner et al 1998, Waddell 1998, Gifford 1999). There has been criticism that primary care advisors have failed to give this essential early advice. In fact, there has been failure to ask the most important questions about patients' pain and its effect on their work/social/economic life (Deyo & Phillips 1996, Turner et al 1998, Askew et al 1998). Turner et al (1998) found that patients who had received early support gained confidence and improved more quickly.

In recent literature particular emphasis is being given to prevention of recurrence and chronic disability as opposed to primary prevention of back pain (Klaber-Moffett et al 1995, Painting et

al 1998). As the analysis of valid trials provides clear evidence that manual therapy can be an effective modality for the treatment of acute LBP (Di Fabio 1992, Deyo 1996), the CSAG and RCGP triage recommends early therapeutic referral for the first two conditions. However, therapists need to be vigilant with regard to the 'Red Flag' or other warning signs of serious pathological conditions which may have been missed earlier (Box 10.4).

Many physiotherapists are now primary contact practitioners. Diagnostic skills and techniques have become of the utmost importance to them and these skills are required not only for primary diagnosis but also for more 'refined' diagnosis of the anatomic origin of back pain or dysfunction (Twomey & Taylor 1994b, Wells 1997).

All guidelines stress that pain and disability are different, although control of pain and overcoming disability go together. Chronic disability can only be prevented if lasting pain relief is achieved and full function is restored. Therefore early treatment for the control of pain, the restoration of function, reeducation of lifestyle and the return to normal activity and work are of major importance in primary care.

EXAMINATION AND ASSESSMENT

Every patient attending for therapeutic treatment must be assessed. This entails taking a

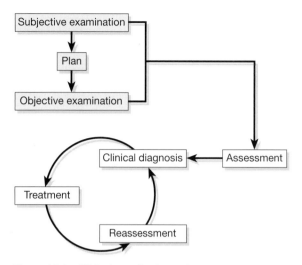

Figure 10.1   Clinical examination and assessment. (Reproduced with permission from Kettle 1999.)

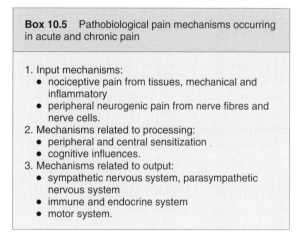

Box 10.5   Pathobiological pain mechanisms occurring in acute and chronic pain

1. Input mechanisms:
   - nociceptive pain from tissues, mechanical and inflammatory
   - peripheral neurogenic pain from nerve fibres and nerve cells.
2. Mechanisms related to processing:
   - peripheral and central sensitization
   - cognitive influences.
3. Mechanisms related to output:
   - sympathetic nervous system, parasympathetic nervous system
   - immune and endocrine system
   - motor system.

careful history, past and present, followed by making a comprehensive active and passive physical examination and finally using clear clinical reasoning for a treatment plan. All therapists should be familiar with assessment described by Petty & Moore (1998), Grieve (1989), Maitland (1986) and McKenzie (1981) (see 'Further reading'). Kettle (1999) uses a clear, simple diagram to demonstrate the processes involved in assessment and treatment (Fig. 10.1).

The scope of the examination is becoming more and more extensive but 'look, feel and move' still remains the overall protocol (Refshauge & Latimer 1995). Within this blueprint there is a need to look not only at articular tests but also at relative flexibility, not only at strength of muscle activity but also at dysfunction, not only at neural conductivity but also at pathodynamics, bearing all mechanisms in mind. Articular tests, neuropraxia tests and sensory-motion tests are all needed to identify any neuromusculoskeletal dysfunction (Mottram & Comerford 1998). Passive movements and palpatory techniques are essential to identify tissue disturbance and may accurately yield the same information as more costly invasive medical equipment (Twomey & Taylor 1994b).

The source of every dysfunction must be addressed, even those that are less obvious: a general physical dysfunction such as an asymmetric walk, which may or may not be relevant to the patient's presentation of pain, should be considered; a general lack of fitness should not be ignored; a musician may present with hand problems but the source of the dysfunction could be the PNS or the CNS (Kember 1997, 1998).

Butler (1999) enlarges on the importance of maintaining the widest possible perspective, stressing the need to think in terms of pain mechanisms related to input, to processing and to output (Box 10.5), all of which may be present in the pain picture under examination. Pain, pathology, sensitized neural tissue and altered proprioceptive input can all influence recruitment of stability muscles, affecting the patterns of movement and functional stability, so function and dysfunction must be assessed in all components of the movement system (Sharma & Yi-Chung Pai 1997, Gill & Callaghan 1998, Mottram & Comerford 1998).

Physiotherapists are trained never to 'assume' anything (Maitland 1986). It is certainly easier to assume that the patient's attitude or emotional stress is the cause of their problem than to acknowledge our own failure to find the source of pain. Care must be taken not to discount a single sign or symptom, no matter how apparently bizarre, until the systems have been carefully examined, incorporating all our present knowledge of neurogenic pain and pain sensitization.

The type of pain that moves, that 'pops up' in various parts of the body in seemingly anatomically impossible ways, requires careful neural pathodynamic examination, not only of the obvious areas but of the entire body. On examination, people with headaches may be found to have limited SLR or in another patient, upper limb tension testing may elicit leg pain; in treatment, mobilization of the thoracic spine can effect change in the cervical and the lumbar areas, and mobilization of C1/2/3 can change SLR. These strange connections cannot be related solely to local 'tissue input' (see 'Neural dynamics' in Chapter 6, p. 92).

Far too many long-term pain problems, previously classed as psychological or even 'psychogenic', have later been found to be complicated patterns of disorders with layer upon layer of dysfunction: for example, degenerative changes with stiffness of the facet joints and, on top, a fall; or intermittent episodes of minor back and neck pain through the years; or a fall off a horse as a child with no pathological changes but thoracic pain recently. The picture of the disorder becomes wider or more layered as chronic dysfunction in an area may eventually cause dysfunction in another area, either by change in gait or habitual movement pattern or on a more pathological level, as with the double crush phenomenon (Kettle 1999).

TREATMENT OF ACUTE PAIN

It is beyond the scope of this book to discuss the treatment of specific disorders such as discogenic pain, nerve root pain or pain from any particular pathology. For this reason only dysfunctional LBP, which may be part of any other lesion, will be discussed.

On assessment, every therapist needs to be aware of symptoms and signs which do not 'fit the picture', the signs described in Box 10.4. These all call for careful monitoring or further investigation.

In the same way that 'look, feel and move' remains the protocol for examination, 'assess,

---

Box 10.6 Evaluating and treating functional problems

1. Look at:
   - feet/knee/hip alignment
   - general dynamic and static posture
   - not only at ROM, but also at relative flexibility
   - joint position and movement in relation to the lengthening/shortening of controlling musculature
   - muscle function: local and global.
2. Evaluate any dysfunction: is it habitual or pain provoked?
3. Examine relevant neural mobility of the whole body: slump in standing and sitting, SLR, PKB, upper limb tension tests.
4. Palpate relevant areas and plan mobilization techniques that may be of relevance
5. Assess and plan treatment relating to:
   - joint/disc dysfunction
   - neural tissue involvement
   - muscle instability.
6. Give a clear, simple and confident explanation of what you believe to be the problem and how both treatment and self-help will work towards solving it.
7. Work towards relieving pain, correcting dysfunction, improving mobility and restoring full activity, using appropriate techniques: antiinflammatory medication, ice or electrical modalities, mobilization, careful neural mobility exercises, muscular reeducation, advice regarding work and recreational activities.
8. Provide support and give clear back care advice in daily activities with written exercises or postural correction instruction.

---

treat and reassess' is the protocol for treatment. After examination, clinical reasoning will determine the priority of technique application and the degree of intervention in the management of dysfunction. Soft tissue techniques, biomechanical intervention and psychosocial intervention may all be necessary (Mottram & Comerford 1998) and treatment will encompass changing techniques and approaches (Box 10.6). When treating the seemingly bizarre pains mentioned above, it is the repeated 'treat and reassess' process that guides the therapist through the necessary changes and evaluates the efficacy of what is being done. There can never be 'rules' about what area to treat or how to treat it but treatment *must always be based on clinical reasoning*, which to date has received little 'evidence-based' research. Validation can only come from measurable subjective and objective improvement.

The importance of aiding full recovery or, if this is not entirely possible, the importance of teaching the management of pain cannot be overemphasized. People with acute back pain may proceed to either coping wellness or chronic illness (Hill 1999) and the progression of this lies very much in our hands. Iatrogenic disability (symptoms induced in a patient by the treatment or comments of physicians) can be fertilized by our misuse of words and pain-centred attitude (Rose 1999). Patients have a strong desire to receive a credible explanation of their pain. It is important to give a clear but unfrightening description of their problem, avoiding words like 'crumbling spine' or 'bad arthritis', explaining that extremely severe symptoms can be caused by benign conditions. 'Arthritis', for example, is a term that needs careful clarification. Understanding their pain may significantly reduce the patient's anxiety and allay their fears in relation to serious disease (Nicholas et al 1992, Klenerman et al 1995, Deyo & Phillips 1996, Klaber-Moffett & Richardson 1997).

During treatment it is important to talk to the patient about what you are doing. Quite simple comments are often the most helpful; for example, during mobilization of a painful, stiff facet joint, as you feel it clearing, speak about it:

'Is the pain changing at all?'

'Yes! It's getting less!'

'I thought so, I could feel the vertebra moving more freely. I'll just go on doing this for a little longer, let me know when it is OK.'

And you invariably reach the moment about 60 seconds later when they say with surprise 'It's OK now!' A move has been made to show that pain is changeable.

As the pain improves, we must avoid equating hurt with harm; the expectancy of pain creates fear that instigates avoidance activities, leading to a passive lifestyle and disability (Painting et al 1996, Gifford 1999). Gifford (1999) points out that clinicians need to accept the complex biology of pain and sometimes the poor healing potential of injured tissues (for example, in whiplash) and this requires a modest shift in therapeutic emphasis from 'fix' and 'relieve' to achieving the best possible physical and mental recovery.

People with complicated pain patterns may need to receive treatment periodically, a bit like a regular car service, to set them once again on the road. This is possible in private practice but the tragedy is that in the NHS there is little time to see even the first course of treatment through, let alone repeat it in 6 months time. So in the limited time available for treatment, there is a need to ensure that we do not waste time. Comerford et al (1998) suggest three reasons for failing treatment in LBP.

1. *Incorrect treatment*: too often a mechanical problem is still treated with ultrasound, heat, TENS, acupuncture and antiinflammatory medication (NSAIDs), ignoring the need to mobilize, restore function and promote activity.

2. *Insufficiently specific treatment*: the analysis of dysfunction is often inadequate, with insufficient attention paid to segmental hyper- or hypomobility. A stiff pain-free segment can be inducing pain in a hypermobile segment.

3. *Inadequate correction and reeducation*: in relation to lifestyle, job activity, posture at work and during leisure.

Treatment should look at every aspect; for example, although NSAID administration is a waste of time for mechanical pain, the modification of pain with analgesia or NSAIDs in the early stages of an acute, inflammatory, non-mechanical condition may have a profound effect on the prevention of centralization and chronicity (Deyo 1996, Siddall & Cousins 1997). We should ensure that medication is used appropriately.

In accepting the importance of the multifactorial problems of pain, it is important not to confuse the new concepts of pain sensitization with the old, vague idea of a 'holistic' approach. The approach now is truly holistic but in a much more scientific way. It is vital for therapists to avoid simplistic thoughts and words like 'tension' which suggest a stress-related, 'psychological' cause for the patient's pain. How many of us have heard patients with long-standing headaches use the term apologetically and almost hopelessly – 'I know it is all tension' – and they probably are tense, who wouldn't be with daily headaches! However, tense or not, the important point is: they do not know what to do with their 'tension'. Blaming tension is a negative and unhelpful approach.

The responsibility for getting pain better is finely balanced between us and the patient and we must be careful not suggest something that they cannot cope with. The patient has come with a burden of pain, anxious to pass it on to someone else to cure. Initially, we have to accept this burden, turning it into a 'working together' partnership before gradually passing it back to them, but only after they have fully understood the meaning of their problem and after we, hopefully, have found a way to affect both the nociceptive and neuropathic input of their pain. In fact, the process starts quite naturally at the very first treatment when we discuss daily activities in relation to relieving or aggravating their pain. Finally, we must give patients the power to continue improvement, to manage their pain if some remains and hopefully to prevent recurrence.

Believing the pain to be 'tension' based can also prevent the patient from looking at the real aggravating or relieving factors: that they are sitting daily with their heads turned to one side at the computer; that they are sleeping on too high pillows at night; that they are lying on the settee watching TV with their head propped up on an arm for hours every evening; that they are taking no general aerobic or physical exercise and in fact, *they are not moving*!

Pain, dysfunction and negative afferent input initiate sensitization and continuing pain. The aim of treatment has to be the restoration of functionally accurate body movements and the right patterns of movement, reinstating positive proprioceptive input to the CNS with the possibility of changing what is going on in the whole system. Patients need local treatment, global treatment, positive advice about the relationship between body postures and pain and between movement and pain, and all this related to their lifestyle.

Having thoroughly treated pain and dys-

Box 10.7   Advice to patients about pain

- Describe the relevant nerves and their pathways.
- Explain that when they have limb pain they need to think more about the position of their vertebrae than the position of their limb, e.g. when a patient stoops to rub his lower leg because of pain in that area, what is he doing to the back while in this position?
- Explain that nerves need a good blood supply for the nourishment of their tissues.
- Therefore movement is essential.
- Give careful postural reeducation and back care advice.
- Give specifically designed exercises for their condition.
- Explain the need for general aerobic activity not only for their general health but also for relieving pain by increasing their own endogenous opioid peptides.

---

function, we must 'demedicalize' pain by giving our patients the right tools and the confidence to know that they *can* manage and, hopefully, prevent their pain with postural care, movement, general activity and awareness (Zusman 1997) (Box 10.7).

TREATMENT OF CHRONIC LOW BACK PAIN (CLBP)

Chronic musculoskeletal disorders include vertebral pain with shoulder/arm or hip/leg pain referral or pain associated with diseases such as rheumatoid arthritis and ankylosing spondylitis, degenerative diseases such as osteoarthritis and spondylosis, and anomalies such as spondylolisthesis and stenosis (Gass 1995). Neurogenic pain may be part of any of these disorders.

All these patients are likely to have long-term, intermittent pain and may need periodic treatment and appropriate advice on pain management but they do not have intractable problems with associated behavioural changes (Gass 1995). Nevertheless, they present with multifactorial dysfunctions which all need addressing, for example in the L4–5 long-standing problem of Figure 10.2. Here the approach may involve more widely spaced treatment sessions with the aim of not only improving their dysfunction but also perhaps influencing their very mode of living, encouraging them to walk instead of

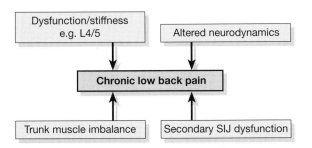

Figure 10.2 Assessing components of the movement system. (Reproduced with permission from Kettle 1999.)

driving, to be active instead of sitting, to take up some form of gentle sport to fit their abilities, the need to *move* being the vital message.

However, the main clinical elements of the problematic 2–5% of patients with non-specific CLBP (pain for which there appears to be 'no diagnosis') are pain with *disability*, physical impairment, psychological distress (with heightened awareness and depression), fear avoidance beliefs and illness behaviour (Fordyce 1995, Rose et al 1997).

Maladaptive fear avoidance beliefs and deconditioning behaviour often arise because of convictions about some structural-anatomical-biomechanical basis for their pain (Fordyce 1995, Zusman 1997). These beliefs may receive neurophysiological endorsement from peripheral input that is normally not registered as being 'pathologically'/clinically painful (Gatchel et al 1995, Greening & Lynn 1998). An important point is made by Gatchel (1995) who found that the high rates of psychopathology seen in chronic pain disability develop as a *result* of the chronicity and do not *cause* it.

Although it is important that pain is not thought of solely in terms of nociception, the fact that pain persists 'beyond normal healing time and there is no longer evidence of tissue damage' does not suggest that patients are imagining their pain (Waddell 1998) or that there is no nociceptive sensory component to the pain (Gifford 1999). There is a danger of 'blaming' the patient and considering them to be 'psychogenic'; instead they need to be helped to cope with their pain both physically and mentally (Gifford 1999).

For these reasons non-specific CLBP disability is managed best within the framework of an interdisciplinary approach. The basic rationale of back pain management programmes can be defined as the alteration of behavioural, cognitive and affective variables which interfere with adaptive functioning.

Pain clinics, back schools and rehabilitation centres

Pain clinics

Rovenstine started the first pain clinic in 1936 at the Bellevue Hospital, New York. In Europe, the first pain clinics were established in the UK in 1986 (Sweet 1997). Pain clinics are now attached to most major hospitals and usually consist of a multidisciplinary team with a pain consultant, psychiatrist or psychologist, physiotherapist, occupational therapist, nurse and social worker. As chronic pain is a multifactorial problem, a diagnosis is reached by a compilation of the assessments of some or all of the team (Gass 1995, Sweet 1997).

Treatment can be managed individually or in groups of 4–6 patients, with each member of the team providing help on self-management: the pain consultant on self-medication; the psychologist on stress reduction and cognitive-behavioural therapy; the psychiatrist on auto-hypnosis or imagery; the physiotherapist on automobilization, isometric muscle strengthening and posture; the occupational therapist on relaxation methods, pacing and goal achievement and the social worker on distraction techniques, self-help groups and domestic issues (Sweet 1997).

Back schools

The first back school was started in Sweden by Zachrisson-Forsell in the 1970s (Waddell 1998). They are now a common facility. Their main aim is education and understanding, giving simple functional anatomy, applied body mechanics, ergonomic advice and postural advice for daily living, relaxation techniques and some form of exercise programme. Back schools work well if they are incorporated into a fitness programme (Frost et al 1995, Waddell 1998).

Rehabilitation/fitness centres or work hardening

In aiming to reduce disability, Frost et al (1995) believe that more aggressive rehabilitation programmes are necessary for CLBP and that fitness programmes are more effective than home programmes, back schools or prevention.

Intensive treatment programmes with a multi-disciplinary approach have been used extensively in the US and Scandinavia and are increasing in number in the UK and elsewhere. These initially assess the back function, fitness and pain levels of patients attending before placing them into a programme of intensive physical therapy appropriate to their physical state. This includes a behaviour modification programme aimed at rapid functional restoration and a return to work as soon as possible (Edwards et al 1992, Twomey & Taylor 1994a, Frost et al 1995, Jones & Thomas 1997).

Each programme is carefully tailored to meet the requirements of participants and is closely monitored by trained staff. There is a mix of weight training, aerobic activity, functional activity, relaxation and stress training, work hardening in relation to the person's particular job, back educational instruction and behaviour modification (Twomey & Taylor 1994a).

Patients are encouraged to feel like sports people who want to improve their fitness rather than people who are disabled. Pain is not discussed in class except to ask patients to advise the therapist if leg pain or neurological symptoms increase. The treatment focus in management of CLBP includes training of muscles surrounding the lumbar spine whose primary role is provision of dynamic stability and segmental control: transversus abdominis, lumbar multifidus and the internal obliques (O'Sullivan et al 1997).

Frost et al (1995) report that the success of these treatment programmes has been greater than expected. Several factors may be responsible: pain reduction from the increase of endogenous opioid peptides in response to aerobic activity; an increase in confidence to carry out physical activities; and an improvement in functional ability. Patients who attribute their improvement to their own efforts are less likely to relapse. Self-reward and self-motivation are the ultimate goals of the programme, thus reinforcing the **locus of control**, a theoretical construct which refers to a person's belief in control over illness (Edwards et al 1992, Frost et al 1995, Jones & Thomas 1997).

Psychological approach to pain management

The way people cope with pain, the methods they use to control their emotional arousal and reactions to a pain episode, can be adaptive and active or maladaptive and passive (Weisenberg 1994). The rationale of back pain management is the alleviation of behavioural, cognitive and affective variables which interfere with adaptive functioning (Rose 1999).

The cognitive-behavioural approach to pain control is being used as part of the more comprehensive programmes described above to teach the relationship between thoughts, feelings, behaviour, environmental stimuli and pain. The procedures relate to the way patients perceive, interpret and relate to their pain rather than to the elimination of the pain *per se* and this becomes the basis for therapy (Weisenberg 1994). Self-appraisal is central to the method and the aim is for patients to be in control of their own pain (Craig 1994).

The cognitive-behavioural approach is part of many treatment programmes and in this context, patients are usually part of a group with multidisciplinary team management. The intensity of treatment ranges from a few hours' outpatients attendance per day to several weeks in patient admission (Rose 1999).

The principles most useful for physiotherapists to teach are as follows.

Pacing. Breaking up the day to balance rest with activity to avoid severe exacerbation of patients' symptoms (Sweet 1997). It achieves control by stopping the activity *before* the pain increases; that is, quota-led rather than pain-led activity (Shoreland 1999).

Goal setting. This provides a focus on improving function and aids return to the patient's desired activity (Shoreland 1999).

Reinforcement. A positive approach to help patients change unhelpful behaviours and habits by rewarding success and playing down failure (Shoreland 1999).

Coping strategies. For example, relaxation techniques and exercise routines which can be allocated to times of the day when the patient can slow down and be tranquil instead of continuing with unbroken work or stress (Sweet 1997, Shoreland 1998).

Cognitive-behavioural rehabilitation has been demonstrated to be an effective means of reducing psychological distress, changing cognition and improving the function of patients with CLBP (Rose et al 1997).

Hypnosis and relaxation

Hypnosis and relaxation are being used successfully in the treatment of chronic pain. These techniques make use of the altered states of consciousness that are known to be attained through practices such as meditative prayer, transcendental meditation, some forms of yoga and autogenic therapy (Benson et al 1977, Melzack & Wall, 1996). It is believed that in these states of consciousness a physiological response, termed the 'relaxation response', takes place which is distinctly different from that observed during quiet sitting or sleep and involves changes consistent with decreased sympathetic nervous system reaction. Relaxation may have physiological significance in countering overactivity of the sympathetic nervous system.

Benson et al (1977) point out that four elements seem to be integral to the many ways of practising relaxation: a quiet environment; decreased muscle tone; a mental device such as a word or voice or phrase repeated audibly or silently to oneself; and a passive attitude.

Several different techniques used for teaching relaxation range from a meditative form described by Benson et al (1977), to a method described by Laura Mitchell (1987) which uses contractions of groups of muscles in order to promote relaxation in the antagonist group, to a technique devised by Edmund Jacobson (1970) which is based on strong muscular contractions followed by their relaxation throughout the body. Both yoga and the Alexander technique teach relaxation and there are various forms of meditation, especially transcendental meditation which is taken from one of the yoga systems (Hare 1986). There are also several commercial relaxation tapes available.

PREVENTION

Care of the back requires an understanding of its structure, an awareness of potential injury and, finally, a resolve to prevent any detrimental occurrences. Chapter 9 has looked at the direct and indirect causes of back pain. Prevention has to lie in avoidance of these.

Twomey & Taylor (1994b) list some important points to aid prevention: correct lifting techniques; the avoidance of unnecessary hazards at work or in sport by acquiring sound techniques and ensuring adequate preparation; good ergonomic advice and installations; correct postural function in all activities and good muscular fitness. The hazards of a sedentary lifestyle, with poor muscle tone, lack of aerobic fitness and poor posture, predispose to dysfunction and possible pain.

Movement and active exercise are unlikely to prevent episodes of back pain but they will ensure that those affected will be better able to cope with the problem, to recover from it more rapidly, to remain at or return to productive work more quickly and to have a much improved quality of life (Waddell 1987).

REFERENCES

AHCPR 1994 Clinical practice guidelines number 14. Acute low back pain problems in adults. Agency for Health Care Policy and Research, US Department of Health and Human Services, Rockville, MD

Askew R, Kibelstis C, Overbaugh S et al 1998 Physiotherapists perception of patients' pain and its effect on management. Physiotherapy Research International 3(1): 37–52

Benson H, Hotch J B, Crassweller K D, Greenwood M M 1977 Historical and clinical considerations of the relaxation response. American Scientist 65: 441–445

Butler D 1999 Integrating pain awareness into physiotherapy – wise action for the future. In: Gifford L (ed) Topical issues in pain. Physiotherapy Pain Association Yearbook 1998–1999. NOI Press, Falmouth, Adelaide

Clinical Standards Advisory Group (CSAG) 1994 Report on back pain. HMSO, London

Comerford M, Kinetic Control 1998 Dynamic stability and muscle balance of the lumbar spine and trunk. Course notes, Kinetic Control Ltd

Craig K 1994 Emotional aspects of pain. In: Wall P, Melzack R (eds) Textbook of pain. Churchill Livingstone, Edinburgh

Deyo R 1996 Acute low back pain: a new paradigm for management. British Medical Journal 313: 30B

Deyo R, Phillips W R 1996 Low back pain. A primary care challenge. Spine 21(24): 2826–2832

Di Fabio R P 1992 Efficacy of manual therapy. Physical Therapy 171(12): 853–864

Edwards B C, Zusman M, Hardcastle P et al 1992 A physical approach to the rehabilitation of patients disabled by chronic low back pain. Medical Journal of Australia 156: 167–172

Fordyce W E 1995 Back pain in the workplace. In: Fordyce W E (ed) Task force on pain in the workplace of the International Association of the Study of Pain. IASP Press, Seattle

Frost H, Klaber Moffett J A, Moser J S, Fairbank J C T 1995 Randomised controlled trials for evaluation of fitness programme for patients with CLBP. British Medical Journal 310: 151–154

Gass E 1995 The challenging role for physiotherapy in chronic musculoskeletal disorders. In: Refshauge K, Gass E (eds) Musculoskeletal physiotherapy Butterworth Heinemann, Oxford

Gatchel R J, Polatin P B, Mayer T G 1995 The dominant role of psychosocial risk factors in the development of chronic low back pain disability. Spine 20(24): 2702–2709

Gifford L 1999 Output mechanisms. In: Gifford L (ed) Topical issues in pain. Physiotherapy Pain Association Yearbook 1998–1999. NOI Press, Falmouth, Adelaide

Gill K P, Callaghan M J 1998 The measurement of lumbar proprioception in individuals with and without low back pain. Spine 23(3): 371–377

Greening J, Lynn B 1998 Minor peripheral nerve injuries: an underestimated source of pain? Manual Therapy 3(4): 187–194

Grieve G P 1989 Common vertebral joint problems, 2nd edn. Churchill Livingstone, Edinburgh

Hare M 1986 Physiotherapy in psychiatry. Heinemann Medical, London

Hill P 1999 Fear-avoidance theories. In: Gifford L (ed) Topical issues in pain. Physiotherapy Pain Association Yearbook 1998–1999. NOI Press, Falmouth, Adelaide

Jacobson E 1970 Modern treatment of tense patients. Charles C Thomas, Springfield, Illinois

Jones F, Thomas G 1997 A rehabilitation approach for chronic disabling low back pain. In: Wells P E, Frampton V, Bowsher D (eds) Pain management by physiotherapy. Butterworth Heinemann, Oxford

Kember J 1997 Focal dystonia in a musician. Manual Therapy 2(4): 221–225

Kember J 1998 The physical therapist's contribution: neck and shoulders. In: Winspur I, Wynn Parry C B (eds) The musician's hand: a clinical guide. Martin Dunitz, London

Kettle D 1999 Personal communication

Klaber-Moffett J, Richardson G 1997 The influence of the physiotherapist-patient relationship on pain and disability. Physiotherapy Theory and Practice 13(39): 90–96

Klaber-Moffett J, Richardson G, Sheldon T, Maynard A 1995 Back pain. Its management and cost to society. Discussion paper 129. Centre for Health Economics, University of York, York

Klenerman L, Slade P D, Stanley M et al 1995 The prediction of chronicity in patients with an acute attack of low back pain in a general practice setting. Spine 20(4): 478–484

Maitland G D 1986 Vertebral manipulation, 5th edn. Butterworths, London

Malmivaara A, Hakkinen U, Aro T et al 1995 The treatment of acute low back pain – bed rest, exercises or ordinary activity? New England Journal of Medicine 332(6): 351–353

Melzack R, Wall P D 1996 The challenge of pain. Penguin, Harmondsworth

Mitchell L 1987 Simple relaxation. John Murray, London

Mottram S, Comerford M 1998 Stability dysfunction and low back pain. Journal of Orthopaedic Medicine 20(2): 13–18

Nicholas M K, Wilson P H, Goyen J 1992 Comparison of cognitive behavioural group treatment and alternative non-psychological treatment for chronic low back pain. Pain 48: 339–347

O'Sullivan P, Twomey L T, Allison G, Sinclair J, Miller K, Knox J 1997 Altered patterns of abdominal muscle activation in patients with chronic low back pain. Australian Physiotherapy 43(2): 91–98

Painting S N, Chester T, McCrann K H 1996 The effect of positions and movement on low back pain. Proceedings of Spring Meeting, Society of Back Pain Research, Bristol

Painting S, Favarin I, Swales J 1998 The management of acute industrial low back pain. Physiotherapy 84(3): 110–117

Refshauge K M, Latimer J 1995 The physical examination. In: Refshauge K, Gass G (eds) Musculoskeletal physiotherapy. Butterworth Heinemann, Oxford

Rose M 1999 Iatrogenic disability and back pain rehabilitation. In: Gifford L (ed) Topical issues in pain. Physiotherapy Pain Association Yearbook 1998–1999. NOI Press, Falmouth, Adelaide

Rose M, Reilly J P, Pennie B et al 1997 Chronic low back pain rehabilitation programmes. Spine 22(19): 2247–2251

Royal College of General Practitioners (RCGP) 1996 Clinical guidelines for the management of acute low back pain.

Royal College of General Practitioners, London

Sharma L, Yi-Chung Pai 1997 Impaired proprioception and osteoarthritis. Current Opinion in Rheumatology 9: 253–258

Shoreland S 1999 Management of chronic pain following whiplash injuries. In: Gifford L (ed) Topical issues on pain. Physiotherapy Pain Association Yearbook 1998–1999. NOI Press, Falmouth, Adelaide

Siddall P J, Cousins M J 1997 Spine update. Spinal pain mechanisms. Spine 22(1): 98–104

Spitzer W O, Leblanc F E, Dupuis M et al 1987 Scientific approach to the assessment and management of activity-related spinal disorders. A monograph for physicians. Report of the Quebec Task Force on spinal disorders. Spine 12(7S): s1–59

Sweet C 1997 The role of the physiotherapist in the pain clinic. In: Wells P E, Frampton V, Bowsher D (eds) Pain management by physiotherapy. Butterworth Heinemann, Oxford

Turner J A, LeResche L, Von Korff M, Ehrlich K 1998 Back pain in primary care. Spine 23(4): 463–469

Twomey L T, Taylor J R 1994a Intensive physical rehabilitation for back pain. In: Twomey L T, Taylor J R (eds) Physical therapy of the low back, 2nd edn. Churchill Livingstone, Edinburgh

Twomey L T, Taylor J R 1994b Back and joint pain: a rationale for treatment by manual therapy. In: Twomey L T, Taylor J R (eds) Physical therapy of the low back, 2nd edn. Churchill Livingstone, Edinburgh

Waddell G 1987 A new clinical model for the treatment of low back pain. Spine 12(7): 632–644

Waddell G 1998 The back pain revolution. Churchill Livingstone, Edinburgh

Weisenberg M 1994 Cognitive aspects of pain. In: Wall P, Melzack R (eds) Textbook of pain. Churchill Livingstone, Edinburgh

Wells P E 1997 Introduction. In: Wells P E, Frampton V, Bowsher D (eds) Pain management by physiotherapy. Butterworth Heinemann, Oxford

Zusman M 1997 Instigators of activity intolerance. Manual Therapy 2(2): 75–86

FURTHER READING

Edwards B C 1992 Manual of combined movements: their use in the examination and treatment of mechanical vertebral column disorders. Churchill Livingstone, Edinburgh

Grant R (ed) 1994 Physical therapy of the cervical and thoracic spine, 2nd edn. Churchill Livingstone, Edinburgh

Grieve G P 1991 Mobilisation of the spine, 5th edn. Churchill Livingstone, Edinburgh

Lewit K 1991 Manipulative therapy in rehabilitation of the locomotor system, 2nd edn. Butterworth Heinemann, Oxford

Maitland G D 1986 Vertebral manipulation, 5th edn. Butterworths, London

McKenzie R 1981 The lumbar spine: mechanical diagnosis and therapy. Spinal Publications, Waikanae, New Zealand

Mulligan B R 1995 Manual therapy 'nags', 'snags', MWMs, etc, 3rd edn. Plant View Services, Wellington

Petty N J, Moore A P 1998 Neuromusculoskeletal examination and assessment: a handbook for therapists. Churchill Livingstone, Edinburgh

Twomey L T, Taylor R (eds) 1994 Physical therapy of the low back. Churchill Livingstone, Edinburgh

11

Posture in standing

Precise postural rules are open to dispute as familial characteristics are variables which any theory needs to take into account. Certain familial tendencies incline towards a greater lordosis whilst others have a flatter back; in both instances correction might be quite unwarranted. In addition, all physical disability will be unique to the particular person and adjustment as described here might not be in any way applicable.

However, as in all testing, there must be a standard when evaluating postural alignment. The ideal skeletal alignment used as standard is consistent with sound scientific principles, involves a minimal amount of stress and strain and is conducive to maximal efficiency of the body (Kendall et al 1993).

The three main curves of the S-shaped spine described in Chapter 1 are the link in postural alignment. Alteration of one curve affects the other two. For this reason correction of one curve without looking at and correcting the entire posture is of little value. Standard or ideal posture should require a minimum of effort to maintain but provide maximum mobility and function. Ideal posture should contain no tension and any postural correction which demands excessive muscle activity is unsustainable and incorrect.

Postural correction should never involve pulling, pushing or forcing parts of the body into a new shape. It is a repositioning not of one isolated section but of one part on the other, gently, all the way up from the feet to the head – a realignment of the whole body. For example,

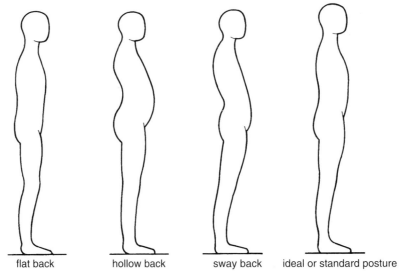

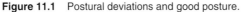

flat back   hollow back   sway back   ideal or standard posture

Figure 11.1   Postural deviations and good posture.

the most misguided advice ever given to amend a dorsal kyphosis is to 'pull your shoulders back!'. Shoulder retraction has no influence on the spinal curves. For this reason arms and shoulders have been omitted from most illustrations of postural correction, except where relevant.

The three most common deviations from ideal posture are shown in Figure 11.1 (Braggins 1994). For the sake of definition they are referred to as the **flat back posture**, the **hollow back posture** and the **sway back posture**. The hollow back may also have a thoracic kyphosis when it is known as the **kyphosis/lordosis posture** (Kendall et al 1993). Each posture should be evaluated from all views, anterior, posterior and lateral. This book will describe only the lateral view in detail; see 'Further reading' for wider information. Laterally, the entire bodily alignment is centred around an imaginary plumb line dropped to the ground from just behind the ear (Braggins 1994). Kendall et al (1993) describe a line the other way up with a fixed point starting at the base, anterior to the lateral malleolus. However, when visually describing postural correction to a patient, the suspended plumb line is a more easily acceptable image (Box 11.1, Fig. 11.2).

Box 11.1   Postural assessment

Look at overall alignment and assess 'type' of posture, noting alignment of lumbar, thoracic and cervical spines.
    Then look at:
1. foot position:
   - increased pronation/abduction (eversion) or with supination/adduction (inversion)
   - valgus or varus position of the forefoot
2. leg/heel alignment
3. tibial torsion
4. femoral medial/lateral rotation
5. hip: increased flexion/extension
6. pelvis:
   - check levels of PSIS and ASIS
   - anterior/posterior rotation
7. abdominal muscle length/strength
8. shoulder girdle: position of scapulae; possible increase in tension of upper trapezius and inefficiency of lower trapezius
9. shoulder/arm: protraction/retraction, elevation/depression; medial/lateral rotation

---

IDEAL OR STANDARD POSTURE

Standard posture should be a position of easy balance, in which the spine presents the normal curves and the bones of the lower extremities are in ideal alignment of weight bearing

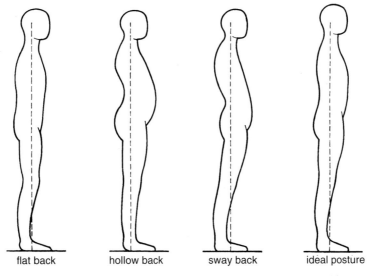

| flat back | hollow back | sway back | ideal posture |

Figure 11.2 Deviations from the centre of gravity (plumb line dropped from behind the ears).

(Kendall et al 1993). The plumb line should fall through the centre of the shoulder joint, through the centre of the hip joint, slightly towards the front of the knee, to end up just anterior to the lateral malleolus. This gives the body a slightly forwards inclination, the weight more towards the ball of the foot than the heels (Fig. 11.2) (Braggins 1994). The 'neutral' position of the pelvis is conducive to good alignment of the abdomen and trunk, while the chest and upper back are in a position that favours optimal function of the respiratory organs. The head should be erect in a well-balanced position with no flattening or exaggeration of the normal cervical lordosis (Kendall et al 1993).

A visually helpful point for patients to note is that in ideal posture, the chest is the farthest point forwards, the buttocks and heels the farthest points backwards with the body aligned evenly around the plumb line. In the sway back posture and the hollow back posture, the farthest point forwards is the abdomen with the thoracic spine the farthest to the rear. Standard posture allows the skeletal components to balance in a way that requires the smallest degree of stabilization to maintain the three vertebral curves in the ideal position.

In standard posture the heels should be about 8 cm apart and the forepart of the feet separated so that the angle of out-toeing is about 8–10° from the midline (Kendall et al 1993); the knees should face anteriorly. In the neutral pelvis position both anterior superior iliac spines (ASIS) are in the same horizontal plane and the ASIS are in the same vertical plane as the symphysis pubis, with a normal anterior curve in the low back (Kendall et al 1993). The thoracic spine should curve slightly in the posterior direction with the scapulae settled flat against the upper back. The scapulae should be level and should function equally and rhythmically with shoulder movement. Upper trapezius should be relaxed at rest. The cervical spine should be in the natural slight lordosis with chin in neutral and head held in well-balanced position.

THE FLAT BACK

The flat back may be the result of sustained sitting, often acquiring an added thoracic kyphosis. It can be the office worker's posture or the elderly person's hazard, both unaware of the need to constantly restore the lordosis on standing. In the adolescent it can result from an attempt to reduce the apparent size of the buttocks and breasts.

The lordosis is lost as a result of a posterior pelvic tilt and flattening of the lumbar spine. The thoracic kyphosis usually has a forward head posture with increased lower cervical flexion and upper cervical extension. However, correction of the pelvic tilt without looking further would neglect a fundamental point: the knees. In this posture the knees and hips can either be held in flexion (more common), leading to tight hip flexors and tight, often overactive hamstrings (Kendall et al 1993), or in hyperextension, leading to long and inhibited iliopsoas and glutei (Comerford et al 1998). Knee hyperextension is more unusual and is often actually a sway back.

THE HOLLOW BACK

The hollow back has a long, increased lordosis encompassing the lumbar and lower thoracic spine, a large abdomen with long, weak abdominal muscles and short, overactive back extensors. There is a marked anterior pelvic tilt with buttocks thrust well back. The knees can be flexed, with increased hip flexion and short overactive hamstrings (often the adolescent posture) or hyperextended (the toddler's hollow back, the pregnancy hollow back or the beer-belly hollow back). The upper thoracic spine can be pulled back or rounded with a thoracic kyphosis (the kyphosis/lordosis posture). The overall weight is thrust back towards the heels. Surprisingly, the hollow back is often found in female gymnasts (Mulhearn & George 1999).

THE SWAY BACK

The hollow back and the sway back have a certain similarity which sometimes causes confusion over postural correction. Both postures have what is mistakenly considered to be an increased lordosis. In the sway back the thoracic kyphosis is increased in length with the lumbar lordosis shortened. The misleading factor is a sharp angle in the lower lumbar spine created by the increased lower thoracic kyphosis; this is not an increased lordosis.

The sway back has come about by allowing the hips to sway forwards into hyperextension with a posterior pelvic tilt. The chest collapses inwards as the thoracic spine sways back into a kyphosis in order to compensate for the pelvic swing forwards, creating the sharp, low, angled curve at the lower lumbar spine while the upper lumbar spine is almost kyphotic; finally, the neck scoops forwards, creating a poking chin.

The sharp angle is often the source of low back pain as the weight of the trunk is thrust into L5–S1 level. The knees are pressed into hyperextension. The overall weight is usually towards the toes. It is the most common postural fault in occupations that involve prolonged standing, the 'hands-in-pocket slouch', and is common in male gymnasts (Mulhearn & George 1999).

So, in the sway back the lower lumbar spine is sharply angled into a shortened lordosis, while in the hollow back the lumbar spine makes a long, exaggerated lordotic sweep from sacrum to lower thoracic spine. The sway back has a posterior pelvic tilt and the hollow back an increased anterior pelvic tilt. If the two postures are corrected in the same manner, by correcting the pelvic tilt, the sway back will be heading for an untenable pose with possibly increased trouble rather than relief.

POSTURAL CORRECTION

Deviations from the ideal posture start from different points. When correcting posture it is therefore essential to find the lowest point at fault, even if it is not the most obvious, correcting from the feet upwards. The final correction must be the adjustment of the centre of gravity plumb line.

Feet play a vital role. Alteration of foot position can affect knee and hip alignment and finally the back. **Orthotics** should be considered for any foot abnormality that is affecting posture or gait, with referral to a podiatrist if necessary.

Certain muscles may be dysfunctional in each posture. Stabilizer muscles can be considered dysfunctional when they are either long and overstretched or inhibited and underused and

> **Box 11.2** The principles of reeducating muscular dysfunction
>
> 1. Retrain the tonic, low-threshold activation of local stabilizers.
> 2. Rehabilitate the global stabilizers to actively shorten and control limb load with low-effort sustained holds in the shortened position.
> 3. Actively lengthen and inhibit the overactive global stabilizers.

mobilizers can be considered to be dysfunctional when they are either short or overactive (Comerford et al 1998). Trunk muscles (abdominals and back extensors), glutei, iliopsoas, tensor fascia latae (TFL), iliotibial tract (ITB), hamstrings and muscles of the cervical spine all need consideration (see Chapter 17).

Full assessment must be made of muscular dysfunction before reeducation can be started. Reeducation should be carried out in a particular order (Box 11.2) (Comerford et al 1998).

Comerford (1993) suggests that it is helpful for the patient to be given little adhesive red dots to stick at strategic places all over the home or workplace. When they see the dot, they correct their posture, perform the setting action or do a stretch, whatever they have been advised to do, throughout the day.

At the end of each postural correction below, there will be advice about corrective exercises and a suggestion for the 'red dot' hold. None of the corrective exercises should produce or provoke any symptoms. All corrective movements must be totally pain free (Comerford et al 1998).

In the Figures, the faulty posture is drawn in continuous line with perfect posture superimposed in dotted line.

Teaching flat back correction

Salient points

Flexed knees, flattened lumbar spine (without thoracic kyphosis).

Possible dysfunction

Lumbar/thoracic relative flexibility; rectus

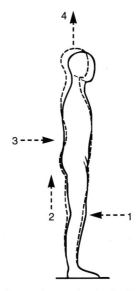

Figure 11.3 Postural correction for the flat back.

abdominis tight; iliopsoas/ITB tight; hamstrings short.

Correction (Fig. 11.3)

1. Straighten the knees. This will immediately help to correct the pelvic tilt.
2. Tip the pelvis forwards gently and increase the lordosis.
3. Straighten the upper back with the head in the upright position. Check that the overall weight is mid-foot.

Exercises

Teach TA with careful differentiation from rectus abdominis or oblique; exercises to correct any lumbar/thoracic spine relative flexibility; strengthen lumbar extensors; trunk stabilization in corrected posture; glutei and quadriceps strengthening; stretch rectus abdominis; stretch iliopsoas/ITB and hamstrings (Chapter 17).

Red dot

Knees straighten, gentle anterior pelvic tilt holds with TA.

Teaching thoracic kyphosis/forward head correction

Salient points

Increased thoracic kyphosis, shoulder protraction, lower cervical flexion and forward head posture.

Possible dysfunction

Shoulder girdle – long and inhibited lower trapezius, short and overactive pectorals; cervical spine flexors – lower short, upper long.

Correction

Figures 9.4, 11.4 and 17.32 with thoracic kyphosis and forward head. Add this correction to any other posture where necessary.

1. Suck in the thoracic spine between the scapulae so that the sternum lifts forwards (but do not lift the chest to do this).
2. Retract the chin in neutral with a feeling of lengthening the upper cervical spine.
3. Lengthen the clavicles out and down to 'set' the scapulae (this should initiate contraction

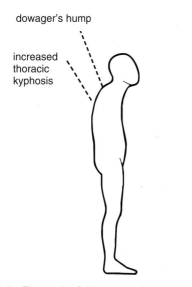

dowager's hump

increased
thoracic
kyphosis

Figure 11.4 The ageing flat back with dorsal kyphosis and forward head posture.

of lower trapezius). Correct any substitution of upper trapezius or rhomboids. The setting should be a gentle movement.

Exercises

Mobilization exercises for thoracic spine (see Figs 17.24–17.26); exercises to correct any relative flexibility of lumbar/thoracic spine; upper quadrant correction, especially lower trapezius; exercises for correcting forward head posture (see Figs 17.31–17.33).

Red dot

Postural correction.

Teaching hollow back correction

Salient points

Knees can be hyperextended or flexed; increased forward pelvic tilt; hips in increased flexion; weight on the heels. In adolescent hollow back there is often foot pronation, femoral medial rotation, tight hamstrings.

Possible dysfunction

Abdominals long and inhibited, especially obliques and rectus abdominis; back extensors short and overactive; iliopsoas/ITB short and overactive.

Correction (Fig. 11.5)

1. Check foot and knee position and correct any dysfunction.
2. If the knees are hyperextended, slacken them slightly which allows the pelvis to tilt posteriorly.
3. Hollow the abdomen, recruiting rectus abdominis, and *gently* tighten glutei to *gently* correct anterior pelvic tilt.
4. Shift the chest forwards and up. This helps to smooth out the lordosis from the top and also brings the centre of gravity forwards to midfoot.

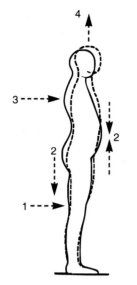

Figure 11.5 Postural correction for the hollow back.

Exercises

If relevant: shorten oblique abdominals and rectus abdominis; stabilization with abdominals in all positions; possibly use two-knee bend if foot/leg correction needs to be combined with stabilization (see Chapter 17, pp. 215–218); strengthen glutei; stretch lumbar spine extensor; stretch hip flexors/ITB; stretch hamstrings. Flexion postures for pain relief may be necessary after any prolonged standing (see Fig. 9.6).

Red dot

Abdominal hollowing with rectus abdominis hold.

Teaching sway back correction

The moves in this postural correction may be difficult to accomplish because of the several unfamiliar shifts of direction but once achieved, it is surprisingly easy to become adept at instantaneous correction.

Salient points

Hips thrust forwards; knees pressed back; chest dropped with resulting rounding of the thoracic spine; poking chin; weight towards the front of the feet.

Possible dysfunction

Erector spinae and LM long and inhibited; TA and oblique abdominals long and inhibited, rectus abdominis short and overactive; upper quadrant – lower trapezius long and inhibited, pectorals short and overactive; cervical flexors – upper long and inhibited and lower short and overactive; iliopsoas long and inhibited, ITB short and overactive; hamstrings often short and overactive.

Figure 11.6 shows a comparison between the sway back and standard posture which may help to clarify the faults.

Correction (Fig. 11.7)

It is important to think in terms of body 'realignment', adjusting one part on the other. It is most important to remain relaxed and to feel this movement rather than force it.

1. Transfer the whole body weight back onto the heels. Do not tilt the pelvis anteriorly.
2. Keep the body steady from the waist down, shift the chest forwards by sucking in the thoracic spine and gently lifting the sternum. Do not extend the thoracic spine by arching back. Do not pull the shoulders back. The shoulders should be relaxed but do not collapse the thoracic spine as the shoulders relax. Or imagine standing facing a chest-high fence; leave the hips and head where they are, then raise the chest forwards and up over the fence. A third image to work on if the other two have failed is to imagine someone is prodding you between the scapulae. Pull the thoracic spine in away from the prod without pulling the shoulders back.
3. TA will often spontaneously react; if not, initiate the setting.
4. Correct the head posture by gentle upper cervical flexion and lower trapezius setting.

In the sway back correction there should be no tension. Every alteration should be a gentle repositioning rather than a forced hold. In a

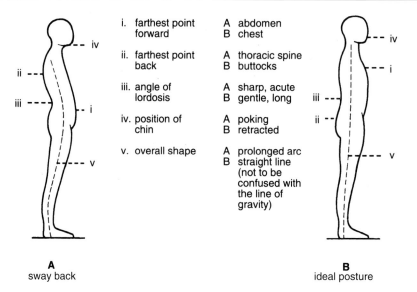

	A	B
i. farthest point forward	abdomen	chest
ii. farthest point back	thoracic spine	buttocks
iii. angle of lordosis	sharp, acute	gentle, long
iv. position of chin	poking	retracted
v. overall shape	prolonged arc	straight line (not to be confused with the line of gravity)

A
sway back

B
ideal posture

Figure 11.6 Comparing the sway back with ideal posture.

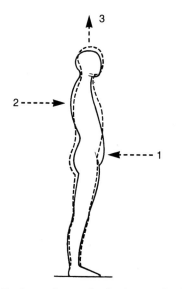

Figure 11.7 Postural correction for the sway back.

good correction the abdominals often spontaneously react.

Exercises

TA/LM in all stabilizing positions with upper quadrant correction (Figs 17.1–17.15); strengthen lower cervical extensors and upper cervical flexors (Figs 17.31–17.33); if short, stretch hamstrings (Figs 17.42–17.43).

Red dot

Constant postural correction

CARE IN STANDING

Standing is one of the most stressful maintained positions. If the lordosis increases, creep occurs with further movement into extension as the soft tissues adjust to fluid loss; the posterior annulus of the disc is compressed and the disc loses fluid; the facet joints lose flow of nutrients across their structures; muscles become fatigued through impaired blood supply. If thoracic slouch increases, creep occurs in flexion with relative changes in tissue fluid content and pain.

Standing with arms folded or hands clasped in front are substitution techniques, using the arms instead of the trunk muscle to support the spine. They should be avoided.

1. Avoid standing in a faulty posture.
2. Correct posture frequently.
3. Constantly initiate TA and hold.

4. Keep a wide base.
5. Change position of feet frequently, shifting the weight from one leg to another, but do not hang on one hip.
6. Sit for 5 minutes if possible.
7. Put one foot up on a step or stool for a short period; this changes the position of the lumbar spine and sacroiliac joint.
8. Slacken the knees occasionally which tends to relax the lordosis; avoid pressing them into hyperextension.
9. Rock the pelvis into anterior and posterior tilt.
10. Stand with the back against a wall and flatten the lumbar spine for a few minutes.
11. Move around as much as possible, if only to shift position.
12. Wear good shoes.

WALKING

The most important aspect of postural correction to pass on to patients is the need for trunk stabilization whilst the limbs do the work. The trunk stabilizes, while the arms at the top defend the body and manipulate objects and the legs below transport the body forwards, upwards and downwards. Stress is placed on the vertebral column when the trunk is used to perform work which the limbs should do, for example incorrect lifting, but even sloppy walking may destabilize the muscular system.

Correct walking pattern

The trunk should be stabilized, allowing a natural arm swing, which activates gentle trunk rotation; the push-off of the rear leg should propel the body forwards with minimal accent on the forward step.

Common incorrect walking patterns

- Excessive upper thoracic rotation with stiff, bent arm swing used for propulsion.
- Excessive pelvic dorsolumbar rotation with pelvic roll on the forward leg and drop on the back leg (the model's walk).

- Overpull of hamstrings on the forward leg to drag the body forwards, with lack of gluteal contraction and toe push-off on the rear leg.
- Increased alternate lateral flexion with minimal leg/foot activity (the older person's walk).

Correction

Teach weight transference with the sternum leading; stabilize the trunk and consciously activate the rear leg gluteal muscles to push the body forwards with a strong plantarflexion push of the rear foot (Comerford et al 1998).

Exercise

Stand with one foot in front of the other with full weight on rear foot. Palpate multifidus on the rear foot side and move the body weight forwards onto the front foot. Control pelvic rotation. Multifidus should activate just after heel lift (Comerford et al 1998). Repeat if dysfunctional. Constantly correct walking at all times. Teach functional stabilization from page 214.

FOOTWEAR
Shoes

Shoes must be wide enough to allow all toes to function freely, otherwise postural balance cannot be maintained. Shoes should grip the heels well so that they remain in place on toe push of the rear leg; if the shoe is loose the foot is held in a cramped position in order to hold the shoe on. This will alter the movement pattern of walking.

High heels

High heels affect posture in different ways depending upon postural type and ankle mobility. Good plantarflexion ROM allows the foot to be comfortable in a high heel whilst the knees remain straight and the lumbar lordosis is unaffected, though there might be a tendency towards an increased lordosis. With restricted plantarflexion, the knees are unable to straighten and the body tends to tip forwards with flexed knees and a flattened lordosis. High heels should be avoided when standing or walking for long periods. However, with shortened calf muscles a slightly heightened heel may be more comfortable.

REFERENCES

Braggins S 1994 The back: functions, malfunctions and care. Mosby Yearbook, London
Comerford M 1993 Personal communication
Comerford M, Kinetic Control 1998 Dynamic stability and muscle balance of the lumbar spine and trunk. Course notes, Kinetic Control Ltd, Harrow

Kendall F P, McCreary E K, Provance P G 1993 Muscle testing and function, 3rd edn. Williams and Wilkins Baltimore
Mulhearn S, George K 1999 Abdominal muscle endurance and its association with low back pain. Physiotherapy 85(4): 210–214

FURTHER READING

Kendall F P, McCreary E K, Provance P G 1993 Muscle testing and function, 3rd edn. Williams and Wilkins, Baltimore

12

Posture in sitting

Every day people sit for hours, both at work and at leisure. Body language plays a big role in sitting postures with the open-legged, laid back macho image on the one hand and the cross-legged, weight on one hip seductive pose on the other. There is also the 'gorilla' pose of resting both hands on the thighs, arms medially rotated and elbows abducted, substituting the arms for trunk stabilization. A number of patients use a similar substitution when sitting on the plinth – hands on either side, pushing hard with their elbow extensors; this is excusable when used to protect an acute LBP but should be corrected as a habitual pose.

Most people sit badly, either from lack of physical awareness or because it is impossible to sit well in a poorly designed chair. Sitting in the lordotic posture results in less back pain than sitting in a kyphotic posture (Williams et al 1991). However, the critical factor is the length of time the position is maintained. Any static posture is detrimental but sitting badly for long periods is more abusive than sitting well.

Good posture in sitting should not have to be an effort; the chair should be designed to maintain the correct position. Manufacturers are producing ergonomically designed car and office chairs but easy-chair design lags behind, accentuating the luxurious feel and appearance rather than ergonomic efficiency.

In sitting the pelvis tends to rotate posteriorly with the lumbar spine falling into flexion. In flexion, the lumbar intervertebral discs are compressed anteriorly and stretched posteriorly

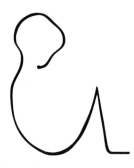

Figure 12.1 Sitting with knees high.

with increased intradiscal pressure exerted towards the posterior annulus (see Fig. 3.5). The soft tissues of the posterior element of the motion segment are all on stretch and creep occurs, allowing the vertebrae to move further into flexion as the tissues readjust to fluid loss. The longer the position is maintained, the greater are the changes (Twomey & Taylor 1994).

Intradiscal pressure in sitting is least in the supported, upright or slightly inclined backwards posture but it increases with removal of the support and further increases when leaning forwards with a flexed lumbar spine (Andersson et al 1975, 1979).

The position of the knees is crucial to the degree of flexion in the lumbar spine (Keegan 1953). The higher the knees are raised, the greater is lumbar flexion (Fig. 12.1). This is relevant to the slope of chair seats: the further the seat is tipped backwards, the higher the knees are raised and the more the lumbar spine is forced into flexion. The lower the thighs are placed, the easier it is to maintain the lumbar lordosis. The optimum comfort of the lumbar spine is achieved when the legs are placed at about 45° of hip flexion (Keegan 1953). A forward-sloping seat mimics this position.

An example of the influence of leg position upon the lumbar spine can be seen when comparing a normal riding position with the position used by the racing jockey (Fig. 12.2). In the former the legs are supported in stirrups in 45° hip flexion and the lumbar lordosis is well maintained; in the latter the shortened stirrups bring the hips and knees into almost complete flexion, forcing the spine into a curve.

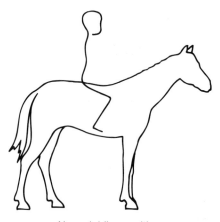

Normal riding position

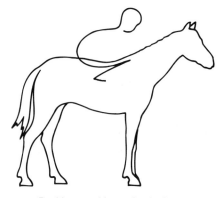

Position used by racing jockeys

Figure 12.2 The effect of change of leg position on the lumbar spine.

The comfort of the sloping thigh position has been used for generations by children who spontaneously tip their chairs forwards when working at a desk or table (Mandal 1984). The principle was adopted by the Balans chair, designed and manufactured in Norway (Fig. 12.3). Although this design puts pressure on the knees and is not necessarily comfortable for many people, the principle is now being incorporated into the design of office chairs with seats that can be tilted forwards.

GENERAL CHAIR DESIGN

The ideal chair should be one in which the hips can be placed right at the back of the seat whilst

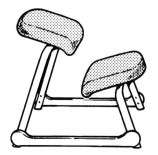

Figure 12.3   The Balans chair – basic design.

the thighs are well supported but with no up-ward pressure against the thighs and no pressure behind the knees. Both feet should rest easily on the floor. There should be good support in the backrest, especially in the lumbar area, maintaining the lordosis and preventing a slump into flexion. The chair should be easy to rise from without effort.

The basic principle is that sitting as in Figure 12.4 should be avoided whilst sitting as in Figures 12.5 and 12.6 gives correct back support. A particularly bad backrest can be found in some rail carriage seats or some particularly expensive-looking office chairs, those that have a high, heavily padded backrest. In both these examples the lumbar support is too low, causing a thrust forwards on the sacrum which forces the low lumbar spine to float back into flexion above the support (Fig. 12.7).

The principle of providing good support for the lordosis applies to all backs apart from

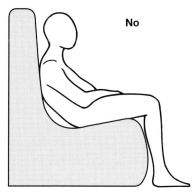

Figure 12.4   Unsupported sitting in the wrong chair.

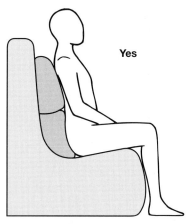

Figure 12.5   Support with cushions.

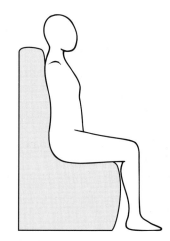

Figure 12.6   Sitting – the right way.

people with certain upper lumbar lesions or with spondylolisthesis who are more comfort-able sitting in slight lumbar flexion.

All chairs should be on good castors for easy moving.

The easy chair

The most common fault of easy-chair design is the exaggerated seat depth. In many chairs it is impossible to sit both with the hips at the back of the chair and the feet flat on the floor (Fig. 12.4). If using a chair like this cannot be avoided, then the back should be supported with cushions as in Figure 12.5.

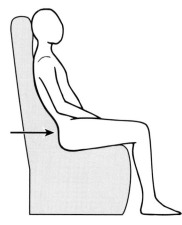

Figure 12.7   Seat with lumbar support too low.

Guidelines for choosing an easy chair

- The depth of the seat should be less than the length of the sitter's thigh.
- The chair should be large enough to allow easy change of position yet small enough to give support where necessary.
- The backrest should provide good lumbar support.
- The backrest should be at an angle of 105–110° to the seat.
- The chair should not be too low.
- The seat should not slope backwards excessively.
- Armrests should be high enough to support the arms with elbows bent at a right angle, avoiding upward pressure on the elbow. All knitters and needleworkers should be careful to avoid using chairs where the armrests get in the way of their elbow movement; if the armrests are too high or if the chair is too narrow, the lack of freedom will encourage hunched shoulders and tension in the neck and shoulder area.

When purchasing easy chairs people should be discouraged from being attracted merely by the appearance or the initial luxurious feel. It is important to sit in a chair for some time to test the comfort. Some easy-chair manufacturers are now offering a range of measurements for the depth of seats and the height of backrests for differing sizes in one family. This should be considered.

The working/office chair

Chair design should be considered as an integral part of task and workshop design (Brunswick 1984) (Fig. 12.8).

The seat

- The seat depth should be less than the length of the user's thighs.
- The seat should be rounded on the front edge to avoid upward pressure.

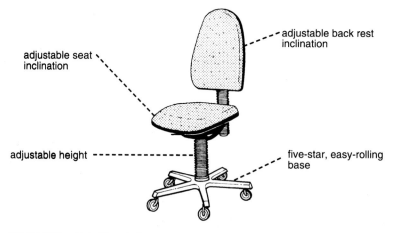

Figure 12.8   The office chair.

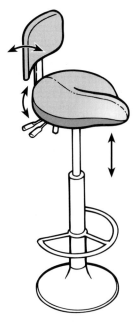

Figure 12.9 The saddle seat. (Reproduced from HMSO 1998, after Vezina N, Geoffrion L, Lajoie A et al 1993 Les contraintes du poste de caissière du supermarché et l'essai de bancs assis-debout. Cinbiose – UQAM November: 1–44. Crown copyright material is reproduced with permission of Her Majesty's Stationery Office.)

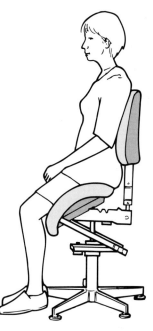

Figure 12.10 A prototype sit-stand seat with backrest. (Reproduced with permission from HMSO 1998, after Corlett & Gregg 1994. Crown copyright material is reproduced with permission of Her Majesty's Stationery Office.)

- A saddle-shaped seat has been found to be of help in certain sit/stand occupations (HSE 1998) (Fig. 12.9). The seat should be adjustable to facilitate variation in the slope from front to back. In office chairs, the angle of inclination should be adaptable from 5° to 15° forward slope (Mandal 1984). For occupations involving a frequent change of position from sitting to standing, a particular sit/stand chair allows a curved-down seat which rotates further forwards as the chair is raised (Fig. 12.10). Portable wedges which create the downward slope can be used in any chair (see Patient Handouts).
- The seat should be upholstered in non-slip, comfortable material.

Height from the floor

Office chairs should have a height adjustment facility to accommodate changes in worktop levels. Footrests should be used if the seat is too high and cannot be adjusted. For occupations which involve frequent change of position, higher, more adjustable sit/stand chairs offer a solution (Fig. 12.10) (HSE 1998).

The backrest

- The backrest should be firm but not hard, with a convex curve to provide lumbar support at waist level.
- The height of the backrest should be adjustable. There is a maze of conflicting recommendations about the positioning of lumbar supports and people choose varying heights; fat people seem to prefer high supports and slim people lower (Coleman et al 1998). People often fail to use them at all but when made aware of them and after experimenting, they tend to adjust supports higher (Coleman et al 1998).
- The correct inclination depends upon the position of the head and the angle of work in relation to the eyes. The angle should be

adjustable between 90° and 100° (Boyling 1992), though some visual display unit (VDU) operators have chosen inclinations varying from 104° to 110°, depending upon the position of their screens (Hayne 1984) (see VDU operation, p. 190).

The base of the chair

Office chairs should be on a five-star, swivel base to allow for quick change of direction without awkward movement. The base should be wider than the seat for stability.

Lever adjustments

All lever adjustments should be comfortable to use and easy to operate.

Armrests

Armrests must support the arms with the elbows bent at a right angle. Care must be taken that they are not too high, pushing up the shoulders. The advantage of armrests in providing support has to be weighed against the disadvantage of them getting in the way as the office worker swings the chair round between computer and other desktop work. In some offices it is preferable to remove them in order to prevent workers twisting repeatedly.

Car seats

All previous guidelines for sitting apply to car seats. Some manufacturers are now designing fully adaptable seats with individually adjustable lumbar supports in the backrest. Driving is a stressful activity, causing postural awkwardness in wheel turning and gear changing, to say nothing of the emotional tension of motorway madness (Twomey & Taylor 1994).

- Sit as far from the pedals as possible, with the legs as straight as it is safe to drive (Fig. 12.11).
- The backrest should be inclined at about 100–110° so that driving can be performed with comfortably bent arms. Leaning back and steering with straight arms puts strain on the upper thoracic area.
- A wedge can be used to correct increased hip flexion from a backward sloping seat and is helpful with leg pain.
- Adjust the headrest close to the back of the head, level with the top of the ears.
- When buying a car, make sure that the height of the interior allows the driver to sit upright, looking straight out of the windscreen, without having to slouch into a forward head posture.

Casual chairs

If a particular lifestyle entails frequent changes of environment with different chairs, some lack-

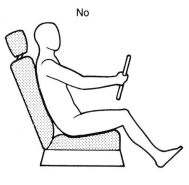

No

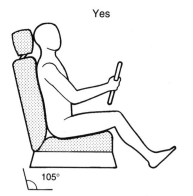

Yes

105°

back rest angle of inclination approx 105°

Figure 12.11 Car seats.

ing adequate lumbar support, it is advisable to take a small cushion around, moving it from chair to chair when necessary. There are several different lumbar support cushions or rolls on the market but it is advisable to try to borrow one on approval first to test it thoroughly before buying (see Patient Handouts).

Rocking chairs

Use of the rocking chair is strongly recommended by Wyke (1987) as a therapeutic means of reducing pain. The rhythmical oscillations of the body as it rocks to and fro activate the motion segment mechanoreceptors, modulating the painful input, an example of the gate control mechanism working in everyday life. The rocking chair also assists pulmonary ventilation and augments the venous return from the lower limbs (Wyke 1987).

GUIDELINES FOR CARE IN SITTING

Sitting is a potentially provocative position for the back when maintained for long periods.

1. Hips should be placed right into the back of the seat.
2. The lumbar spine should be well supported in the natural lordosis for each person.
3. Avoid sitting in one position for long periods; shift position or stand up and walk around at intervals.
4. On long car journeys get out and stretch at regular intervals, restoring the lordosis with a good arch (see Fig. 9.4).
5. Avoid rising from sitting with the back still in flexion; always arch the back as in Figure 9.4.
6. Avoid sitting with both legs up on a stool. If this is necessary for medical reasons, a reclining chair must be used, so that the back is resting in a half-lying position. The maintained long-sitting position can prolong or even create sciatica pain (see Patient Handouts).
7. Avoid sitting propped up in bed for the same reason. Raise the TV and lower the pillows.
8. Likewise, avoid sitting for hours on the floor propped against furniture with both legs straight out in front. When this position is used in yoga or other therapy it is an active stretch rather than a passive maintained position and is therapeutically beneficial. If the floor is a favourite spot for sitting, then change poses frequently. Use cushions for extra support.
9. Sitting with the legs crossed is inadvisable with sciatic pain and for venous return. It decreases the activity of the abdominal obliques and could affect sacroiliac pain positively or negatively (see Snijders et al 1995).
10. Avoid sitting with both legs sideways up on the seat for longer than 10 minutes; change position frequently or preferably avoid it altogether. This is another position that can enhance leg pain referral.
11. Get into a car by sitting first and then swinging the legs in. Be especially careful during periods of intermittent LBP.

SCHOOL FURNITURE

School life imposes one of the most sedentary occupations upon children and the sitting habits developed in these formative years can affect their future behaviour and physical structure (Yeats 1997). Caldwell (1994) reported the shortcomings in current classroom design in the US and the possible effects of environment on concentration, behaviour and learning.

In 1997 the NBPA formed a working party to review school furniture and fitness in relation to children in the UK. Taylour (1997), compiling the results of the working party, reported a considerable criticism of school furniture, with 68% of furniture in some schools unfit for use. The total cost of replacing furniture would amount to £500 million.

The British Standards specification for school furniture has been in operation since 1950, with little success (Taylour 1997). However, the European Standard for Educational Furniture is due to be issued in the near future. Innovative design is being encouraged, reflecting the Scandinavian health-driven attitude to furniture (Taylour 1997).

The working posture of children is divided equally between the backward-leaning and forward-leaning positions and this fact should be taken into consideration in designing new furniture (Linton et al 1994). The NBPA report cites Medd (1981) who believes that school furniture should possess the characteristics of variety, versatility, mobility and compatibility. There is no doubt that school furniture should, in a basic and least expensive way, copy the office design of an adaptable chair and an adjustable desktop (see School Pupils in the Patient Handouts).

There is also an educational need for teachers and pupils to understand ergonomics and receive practical help in adjusting and using the furniture correctly (Linton et al 1994).

There is now overwhelming scientific evidence to suggest that the careful selection, use and management of school furniture can play a major part in helping to reverse the back pain epidemic as well as significantly improving behaviour and alertness in the classroom (Linton et al 1994, Storr-Paulsen & Aagaard-Hensen 1994, Taylour 1997, Yeats 1997).

REFERENCES

Andersson B J G, Ortengren R, Nachemson A L, Elstrom G, Broman H 1975 The sitting posture. An electromyographic and discometric study. Orthopedic Clinics of North America 6(1): 105–120.

Andersson B J G, Murphy R W, Ortengren R, Nachemson A 1979 The influence of back rest inclination and lumbar support on lumbar lordosis. Spine 4(1): 52–58

Boyling J D 1992 Personal communication

Brunswick M 1984 Ergonomics of seat design. Physiotherapy 70(2): 40–43

Caldwell B S 1994 The learning-friendly classroom. Ergonomics in Design 1: 30–35

Coleman N, Hull B P, Ellitt G 1998 An empirical study of preferred settings for lumbar support on adjustable office chairs. Ergonomics 4(4): 401–419

Corlett E N, Gregg H 1994 Seating and access to work. In: Weber R, Noro K (eds) Hard facts about soft machines. Taylor and Francis, London

Hayne C R 1984 Ergonomics and back pain. Physiotherapy 70(1): 9–13

Health and Safety Executive (HSE) 1998 Musculoskeletal disorders in supermarket cashiers. HMSO, London

Keegan J J 1953 Alterations of the lumbar curve related to posture and seating. Journal of Bone and Joint Surgery 35: 589–603

Linton S J, Hellsing A-L, Halme T, Kerstin A 1994 The effects of ergonomically designed school furniture on pupils' attitudes, symptoms and behaviour. Applied Ergonomics 25(5): 299–304

Mandal A C 1984 The correct height of school furniture. Physiotherapy 70(2): 48–53

Medd D 1981 Variety, mobility and compatibility. Extract from PEB Exchange, FIRA archives library, Maxwell Rd, Stevenage, Herts. Cited in NBPA 1997

NBPA 1997 Furniture + fitness = healthy attentive pupils. National Back Pain Association, Teddington

Snijders C J, Slagter A H E, van Strik R et al 1995 Why leg crossing? The influence of common postures on abdominal activity. Spine 20: 1989–1993

Storr-Paulsen A, Aagaard-Hensen J 1994 The working positions of schoolchildren. Applied Ergonomics 25(1): 63–64

Taylour J 1997 Furniture and fitness = healthy and attentive pupils. Children's Working Party. National Back Pain Association, Teddington

Twomey L T, Taylor J R 1994 The lumbar spine, low back pain, and physical therapy. In: Twomey L T, Taylor J R (eds) Physical therapy of the low back, 2nd edn. Churchill Livingstone, New York

Williams M M, Hawley J A, McKenzie R A et al 1991 A comparison of the effects of two sitting postures on back and referred pain. Spine 16(10): 1185–1191

Wyke B 1987 The neurology of low back pain. In: Jayson M I V (ed) The lumbar spine and back pain, 3rd edn. Churchill Livingstone, Edinburgh

Yeats B 1997 Factors that may influence the postural health of school children. Work 9(1): 45–55

13

Posture in lying

There are no rules about the correct way to lie. It is best to lie in the most comfortable position. Stretching and moving freely in bed adds movement and change of position to the resting period and should be encouraged. Sleep is part of the natural regenerative process and so is movement.

For acute pain, follow the advice suggested in Chapter 16. Any pillow support used for pain relief should be discarded as soon as possible to restore freedom.

TYPES OF BEDS

Medical opinion used to be in favour of extra firm beds, even to the extent of advocating sleeping on the floor. Gradually we have come to realize that the body contours are un-supported on a hard surface, with gravity tending to influence the direction of the spinal curves; if these curves are without buttress during sleep, they are under stress.

Figures 13.1–13.6 show the effect on the back of hard, soft and firm beds with comments by the side. The firm bed with the undulating surface is obviously the better choice.

BED DESIGN

Fillings

'Fillings' are the many types of materials used for upholstering mattresses and are put together in different combinations. They consist of

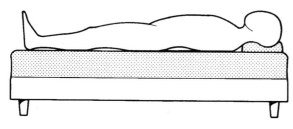

gravity tending to pull the lumbar spine down, the bed giving no support

Figure 13.1   A hard bed.

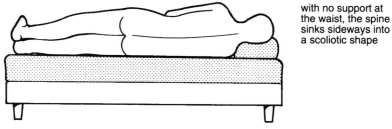

with no support at the waist, the spine sinks sideways into a scoliotic shape

Figure 13.2   A hard bed.

The sagging bed causes the lumbar spine to round into flexion

The sagging bed causes the whole body to lose good alignment

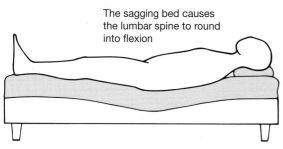

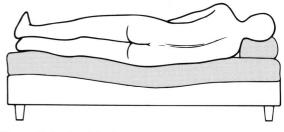

Figure 13.3   A soft bed.

Figure 13.4   A soft bed.

the firm bed with soft surface undulates with the body's curves

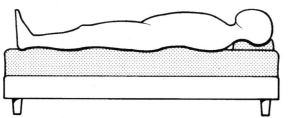

Figure 13.5   A firm bed.

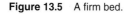

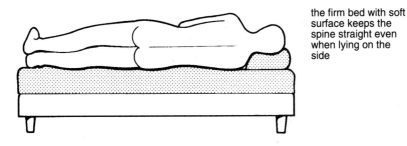

the firm bed with soft surface keeps the spine straight even when lying on the side

Figure 13.6   A firm bed.

approximately three layers and lie immediately under the mattress cover. The variation in combination greatly influences the comfort and finally differentiates one product from another. The choice is a matter of personal taste (Sleep Council 1999).

Mattress construction

Mattresses can be made from springs, foam or latex or they can be water filled. Sprung mattresses are constructed in three different ways: with open springs, continuous springs and pocketed springs. Certain manufacturers combine one or more methods (Sleep Council 1999).

Open springs

The open-spring mattress consists of rows of hourglass-shaped upright springs which are joined to neighbouring springs by a helical wire. The gauge of the wire and the number of springs can vary and on the best units, the edge of the spring unit is strengthened by a heavy-gauge border rod, top and bottom. Open springs of varying quality are used in everything from budget beds to the luxury end of the market, where the spring count is usually higher (Sleep Council 1999).

Continuous springs

The continuous spring is a variation of the open spring, made by forming a single length of wire into coils up and down the mattress. The result is the softest and possibly the most luxurious feel, but with minimal support (NBF 1988).

Pocketed spring

The pocketed-spring mattress has rows of individual upright springs, which are separately housed in fabric pockets, making them better able to operate independently, to give more individual support. At the point of any bony protuberance, the individual springs will give whilst the surrounding springs remain in place supporting the hollows. In this way every part of the body receives constant support regardless of positional change. When two people sleep in a bed, pocketed springs reduce the tendency to roll together towards the middle. The degree of firmness depends upon the number of springs in the mattress, which can be from 500 to 1200 (NBF 1988). So a pocketed-spring mattress can vary from being relatively soft to extremely firm. The more expensive and those with a reputation for particular luxury are the hand-finished products with exclusive fillings (Sleep Council 1999)

Foam and latex mattresses

Polyurethane foams are flexible, versatile and resilient with greatly improved fire retardant characteristics. Latex foam is a natural product of the sap obtained from rubber trees and is considered a luxury quality product. It is distinctive, resilient and provides excellent durability. A major benefit of these mattresses is that they do not need to be turned regularly

(Sleep Council 1999). Heavier mattresses have a greater durability than lighter weight ones and in this type of mattress, price can be a guide to value. The non-allergic properties of these mattresses make them particularly suitable for people who are affected by the natural fillings used in spring systems (NBF 1988).

The 'orthopaedic' mattress

'Orthopaedic' mattresses often combine the open coil and pocketed spring, achieving the firmest possible support, but the label means very little since they have no special medical properties (NBF 1988). This does not mean that people who already have an 'orthopaedic' mattress and sleep well should be put off it; however, when purchasing a new bed, it is worth ignoring all publicity and carefully choosing one that feels right for you.

Water beds

Water beds provide an even distribution of support and are especially important for reducing pressure points for disabled people (Sleep Council 1999). Most water beds rest on a wooden base but some are supported on all sides by springing (NBF 1988).

Summary

With the vast range of mattresses available, the final choice lies with the purchaser, providing the rules of support mentioned earlier are fulfilled. Never buy a bed for its name or solely by recommendation. Test the bed personally. Lie on it in the shop, not just for a second but for several minutes and test it in the way described in Box 13.1. Some firms make custom-built beds especially calculated to accommodate particular weights and heights. If two people are of very different weights, it is worth considering two single beds of different firmness, zipped together. It is important to remember that the best bed is not necessarily the most expensive.

Details of types of bases and padding, and general bed-buying advice can be obtained from

Box 13.1 Buying a new bed
• Take time over the choice – this is one purchase that cannot be returned.
• Make sure the base is firm.
• Choose a pocketed spring or mixed mattress.
• The more springs there are, the firmer it will be, therefore heavier people require more springs and lighter people fewer.
• If two people are sharing a bed, they should lie on it together and should not roll to the middle of the bed.
• If two people of different sizes are sharing a bed, consider a zip-up mattress with different firmness in each bed.
• Lie on the bed to test its comfort – do not prod it or sit on it.
• If you can push your hand into a gap between the lumbar spine and the bed, it is too firm; if you cannot push your hand in at all, the bed is too soft (Sleep Council 1999).
• Turning over on the mattress should be easy.

the Sleep Council, whose address is in the Useful Addresses section.

PILLOWS

People tend to sleep on too many pillows. In any pillow-less lying position, the gap between head and bed is much smaller than one imagines; when side lying, the shoulder accommodates so that the ear is much closer to the bed than the actual gap between ear and shoulder tip when standing. When lying supine, two pillows push the head into flexion and can induce neck problems and head aches; in side lying the head is pushed into lateral flexion unless the person has very broad shoulders.

One soft, malleable pillow is usually sufficient to fill the gap in any position and is all that is required unless the person has a heart condition, a hiatus hernia, asthma or any other state which requires a high pillow rest. If the thoracic spine has acquired an increased kyphosis it may be too late to reduce the pillow height. During an episode of lower cervical or thoracic spine pain it might be necessary to increase pillow height temporarily.

The softest pillows are feather or down but if manmade fibre is preferred, the proviso is that a hollow in the centre should remain indented and that the pillow is not too thick. Foam rubber is not good for this reason, as it resumes its own shape and never adapts to head contours. Similarly, a shaped pillow cannot adapt to change of position. A malleable pillow can be formed into a 'butterfly' shape, with a hollow in the centre and two 'wings' on either side; this allows the head to nestle in the centre, supported by billowing pillow on both sides.

Sleeping prone is bad for the neck if the head is maintained in rotation but it can be a good position for the lumbar spine. The problem can

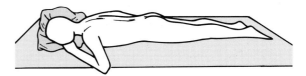

Figure 13.7 Sleeping prone with pillow supporting the head in a non-rotated position.

be solved by bunching up the pillow to form a slope so that the cheek can be rested against it with the face and nose pointing towards the mattress (Fig. 13.7).

REFERENCES

National Bed Federation (NBF) 1988 A selling guide. National Bed Federation London

Sleep Council 1999 Sleep good, feel good. Sponsored by the National Bed Federation. Sleep Council, Skipton

14

Posture in manual handling

Heavy manual labour, repeated lifting of more than 25 lbs, lifting away from the body and twisting while lifting have been verified by epidemiological studies as being major factors for the development of LBP (Kelsey et al 1984, Twomey & Taylor 1994, Fathallah et al 1998).

Since 1992 (HSE 1992) there have been regulations and guidelines for health and safety at work which alerted employers and workers to the dangers of manual handling activities. Employers have been required to avoid manual handling operations where it is practicable to do so and where it is not, to assess the risk and take appropriate action to reduce it (Mcelwaine 1998). Complying with this approach can work, so why are there still 50 000 handling accidents per year? Why does the proportion of manual handling accidents to all accidents remain the same and the number of musculoskeletal disorders caused by work remain the same (Mcelwaine 1998)? Maybe the answer lies in evidence that suggests there is a need to practise back care off duty as well as at work (Blamire 1995).

The previous chapters of this book have emphasized the forces acting on backs which predispose to injury: sustained standing, prolonged stooping, twisting and reaching forward in the flexed position, frequent bending and lifting. These movements are part of the daily routine in the work and domestic life of all people (Straker 1989, Blamire 1995, HSC 1998). Backs must be protected during work but misuse must also be prevented when off duty (Crozier & Cozens 1998).

This should be one of the key elements in manual handling training.

All manual handling represents a hazard but although an episode of pain may appear to stem from one particular incident, it is the cumulative effect of general postural stress that causes the incident to 'trigger' the pain (HSE 1992). Large, obvious weights are not always the most injurious; it is frequently the insignificant movement of adjusting a patient's pillows or lifting a half-filled bag out of a supermarket trolley that provokes back injury (Cholewicki & McGill 1996). These are the moments when for one reason or another the muscles of the trunk fail to stabilize.

The aim of efficient movement is to establish habitual patterns of natural movement which operate with the least effort, while preserving the natural elasticity of the body tissues, with the least amount of cumulative strain (Crozier & Cozens 1998). This applies to occupational and domestic activities at all times. Everyone should learn to function with patterns of movement involving the limbs working with a stabilized back.

Lifting involves a set of movement principles embodied in a 'skill framework' which facilitates variation of safe and effective musculoskeletal function. The principles of good practice should be taught, giving staff the flexibility and responsibility to apply and adapt the principles to situations as they present themselves. Understanding, awareness, motor skill and behaviour are influential factors on the performance of lifting; the whole body is important, not only the back (Crozier & Cozens 1998, Sedgwick & Gormley 1998).

Stress and strain on the back are not solely products of the workplace and for this reason good practice in manual handling must be taught as a 'philosophy for life' applicable to all activities, including non-loading movement and posture (Blamire 1995).

THE PREVENTION OF INJURY

Many university ergonomic research units have investigated back problems, especially in health service workers, continuing to search for answers to the secrets of prevention. Does it lie in careful selection of workers, in diligent training or in ergonomics, designing the job to fit the worker (Snook 1978, Robens Institute 1986, Pheasant & Stubbs 1994, Klaber-Moffett et al 1995)?

Selection

There is no proven strategy for identifying individuals who might be at risk in heavy lifting tasks (Robens Institute 1986) and there is no evidence to associate anthropometric measurement with back pain or injury, with the exception of obesity (Hollingdale 1997). The selection of staff remains a matter of subjective skill and experience of the examiner (Troup 1977).

Training

Although studies have not yet provided clear evidence that training alone reduces the prevalence of back disorders (Robens Institute 1986, Birnbaum et al 1991, Hollingdale 1997), they do show that people can successfully lift heavy objects in any position providing they are well trained to do so (Twomey 1992). So, meticulous, well-monitored training is essential.

Ergonomics

The European Manual Handling Directive of May 1990 (EEC Council 1990), brought into effect in January 1993, gave new legislation based on the ergonomic approach. It requires employers to assess the handling of loads in their organization and to prevent reasonably foreseeable injuries to employees as a result of load handling (Birnbaum et al 1991).

Ergonomics combined with expert and well-monitored training, is the best way to approach the problem of manual handling, looking at the equipment, the task, the load, the environment and the individual. Risk assessment is the first crucial step. The following is a compilation of guidelines drawn up by the Robens Institute (1986), the HSE (1992), the RCN (1996) and the HSC (1998).

Risk assessment

Decide if there is a problem; decide who might be harmed and how; evaluate risks and decide whether existing precautions are adequate or if more should be taken; record findings; review assessment from time to time.

The equipment

- Equipment must be easy to operate and maintain, compatible with other pieces of equipment, compatible with the space required for it, well designed for the task for which it is to be used and well maintained.
- Essential pieces of equipment are: sliding aids for moving patients; hoists; handling belts; special beds for intensive care wards; chairs of various heights with removable arms; trolleys for transport; efficient levers and pulleys attached to machinery.
- Increased space may be necessary – larger toilets and bathrooms, fewer beds in the ward; new uniforms providing greater freedom of movement.

The task

Does it involve:

- prolonged postural stress, e.g. holding the load at a distance from the body, stooping or stretching?
- awkward movements beyond easy reach?
- the load being moved, lifted, lowered over a long distance?
- the risk of sudden movement of the load?
- frequent or prolonged physical effort?
- insufficient rest or recovery periods?
- insufficient provision of stools or chairs to reduce stress?
- insufficient staff, causing one person to perform a task which should be carried out by two?

The load

Is it heavy, bulky or unwieldy, difficult to grasp, unstable or with contents likely to shift or spill; is it sharp, hot or potentially damaging?

The environment

Is or are there:

- space for easy transport of equipment?
- space constraints preventing good posture?
- uneven, slippery, unstable floors, unnecessary stairs or slopes?
- variation in work surfaces?
- adequate heating, ventilation and lighting?
- insufficient storage facilities?

The individual

Does:

- the job require unusual strength, height or other particular physical characteristics?
- the design of the equipment, environment and task fit the abilities of the staff?
- the job put at risk those who are or were recently pregnant, have a history of back trouble or other health problems?
- the job require special knowledge or training if it is to be done safely?
- the job need the use of equipment or assistance from another member of staff?

The conclusion to be drawn from these reports is that no single factor is decisive. The cause of back pain is cumulative stress which is then triggered into an episode of pain by any small or large unmonitored movement, but the risk can be reduced if all these guidelines are taken into careful consideration.

THE BIOMECHANICS OF LIFTING

Forces acting on the spine during lifting may be estimated by using body diagrams and static equations to predict joint reactions and muscle force requirements related to body position, the weight of the lifter, the load and the acceleration of the body, etc. Now state of the art equipment can make these measurements and predictions with increased accuracy (Sullivan 1994). However, this still does not solve the problem of the 'ideal' method of lifting.

Back support mechanisms during lifting

There are three main physiological and anatomical mechanisms for back support during lifting, carrying, pulling and pushing: an increase in intraabdominal pressure, the use of the abdominal muscles to support the spine as 'an arch' and tension in the thoracolumbar fascia (Aspden 1989, Sullivan 1994).

Intraabdominal pressure

Intraabdominal pressure (IAP) is a physiological mechanism created by contraction of the transversus abdominis and the oblique abdominal muscles and the muscles of the pelvic floor. The contraction raises the intraabdominal pressure which then acts upwards on the diaphragm like a balloon, converting the trunk into a more solid cylinder which serves to support the spine by bracing it and transmitting the load over a wider area.

During lifting, increase in IAP occurs as a reflex action, increasing with added load and added flexion of the spine (Aspden 1989, Twomey & Taylor 1994). Increased IAP was thought at one time to decrease the compressive load on the spine but there is now doubt about this phenomenon or even the need for it as normal, healthy vertebrae are sufficiently strong to withstand these compressive loads, but its role as spinal support remains clear (Aspden 1989, Sullivan 1994).

IAP is increased in jumping, pulling and pushing. It is greatest in pushing because the counterpressure created by stress on the arms tends to flatten the rib cage, even making breathing less efficient (Troup 1979, Twomey & Taylor 1994). The increase is less in pulling, especially when facing the load being pulled (Hoozemans et al 1998).

A bracing movement can be performed actively by contracting the abdominal muscles to expel air against a closed glottis, a 'forcing' movement known as the **Valsalva manoeuvre**. This in fact can enhance LBP because of an increase in intradiscal pressure and an increased mechanical load on the lumbar spine produced by muscular contraction (Nachemson & Morris 1964). Hence, in the presence of LBP, pain is often increased with coughing.

The spine as an arch

Aspden (1989) describes the lumbar spine as an arch. An arch is strongest when loaded on its convex surface and thus loading, by means of abdominal muscle contraction, increases the compressive strength along the arch and, by maintaining the lordosis, resists the forces of flexion. In this way IAP and the lumbar lordosis work together to strengthen the spine (Aspden 1989, Delitto & Rose 1992).

The thoracolumbar fascia

The thoracolumbar fascia, described in Chapter 5, was considered to be an important element in stabilizing the posterior ligamentous structures of the spine but its importance has recently been questioned. However, as it surrounds the muscles and ligamentous structures and is tensed by muscle contraction, not only by transversus abdominis and the back muscles but also by the latissimus dorsi, it does have a role to play in resisting spinal flexion and thus supporting the spine during lifting (Sullivan 1994).

THE PHYSICAL MECHANICS OF LIFTING

In examining the physical mechanics of lifting, two main models exist: the spine as a **cantilever** and the spine as an **arch**.

If the spine is viewed as a cantilever, contraction of the back extensors produces an extension moment at the lumbar spine to counteract the flexion moment produced by holding a weight in forward bending (Aspden 1989, Sullivan 1994). Even modest weights can produce a large flexion moment, hence the sharp increase of pain experienced by someone in an acute episode of LBP when merely picking up a teacup from a table whilst standing. The very large muscle forces that are developed, the weight of the upper body and the load all contribute to compression of the lumbar spine (Fathallah et al 1998).

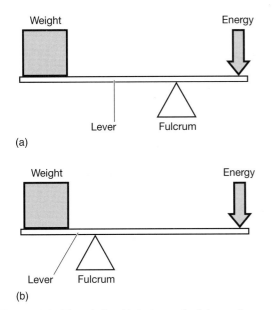

Figure 14.1   The relationship between the fulcrum, the weight and the length of lever.

If the spine is viewed as an arch (see above), the increase of IAP and the maintenance of the lordosis are crucial when lifting heavy weights (Aspden 1989).

Lifting techniques

A practical and pictorially acceptable way for patients to understand the mechanics of lifting is to compare it with the lifting action using a lever, a fulcrum and a weight (Fig. 14.1). Lifting a weight is most difficult when there is a long lever between the fulcrum and the weight (Fig. 14.1a). The closer the fulcrum is to the weight, the easier the lift becomes (Fig. 14.1b).

In Figure 14.2 the body is compared with the above diagram. In Figure 14.2a (similar to a stoop lift) the back and arms become the lever; the fulcrum is at the hips and the energy spread over the whole hips and back. The forces of flexion are high. In the body, it is not possible to move the fulcrum so, to protect the back, it must be secured as part of the fulcrum, with the weight moved as close to it as possible (Fig. 14.2b) (like a squat lift); the legs, with the braced back, provide the energy.

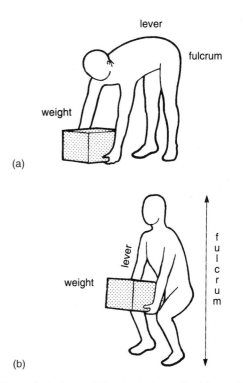

Figure 14.2   The relationship between the fulcrum, the weight and the length of lever in the body.

The two main models for lifting inanimate loads, the stoop lift and the squat lift, can be compared to the mechanisms of the cantilever and the arch.

In the stoop lift, the knees are slightly bent for comfort in reaching the load and the hips flexed. As the spine bends forwards, contraction of the back extensors produces an extension moment to balance a flexion moment produced by the forward inclination of the upper body and a hand-held weight (Sullivan 1994). The lift is initiated by posterior pelvic tilting generated by the hip extensor muscles, with tension in the ligaments and back muscle pulling the spine into extension.

In the squat lift, the trunk is more vertical, the knees more fully flexed and the natural lordosis is maintained in neutral with abdominal stabilization and an increase in IAP. The lift is carried out by knee extension.

Sedgwick et al (1994) carried out an 8-year project to clarify the principles of safe lifting, to develop guidelines for training and to promote

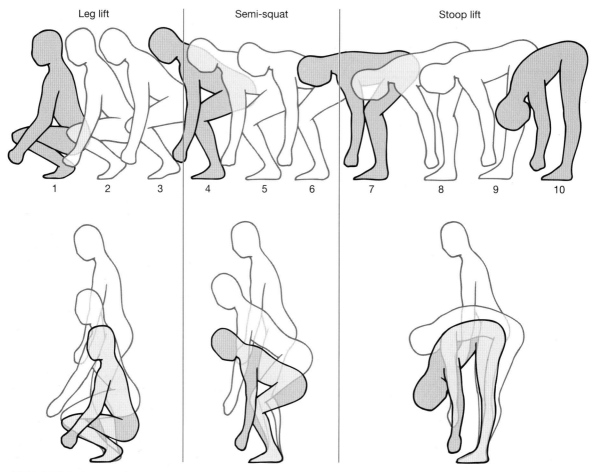

Leg lift   Semi-squat   Stoop lift

1   2   3   4   5   6   7   8   9   10

Major features

(a) Height of centre of gravity is low in 1–3, moderate in 4–7, higher in 8–10

(b) One or both heels is (are) raised in 1–3, both heels are grounded from 4–10

(c) Forward trunk inclination is least in 1–3, moderate in 4–7, most in 8–10

(d) Knee flexion is greatest in 1–3, moderate in 4–7, non-existant in 8–10

(e) Knees protrude in front of vertical line through shoulders in 1–3,
   coincide with that line in 4–7, and are behind it in 8–10

Figure 14.3   A continuum of lifting starting positions and related lifting movements. (Reproduced with permission from Sedgwick & Gormley 1998 and Elsevier Science.)

application of the guidelines. They divided the squat lift into the leg lift and the semisquat (Fig. 14.3). This diagram provides a good analysis of the movements through the various techniques. Sedgwick et al (1994) recommend the semisquat as 'state of the art' training and believe the leg lift should be abandoned as a model for training purposes. The full squat lift (or the leg lift) which is used when lifting an object without handles from the floor requires the heels to be raised and some degree of flexion of the lumbar spine; these lifts need to be made with great care (Sullivan 1994) (Fig. 14.4).

The consensus of opinion seems to be that the squat approach (semisquat) provides the safest and most effective basis for lifting training. The

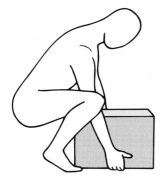

With the lumbar spine in flexion

Figure 14.4   The alteration in back position in a full squat lift.

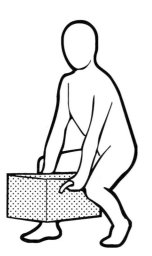

Figure 14.5   A wide-based asymmetric stance in the semisquat lift.

squat lift (Fig. 14.5) eliminates full knee flexion but uses the technique of maintaining a neutral lordosis while avoiding the potentially injurious loaded flexion of the stoop lift. It allows the subject to lift from between the legs, shortening the horizontal distance of load from body which also decreases the flexion moment of the lumbar spine (Delitto & Rose 1992, Pheasant & Stubbs 1994, Sullivan 1994, Gassett et al 1996, Sedgwick & Gormley 1998).

However, as positions can be chosen anywhere between the squat and stoop lifts, there is no such thing as a single, correct lifting technique; separate variables should be used for different work situations (Parnianpour et al 1987, Trafimow et al

---

<table>
<tr><td>Box 14.1   The principles of lifting training</td></tr>
<tr><td>

• Adaptability is the essence of safe and effective lifting.
• The principles of skill learning should be adhered to during training.
• Initial training requires many hours distributed over several weeks.
• Training in workplaces should be applied in the context of 'behaviour modification' and 'adult learning'.
</td></tr>
</table>

1993, Sullivan 1994, Kjellberg et al 1998). The controversy about the 'correct' lift still exists because the rules have to cover so many possibilities: the weight of the object, the strength of the lifter, the position of the object, its cumbersome nature, the speed with which it has to be lifted and how often the lift has to be repeated.

Four major training principles emerged from the research of Sedgwick et al (1994), principles which seem to be echoed by other references (Box 14.1).

Interestingly, Trafimow et al (1993) found that lifters repeating the squat lift would change to the stoop when the quadriceps muscles became fatigued. In certain conditions, for example when the load cannot be brought close to the body, this could create greater risk of injury (Trafimow et al 1993). Also, Sullivan (1994) found that untrained people do spontaneously choose the stoop lift. Could this be because people tend to use knee flexion less and less as life progresses and inevitably lose the ability to squat? Unlike young children who squat spontaneously, adults tend to avoid it. To use a hackneyed colloquialism but a very apt one in relation to the body, 'If you don't use it, you lose it'. In view of this, one of the most important aspects of back care, which therapists should stress, is the need to maintain knee strength and mobility throughout life (Patient advice 14.1).

GUIDELINES FOR MANUAL HANDLING

After a thorough assessment of the problem and following the prevention of injury guidelines above, certain key points are important.

Foot placement

Correct foot placement is in many respects the key to safe lifting (Pheasant & Stubbs 1994). The position of the hands and feet and the direction of exertion are important determinants of strength, strength being limited by the distribution of body weight and the extent of the footbase (Pheasant & Grieve 1981). The strength of the lifting action is greatest when the line of thrust lies within the area of the lifter's footbase (Fig. 14.6). When the load is moved outside this area, the flexion moment is increased and greater muscle activity is needed for stabilization. In lifting a load outside the footbase, the individual is potentially off balance and therefore at risk. A lifting action which commences at a distance and moves into the footbase is probably preferable to one which starts in the footbase and terminates at a distance, but neither is desirable (Pheasant & Stubbs 1994).

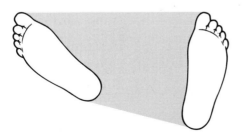

Figure 14.6 The area of footbase. (Adapted from Pheasant & Stubbs 1994.)

Discometric and electromyographic studies of the lumbar spine during lifting have shown that, in relation to changes in disc pressure and back muscle activity, the distance of the load from the body is even more critical than the choice between stooping or squatting (Macintosh & Bogduk 1987, Pheasant & Stubbs 1994).

This links with the research of Hodges & Richardson (1996) which demonstrated that trunk muscles, especially TA, normally react prior to arm movements outside the footbase, creating a spinal 'stiffness' ready for action. Both TA and LM were shown to be inhibited after an episode of LBP and LM did not spontaneously recover (Hides et al 1994, 1996). In view of this, is it possible that some lifting injuries are due to unrecognized muscle instability rather than an incorrect lifting technique? Stabilization is essential for efficient function, so perhaps its absence owing to unrecognized dysfunction or a poor pattern of movement may be the key to understanding musculoskeletal injury.

In situations where the application of external load to the spinal mechanisms can be anticipated, spinal stability can be instantaneously increased and this can be functionally trained (Panjabi 1992). Maybe instability training should be part of all lifting training. Researchers have found that it is the young therapists (Mierzejewski & Kumar 1997) and inexperienced young nurses (Hollingdale 1997) who damage their backs, the older and more experienced nurses being part of a survivor group with stronger backs; have they learned by experience to stabilize?

Jackson & Liles (1994), researching physiotherapists' working postures, reported that students seemed willing to accept unaltered bad habits, even when they caused them to adopt stressful postures. In fact, the optimum postures for patient management are achieved largely at the expense of the therapist's posture (Jackson & Liles 1994).

Care throughout the movement
(Braggins 1994)

- Stand with a firm, wide, adaptable base which allows a shift of weight backwards, forwards or sideways, allowing easy flexion and extension movements of the knees.

- Use the legs to provide momentum and energy for the movement, so that the body moves as a whole.
- Hold the object to be moved with a firm, comfortable hand or arm grip.
- Brace the back with a conscious effort, in the lordotic posture or using abdominal bracing.
- Keep the weight close to the body.
- Avoid sustained holding of the weight.
- Avoid twisting.
- Avoid stooping whilst holding a weight.

Rest pauses during work
(Pheasant & Stubbs 1994)

- Frequent short pauses tend to be more beneficial than infrequent long rests.
- If possible, rest before the sensations of fatigue become pronounced.
- Avoid working to the point of exhaustion.

Guidelines for lifting from the floor

As mentioned above, describing a single 'correct' lift is not practicable but there are certain guidelines.

- *Test the load*: Prior to starting to lift, test the weight; if too heavy, get assistance.
- *Stance*: Stand with a wide footbase, preferably with one foot in front of the other for surer balance. If possible, straddle the object to be lifted. Most 'correct' bent-knee lifts, except those of the professional weight lifter, have an asymmetrical base (Grieve & Pheasant 1982). Stand close to the object, feet firmly in position.
- *Posture*: The shoulders should be symmetrically aligned above the pelvis, neither twisting nor bending in any way.
- *Knees*: The knees should be bent to the half-crouch position if the load is not too low (Fig. 14.5). However, if the weight is on the floor, the full crouch will be needed providing the knees are sufficiently mobile to reach the position and the quadriceps and hip extensor muscles sufficiently strong to rise out of it. Floor lifts of

cumbersome objects are awkward and require good training and care or, preferably, the use of hoists.

- *Back*: A full squat floor lift is difficult to perform whilst maintaining a lordotic back (Fig. 14.4). Lifting in slight flexion is necessary at times; the back should be stabilized and the lift performed quickly. If the lift must be performed with the arms extended, the back must be locked into some degree of lordosis which allows the spine to function as an arch (Sullivan 1994). If the load is too great for the back, the lift must not be performed.
- *Object*: Grip the object firmly with a good hand grip, adding a forearm support if the object is bulky. Get the weight close to the body before starting the lift. Keep the arms close to the body. Use handles whenever possible.
- *Lifting*: Lift the object by straightening both knees and hips smoothly, without jerking, keeping the weight tucked in close to the body within the footbase area.
- *Lowering*: Lower the object into its new place by reversing the procedure: keep the back braced, bend the knees until the required position is reached, then lower carefully. Do not drop the weight suddenly.
- *Mechanical aids*: Always use hoists, pulleys, forklifts or any mechanical aids wherever possible to avoid excessive strain. They should be used at all times when the weight is too heavy to manage; this applies especially to people like nurses, health care workers or manual workers who are constantly faced with difficult loads (HSE 1992).
- *Always* complete the lift. It is dangerous to stop and hold the weight in mid-lift or to suddenly change the direction or rhythm of the movement.
- *Always* keep your hips lower than your head.

Awkward moments in manual handling

Moving other human beings

This book cannot go into the numerous techniques needed for moving and handling people in the many different situations in which this occurs, both in the health care professions and in looking after the disabled in the home. *The guide to the handling of patients* (NBPA 1998a) gives detailed advice in words and diagrams for every kind of lift.

Moving cumbersome loads

When moving cumbersome loads such as full sacks, tip them up on end, try to hug them close to the body and use the body as a prop for carrying.

Long objects

With objects such as stepladders or long planks, pick them up in the middle; if necessary, balance the length of weight by throwing your own body weight further back. Preferably get help.

Lifting with other people

When lifting with other people, make sure everyone coordinates the lift; use 'one, two, three, go!' to be certain.

Lifting from a shopping trolley

Stand close to the side of the trolley, slacken both knees and bend them slightly, lean over with back braced. Get a good grip with both hands well under the box or grip the bag handle. Keep the back braced. Lift with the arms while straightening the legs.

Turning with a load

Having lifted the weight, *never* twist the body leaving the feet still. In order to turn, *always* keep the body in straight alignment and move the feet round.

Lifting in or out of the car boot or a baby's cot

At any time when the obstacle in front prevents free knee bending, use the edge of the obstacle itself for support, propping the thighs against the rear of the car or against the railing of the cot (providing the cot is secure). Brace the back and lean forwards, using the thigh support to shorten the lever of the back.

Fatigue

Everyone should take special care in lifting if tired or unwell.

Clothing

Beware of tight skirts, protective aprons or clothing which may restrict the ability to move freely or to bend the knees.

CARRYING, PULLING AND PUSHING

Guidelines for carrying

- Carry all weights close to the body, even supported by the body (see Patient Handouts).
- Carry heavy loads on the back; for example, young children, rucksacks, sacks of cement. Take great care getting them onto the back. Do not swing them round from the front in a twisting movement. Squat with the weight behind you or lift the weight onto a higher level first or seek assistance.
- Carry with an equal distribution of weight. If possible, split all heavy loads into two, one for each hand, to give balance. Use two suitcases rather than one for holidays.
- Carry a heavy load no further than 10 m without rest (Pheasant & Stubbs 1994).
- Use conveyors wherever possible.

In 1997, in response to the concerns of many parents and increased reporting of back and neck pain in children, the NBPA mounted a National School Bag Survey (NBPA 1998b). As a result they have mounted a campaign to find ways of lightening the loads children are expected to carry (Boxes 14.2 and 14.3). The NBPA have issued a set of bag weight/body weight guidelines, together with an information pack including the findings and recommendations of their survey. They have also launched an ergonomically designed school bag.

Guidelines for pulling and pushing

The strength of pulling and pushing action depends greatly upon foot placement and the

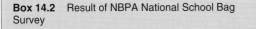

Box 14.2   Result of NBPA National School Bag Survey

- Eighty percent of children are carrying too much weight.
- Most children carry bags in the most harmful way: on one shoulder.
- Only 40% of schools provide lockers and then, not for every child.
- Many children were found to carry books equal to one-third of their body weight in their bags.

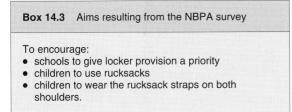

Box 14.3   Aims resulting from the NBPA survey

To encourage:
- schools to give locker provision a priority
- children to use rucksacks
- children to wear the rucksack straps on both shoulders.

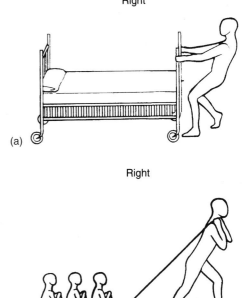

Figure 14.7   (a) Pulling by facing the weight. (b) Pulling turned away from the weight, rope as above or held at waist height.

conditions underfoot (Pheasant & Stubbs 1994, Hoozemans et al 1998). Some research seems to indicate that pulling results in a lower level of spinal loading than pushing and that pushing results in a greater increase in IAP, tending to fix the rib cage, causing breathing to be difficult and making pulling preferable (Twomey & Taylor 1994, Pheasant & Stubbs 1994).

In a comprehensive review of research, Hoozemans et al (1998) point out that risk factors have been found to influence the acceptable degree of push or pull forces as well as the physiological and mechanical strain on the body. These vary in relation to:

- work situation, such as distance, frequency, handle height and cart weight
- working method and posture/movement/exerted forces, such as foot distance and velocity
- worker's characteristics.

Gassett et al (1996) agree that the two primary risk factors related to pulling and pushing are friction and handle height; the greater the friction, the greater the risk of overexertion and injury and a handle height of 35–45″ above floor level is recommended.

Pulling

The head should be further away from the load than the feet. Wherever possible, apply the hands to the load at a height between waist and shoulder. Pull facing the object or turned away from it (Fig. 14.7).

Pushing

The head should always be nearer the object than the feet, facing the object or with back against it (Fig. 14.8).

Awkward moments in pulling and pushing in the home

Drawers

Beware of opening and closing heavy drawers. Avoid doing so whilst sitting, especially if leaning sideways; always get up, stand well back in front of the drawer and bend both knees, one in front of the other, to give easy free access.

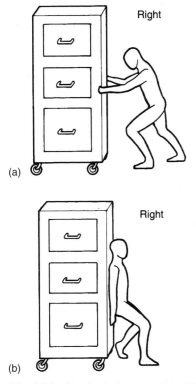

Right

(a)

Right

(b)

Figure 14.8 (a) Pushing by facing the weight. (b) Pushing turned away from the weight.

Furniture

Take care when shifting heavy furniture; try to have good castors on all frequently moved items or fit Glisdomes (hard rubber discs, coated with low-friction Teflon) on each corner.

Floors

Beware of slippery floors and a poor foothold.

NURSES

Nursing is among the high-risk occupations with respect to low back problems. More frequent patient handling appears to correlate with increased incidence of LBP but the traditional approach of training in lifting and handling techniques alone has been shown to be of little help (Hignett 1996). Certain factors predispose to injury (Box 14.4).

The RCN Code of Practice (1996) offers a frame-work for implementing the Health and Safety Executive (1992) Manual Handling Regulations. Its aim is to eliminate manual handling in all but exceptional situations.

Ruszala (1997) believes that the equipment now available enables virtually all patients to be cared for and moved without manual lifting. Patients should be encouraged to assist in their own transfers and handling aids must be used whenever they reduce the risk of injury. Handling patients manually may continue only if it does not involve lifting most or all of the patient's weight and there must be routine assessment before action. Care must also be taken when supporting a patient and pushing and pulling should be kept to a minimum.

Maintaining patient mobility and some rehabilitation programmes may require staff to work at higher risk and assessment must be addressed carefully in these cases. Infrequent, unexpected emergency situations will present the most difficulties (NBPA 1998a). Urgent action is still needed so that adequate measures are implemented to ensure that all routine and reasonably foreseeable lifting activities are eliminated (Ruszala 1997).

CONCLUSION

As lifting ability is a function of body weight, skill and experience as well as of muscle strength (Troup 1979), a single correct lifting technique cannot be the rule (Parnianpour et al 1987, Hignett 1996). The greatest aid to good performance is to understand the many principles involved in good technique and adapt them intelligently for each new problem. Injury usually arises when an action is performed with the wrong force, the wrong speed, the wrong movement or the wrong assessment of the manoeuvre. All these points must be given due attention and workers should understand the need to look after their backs on and off duty.

REFERENCES

Aspden R M 1989 The spine as an arch. A new mathematical model. Spine 14(3): 266–273

Birnbaum R, Cockcroft A, Richardson B with Corlett N 1991 Safer handling of loads at work – a practical ergonomic guide. Institute for Occupational Ergonomics, University of Nottingham, Nottingham

Blamire G 1995 An educational framework for training in manual handling. Physiotherapy 81(3): 149–153

Braggins S 1994 The back: functions, malfunctions and care. Mosby Yearbook Europe, London

Cholewicki J, McGill S 1996 Mechanical stability of the in vivo lumbar spine: implications for injury and chronic low back pain. Clinical Biomechanics 11: 1–15

Crozier L, Cozens S 1998 The neuromuscular approach to efficient handling and movement In: NBPA/RCN (eds) A guide to the handling of patients. National Back Pain Association, Teddington, Royal College of Nursing, London

Delitto R S, Rose S J 1992 An electromyographic analysis of two techniques for squat lifting and lowering. Physical Therapy 72(6): 437–448

EEC Council 1990 Directive No 90/269/EEC. Official Journal of the European Community, No L 156 21.6.90

Fathallah F A, Marras W S, Parnianpour M 1998 An assessment of complex spinal loads during dynamic lifting tasks. Spine 23(6): 706–716

Gassett R S, Hearne B, Keelan B 1996 Ergonomics and body mechanics in the work place. Orthopedic Clinics of North America 27(4): 861–879

Grieve D, Pheasant S 1982 Biomechanics: the body at work. In: Singleton W T (ed) Biological ergonomics. Cambridge University Press, Cambridge

Health and Safety Commission (HSC) 1998 Manual handling in the health services. Health Services Advisory Committee. HMSO, London

Health and Safety Executive (HSE) 1992 Manual handling – guidance on regulations. HSE, Sheffield

Hides J A, Stokes M J, Saide M et al 1994 Evidence of lumbar multifidus muscle wasting ipsilateral to symptoms in patients with acute/subacute low back pain. Spine 19(2): 165–172

Hides J A, Richardson C A, Jull G A 1996 Multifidus muscle recovery is not automatic after resolution of acute first-episode low back pain. Spine 21(23): 2763–2769

Hignett S 1996 Work-related back pain in nurses. Journal of Advanced Nursing 23: 1238–1246

Hodges P W, Richardson S A 1996 Inefficient muscular stabilization of the lumbar spine associated with low back pain. Spine 21(22): 2640–2650

Hollingdale R 1997 Back pain in nursing and associated factors: a study. Nursing Standard 11(39): 35–38

Hoozemans M J M, Van Der Beek A J, Frings-Dresen M H W et al 1998 Pushing and pulling in relation to musculoskeletal disorders: a review of risk factors. Ergonomics 41(6): 757–781

Jackson J, Liles S 1994 Working postures and physiotherapy students. Physiotherapy 80(7): 432–436

Kelsey J L, Githens P B, White A A et al 1984 An epidemiologic study of lifting and twisting on the job and risk for acute prolapsed lumbar intervertebral disc. Journal of Orthopaedic Research 2: 61

Kjellberg K, Lindbeck L, Hagberg M 1998 Method and performance: two elements of work technique. Ergonomics 41(6): 798–816

Klaber-Moffett J, Richardson G, Sheldon T A, Maynard A 1995 Back pain, its management and cost to society. University of York, York

Mcelwaine J 1998 Do we need a new manual handling strategy? HSE manual handling policy co-ordinator. Column 10(4): 8–10

Macintosh J, Bogduk N 1987 The anatomy and function of the lumbar back muscles and their fascia. In: Twomey L T, Taylor J R (eds) Physical therapy of the low back. Churchill Livingstone, New York

Mierzejewski M, Kumar S 1997 Prevalence of low back pain among physical therapists in Edmonton, Canada. Disability and Rehabilitation 19(8): 309–317

Nachemson A, Morris J 1964 In vivo measurements of intradiscal pressure. Journal of Bone and Joint Surgery 46-A(5): 107–1092

National Back Pain Association (NBPA) Royal College of Nursing (RCN) 1998a The guide to the handling of patients, 4th edn. National Back Pain Association, Teddington, and Royal College of Nursing, London

National Back Pain Association (NBPA) 1998b Taking the weight off their shoulders. National Back Pain Association, Teddington

Panjabi M M 1992 The stabilizing system of the spine Part 1. Function, dysfunction, adaptation and enhancement. Journal of Spinal Disorders 5(4): 383–389

Parnianpour M, Beijani F J, Pavlidas L 1987 Worker training: the fallacy of a single correct lifting technique. Ergonomics 30: 331–334

Pheasant S T, Grieve D W 1981 The principal features of maximal exertion in the sagittal plane. Ergonomics 24(5): 327–338

Pheasant S T, Stubbs D 1994 Manual handling, an ergonomic approach. National Back Pain Association, Teddington

Robens Institute, Ergonomic Research Unit 1986 Back pain in nurses. Summary and recommendations. Robens Institute, University of Surrey, Guildford

Royal College of Nursing (RCN) 1996 RCN code of practice for patient handling. Royal College of Nursing, London

Ruszala S 1997 Can patient lifting really be eliminated? Pressure care and manual handling study day, lecture notes

Sedgwick A W, Gormley J T 1998 Training for lifting: an unresolved ergonomic issue? Applied Ergonomics 29(5): 395–398

Sedgwick A W, Glencross D J, Gormley J T, Kitcher D, Smith D S 1994 Training for safe and effective lifting. Unpublished paper

Snook S H 1978 The design of manual handling tasks. The Society's lecture. Ergonomics 21(12): 963–985

Straker L M 1989 Reducing work-associated back problems in the health service. Physiotherapy 75(12): 697–700

Sullivan M S 1994 Lifting and back pain. In: Twomey L T, Taylor J R (eds) Physical therapy of the low back. Churchill Livingstone, New York

Trafimow J H, Schilein O D, Novak G J, Andersson G B J 1993 The effects of quadriceps fatigue on the technique of lifting. Spine 18(3): 364–367

Troup J D G 1977 Dynamic factors in the analysis of stoop and crouch lifting methods. Orthopedic Clinics of North America 8(1): 201–209

Troup J D G 1979 Biomechanics of the vertebral column. Physiotherapy 65(8): 238–244

Twomey L T 1992 Personal communication

Twomey L T, Taylor J R 1994 Lumbar posture, movement, and mechanics. In: Twomey L T, Taylor J R (eds) Physical therapy of the low back. Churchill Livingstone, New York

FURTHER READING

Chartered Society of Physiotherapy (CSP) 1994 Moving and handling. Advice to chartered physiotherapists on manual handling legislation and related issues. Chartered Society of Physiotherapy, London

Health and Safety Executive (HSE) 1998 Manual handling in the health services. HMSO, London

National Back Pain Association (NBPA) and the Royal College of Nursing (RCN) 1998 The guide to the handling of patients. National Back Pain Association, Teddington and Royal College of Nursing, London

Pheasant S, Stubbs D 1994 Manual handling. An ergonomic approach. National Back Pain Association Teddington

Royal College of Nursing (RCN) 1996 Manual handling assessments in hospitals and the community. Royal College of Nursing, London.

15

Posture at work and at home

Ergonomics is the scientific study of the relationship between the person and the working environment (Pheasant 1991, Boyling 1996). It examines the logistics of fitting the person to the task or fitting the task to the person. Since 1993, in compliance with new EEC directives (EEC 1990), all employers have to examine the environment of their workforce, seeking and implementing the advice of qualified ergonomists.

By far the most frequent self-reported work-related illness is that of musculoskeletal disorder (MSD). In 1997, 5.4 million working days were lost as a result and 964 000 people suffered from an MSD believed to be caused or made worse by work (HSC 1998). The risk factors for MSD are a combination of awkward postures, frequency of action, high levels of forces acting on the body, difficult manual handling tasks and exposure to too much bending, stretching or effort (HSE 1998b).

The HSE book *A pain in your workplace* (1998b) is a clear, comprehensive job-by-job description of case studies in 90 different occupations, giving body areas affected, risk factors and solutions to the problems.

THE WORK SPACE

Examination of the work space begins at the entrance: do the doors of the house, office, shop, hospital, ward, treatment room or factory open without undue force and, if they are doors for the public, do they provide easy access for all, including wheelchair users and their attendants?

Stairs provide a commendable form of exercise but do they present an obstacle to the efficient transportation of items or people within the building? Are people having to carry heavy loads up the stairs? Should a lift be installed?

Inside the building, are the rooms well ventilated, with easily adjusted air and heat? Heat, cold and lack of air can have an effect on the whole body. Is the lighting adequate and well placed for good visibility, especially for writing, reading, fine working and VDU operating? Poor lighting affects eye position which in turn influences head and neck posture (HSE 1999).

Is the furniture well placed for efficient and unstressed movement? Are the storage shelves low enough to allow items to be reached without strain? Is there enough storage space? Are the cupboards and their contents arranged to minimize the time and effort spent walking backwards and forwards to collect items from them? In the hospital ward, if the bedside table were moved, would it be easier to lift the patient? Is there enough space to move the bedside table anywhere? Could the cartons that are always stacked by the window be stored out of the way? At home, if you put the bucket at the back of the store cupboard, would it save lifting the vacuum cleaner over the top of it ... and so on.

Whenever anything appears difficult or clumsy, stop and consider if there is a better way of arranging it or handling it or getting around it. Make sure that work is not made more stressful by surroundings that can be improved.

It is important to become alert to the relationship between the body and the patterns of movement involved in lifting, carrying, pushing, pulling and manipulating all objects, animate or inanimate.

THE WORK SURFACES

Height

Many work situations involve standing or sitting in front of a desk, table, bed, drawing board or some other surface while manipulating tools on those surfaces.

If the work surface is too low it becomes necessary to stoop; if the work surface is too high, shoulder elevation causes arm position to become awkward and tension develops in the upper trapezius and cervical area.

Standing at a worktop

When standing, the work surface should be waist high or slightly below so that the elbows are bent no more than 10–15° below the right angle when hands are resting on the surface (Fig. 15.1). If the surface is too low, either sit or raise the work surface (Fig. 15.2).

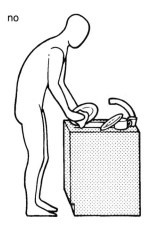
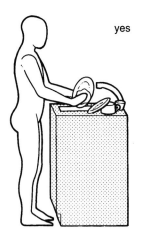

Figure 15.1 Correct worktop height.

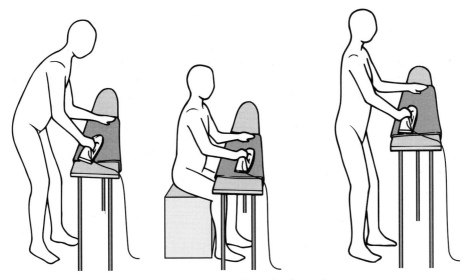

Figure 15.2   Worktop too low. Either lower yourself or raise the worktop.

Working at a bed or couch

All therapeutic couches or patients' beds should be either electrically or hydraulically adjustable in height to fit postural adjustment of health care workers.

Sitting at a desk or table

The top should be high enough to support the forearms comfortably with the elbows bent to a right angle without having to slump forwards onto the desk (Fig. 15.3). If the chair cannot be adjusted to meet these requirements, then the table should be raised or lowered as necessary. If objects such as typewriters or keyboards raise the level of work, the top must be lowered or the chair raised to adjust to the required forearm position.

The chair should be close to the desk, pulled well in to the desk to support the back, and workers should avoid sitting on the edge of the chair and then slouching back when resting.

An adjustable office chair should be used whenever possible if working at a desk; other

no   yes

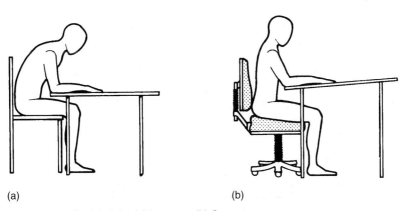

(a)   (b)

Figure 15.3   Desk height. (a) Incorrect. (b) Correct.

occupations which require moments of sitting whilst supervising, such as nurses' workstations, need well-designed, supportive chairs, possibly with armrests. Refer to Chapter 12.

Slope

If the worktop is being used for writing or reading, the top should slope upwards 10–15°. This is based on the fact that we tend to work with our eyes 30 cm from any paper or book (Mandal 1984) (Fig. 15.3b). Portable, adjustable, sloping desktop stands for reading or drawing are now obtainable.

Artists or designers should have an easel-type sloping work surface to draw on.

Depth

No work surface should be deeper than the reach across it.

Worktop objects

Everything on the worktop should be easily accessible. Implements on the desk, counter or kitchen surface should be organized in relation to frequency of use, weight of object and ease of operation. Heavy articles should be placed so that they do not need to be moved for easy access. All work tools should be placed in a good functional position, so that access to them utilizes a variety of normal, free body movements with easy change of position. Reaching for objects should be avoided, especially if they are heavy.

The position of objects in relation to eyes is an important consideration when organizing the placing of equipment on the worktop. Looking at the keyboard, watching the screen, looking sideways at the copy all have a direct effect on head and neck posture. All copy material should be on an adjustable stand (Fig. 15.4) which should be placed centrally or alternated from side to side every other day.

Neck pain and headaches may originate from stress on the joints of the cervical spine after being held in sustained head postures, either maintained in rotation or in the forward head position.

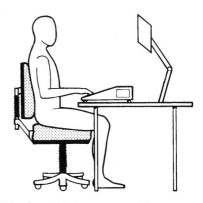

Figure 15.4 Correct typing posture, with a copy stand.

VISUAL DISPLAY UNIT OPERATION

An EEC directive (EEC 1990) has laid down minimum safety and health requirements for work with display screen equipment (Fig. 15.5) because the bulk of research evidence suggests that VDU workstations are not ergonomically sound and workers will experience physical symptoms (Scheer & Mital 1997).

However, given a well-designed workstation, a good management philosophy, rest breaks and pause exercises, a VDU worker should have no more health complaints than any other worker (Scheer & Mital 1997).

The screen

The VDU screen should be flicker, glare and reflection free, with clear, well-defined characters; it should be adjustable in height, tiltable and on a swivel stand (EEC 1990, Boyling 1997). The top of the screen should be level with the forehead so that the eyes move through an angle of 0–15° downwards from the horizontal (Boyling 1997, Bauer & Wittig 1998). The distance of eye to screen should be between 50 and 90 cm (Glazer & Glazer 1991). The screen *must* be directly in front of the operator.

Chairs

All VDU chairs must be fully adjustable office chairs with variable seat and back inclinations and variable height adjustment (EEC 1990) (see

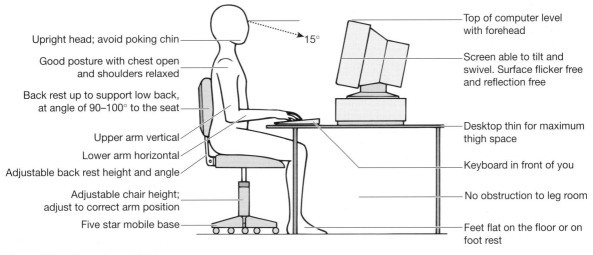

Upright head; avoid poking chin

Good posture with chest open and shoulders relaxed

Back rest up to support low back, at angle of 90–100° to the seat

Upper arm vertical

Lower arm horizontal

Adjustable back rest height and angle

Adjustable chair height; adjust to correct arm position

Five star mobile base

15°

Top of computer level with forehead

Screen able to tilt and swivel. Surface flicker free and reflection free

Desktop thin for maximum thigh space

Keyboard in front of you

No obstruction to leg room

Feet flat on the floor or on foot rest

Figure 15.5   Computer workstation.

Chapter 12). The height should be adjusted in relation to the keyboard so that the upper arms hang vertically, with the forearms horizontal, the wrists level and hands straight on the keyboard. The feet should be flat on the floor or a footrest should be provided (EEC 1990). The seat can be tipped forwards 5–15° if the operator works in a very upright position or conversely inclined 5° back if the operator find this more satisfactory (Boyling 1996). Chair arms should be removed if they prevent freedom of chair movement either in relation to distance from the desk or ability to rotate the chair.

The keyboard and mouse

Keyboards

Keyboards have been deemed the culprit in many ergonomic problems faced by keyboard operators. The sensitivity of pressure allows the user to strike an average of 240 times each minute, creating a highly repetitive task (Gassett et al 1996). All keyboards should be detached and tiltable, so that the worker can find the best position to avoid arm or hand fatigue (EEC 1990). The parallel keyboard rows require 20° of ulnar deviation and overpronation of the forearm; several innovative designs have been developed to replace the standard shape (Gassett et al 1996). The keyboard must be at the right height for performance with

the upper arms vertical, lower arms horizontal and wrists/hands level, with the keyboard in front of the operator (Boyling 1996) (Fig. 15.5).

The space on the work surface in front of the keyboard must be sufficient to provide supportive rest for the hands and arms of the operator, that is, between 6 and 8 cm (EEC 1990, Boyling 1996), or wrist rests, equal in height to the keyboard, can be used to support the wrists in a neutral position. The symbols on the keys should be adequately contrasted and legible from the design working position (EEC 1990).

The mouse

The mouse, trackball or similar pointing device must be comfortable for the worker to use. It should be positioned as close to the keyboard as possible so that the mouse arm is relaxed, with the wrist held straight. The keyboard can be moved out of the way if it is not being used. The mouse should not be gripped tightly and the finger should rest lightly on the buttons. Workers should relieve the working hand by changing from right to left or vice versa, taking short breaks and exercising the arm (HSE 1999).

Many varying designs of mouse and keyboard can be obtained to help people achieve better alignment of finger, hand and wrist whilst working.

Copy stand

The document holder should be stable and adjustable, either propped in front of the computer or, preferably, at the side, at easy eye level, and should be positioned to minimize the need for major head and eye movements (EEC 1990, Bauer & Wittig 1998). If at the side, it should be changed from left to right daily or at least every week.

Desktop material

The desktop should be no more than 30 mm thick to allow for maximum thigh space (Boyling 1996). The surface should be of low reflectance and large enough to allow flexible arrangements of equipment (EEC 1990). The depth of the surface from front to back should be 80–100 cm (Boyling 1996).

Lighting

The VDU screen should be at right angles to the windows or main lighting. This avoids reflection on the screen and protects the operator from glaring light (EEC 1990, Boyling 1996).

Leg room

There should be no obstruction to free leg room and there should be adequate space for change of position and movement. A foot rest should be available if required (EEC 1990, Boyling 1996).

Reading glasses

No one should work on a VDU with bifocal reading glasses. In order to look through the reading lenses, the person has to tip the head back into extension. Reading glasses with the focal length measured for the computer are the ideal but workers who have to move and look around the office intermittently should discuss this with their optician, as special variable-focus glasses can be made.

The telephone

Avoid holding the telephone between ear and shoulder. This can cause cervical spine problems and upper limb disorders. Anyone who uses the telephone consistently throughout the day should use earphones.

SUPERMARKET CASHIERS

Supermarket cashiers have similar workstation problems to VDU operators and the reports of disability attributed to musculoskeletal symptoms are increasing (HSE 1998a).

There is a wide variety of checkout designs ranging from the simple to the complex. The basic unit has to contain: a location for the cashier, some form of goods delivery to the cashier, a method for the cashier to record transactions, a receptacle for cash, a location of ancillary equipment such as weighing scales and an area for return to the customer (HSE 1998a). But many checkouts have unsuitable chairs, lack of space and a mismatch between checkout height, set design and working postures, especially for particularly small or large people (HSE 1998a).

The ergonomic approach emphasizes the need for an acceptable fit between operator and equipment or tasks and for the operator to feel comfortable in the workstation (HSE 1998a).

- The cashier should be able to sit or stand.
- The checkout should fit the user's requirements.
- The cashier should be able to avoid twisting, bending and reaching.
- The cashier should not be expected to work for long, unbroken stints.
- The environment should contain no conditions that lead to discomfort or irritation.
- Good training should be provided.
- Employees should be encouraged to report any symptoms.
- Management should be sympathetic in approach.

WORK-RELATED UPPER LIMB DISORDERS

Upper limb pain, described variously as work-related upper limb disorders (WRULD), overuse syndromes, repetitive strain injury (RSI), cumulative trauma disorders (CTD) and others, consists of a number of well-defined soft tissue disorders of the upper limb and a less well-defined condition of non-specific arm pain (Boyling 1996, Helliwell 1996). The well-defined tissue disorders (nerve – carpal tunnel; tendon – trigger finger; fascia – Dupuytren's) are easily diagnosed but the non-specific arm pain presents more of a diagnostic problem. Non-specific arm pain has been in existence for many years but has only recently been recognized as including other syndromes (for example, 'tennis elbow' and 'frozen shoulder').

WRULD is often characterized by diffuse upper limb pain, sometimes described as burning in character, and may be of such intensity that hand function becomes limited (Greening & Lynn 1998). RSI patients have objective signs of minor polyneuropathy, the median nerve being more affected than the ulnar or radial nerve, with clear changes being apparent in the median nerve vibration threshold of office workers who use computers intensively (Greening & Lynn 1998). Quantitative measurement of the vibration threshold may be useful in patient assessment and may also be a means of detecting early neural deficits and possibly instigating early treatment (Greening & Lynn 1998).

WRULD may arise from postures in which the hands move slightly and repetitively whilst the head, neck and shoulders are held in a static pose, possibly in thoracic flexion, with protracted shoulders and a forward head posture (Pheasant 1991, Cohen et al 1992, Griegel-Morris et al 1992, Grant et al 1997). VDU operators and checkout cashiers are vulnerable, as are musicians.

At least part of the cause of the apparent epidemic of WRULD is the attempts of industry to remain competitive by increasing the efficiency of workers (Scheer & Mital 1997).

Treatment

All upper limb pain and dysfunction needs to be assessed in the usual way, looking at the articular, neural and myofascial elements, never forgetting the extensive range of vertebrae that may refer into the area and the changes in neural sensitization discussed in Chapter 7 (Elvey et al 1986, Boyling & Palastanga 1994).

People who suffer from upper limb problems are also more likely to have LBP and headaches (Pheasant 1991) so treatment needs to be based on accurate examination of all neurodynamics. Without this, any treatment is doomed to failure or, worse, the prolonging of the patient's problem (Boyling 1997).

The ability to position and control movements of the scapula is essential for optimal upper limb function and the inability to achieve this stable base frequently accompanies the development of shoulder and upper limb pain and pathology (Mottram 1997). Addressing the dynamic stabilization of the scapula with progressive setting and stabilizing techniques is an essential part of the management of shoulder girdle neuro-musculoskeletal dysfunction (Grant et al 1997, Mottram 1997, Kember 1997, 1998).

As in all musculoskeletal conditions, early return to work should be considered but this will depend on the severity and irritability of the condition. If the mobility of neural tissue has not been restored, stretch or movement of that tissue under load at work will exacerbate the symptoms (Boyling 1997). So accurate treatment, the restoration of full movement and the education of the patient in the management of their problem are all essential.

Prevention

Acceptance that WRULD or work-related musculoskeletal disorders (WMSD) in general arise from sustained positions offers a practical approach to prevention and control (Turner 1998). Prevention is a mutually shared responsibility between employer and employee.

Employer

The employer has a responsibility to comply with all health and safety guidelines. The condition is avoidable by using ergonomically designed work stations, by appropriate education and training, and by attention to task, design and work rates, rest breaks and support, including stress management (Turner 1998).

Box 15.1 Prevention of musculoskeletal disorders in VDU operators

- Correct workstation layout.
- Adjust chair/keyboard/screen into position of least postural stress.
- Vary the rhythm of work if possible, e.g. work on VDU for a short time, then on files for a short time.
- Get up and move around every half an hour.
- Stretch and do one or two pause exercises intermittently all day.

Employee

Workers should be meticulously aware of posture, correcting any position or activity that may lead to stress and dysfunction. Movement is *essential* and as therapists, we cannot stress this too much. Workers should move every 30 minutes, exercising and stretching all joints of the neck, upper limbs and low back (Box 15.1) (Gifford 1992, Boyling 1996, HSE 1999) (see 'Pause exercise' in the Patient Handouts).

NURSES, PHYSIOTHERAPISTS AND HEALTH CARE WORKERS

Work-related musculoskeletal disorders (WMSD) are common in all health care workers but nurses and any carers who look after ill or disabled people are particularly vulnerable. Chapter 14 discusses manual handling in the broad concept and *The guide to the handling of patients* (NBPA 1998) gives extensive instruction in the manual handling of patients for nurses in particular.

Physical therapists are also at risk from WMSD (WMD in the US) in the upper limbs and low back (Bork et al 1996, Mierzejewski & Kumar 1997). Lifting patients is cited as the most common mechanism of injury, especially lifting with sudden maximal effort, bending or twisting and lifting while transferring patients. Work-related wrist and hand symptoms are also a problem, especially for manual therapists. Therapists should be in a good position to recognize the need for breaks, change of position and possible modification of techniques to reduce the amount of stress placed on all parts of the body.

GUIDELINES FOR EVERYDAY WORKING HAZARDS

These common situations and daily activities are listed alphabetically.

Bath cleaning

Kneel by the bath or half-squat with both knees pressed against the side of the bath for extra support. Use long-handled brushes for the far corners. Arch the back to restore the lordosis after finishing the job (Fig. 15.6).

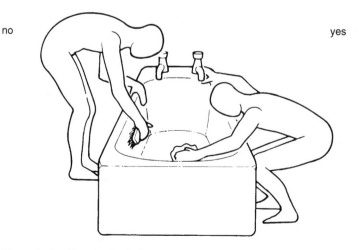

no   yes

Figure 15.6 Cleaning the bath.

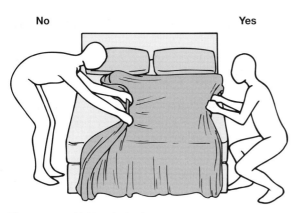

No   Yes   Yes

Figure 15.7 Making the bed.

Bed making

In domestic situations either bend both knees to a half-squat or lean forwards with a braced back, taking the weight on one arm while the other moves the bed clothes. If using sheets and blankets, care must be taken when throwing them up the bed. Duvets are easier for bed making and should be adopted by all back pain sufferers (Fig. 15.7).

In all health care, the bed should be raised to eliminate a stoop position so that sheets and blankets can be manipulated with minimal back stress. Two people should work together wherever possible. All beds should have good castors for easy mobility.

DIY

- The height of the workbench should be adjustable for efficient, stress-free operation.
- Use a wide-based stance for sawing. Rest one foot up on a low footstool of 10–16 cm occasionally to relieve the back if it is painful.
- Take care when lifting ladders, planks, etc. (see Chapter 14).
- Stand on firm planks or trestles when painting high surfaces and get close to the job without stretching up. Avoid reaching whilst off balance.

Gardening

Gardening is one of the most common back hazards. Encourage people to:

- remember the back is especially vulnerable where heavy work is involved
- avoid prolonged stooping. Bend the knees and get down as close as possible to whatever is being done. If squatting is difficult, use a kneeling pad or sit on a low stool. Stools on wheels are now available
- use long-handled tools. Hang them up or prop them up when not in use in order to avoid stooping to pick them up and so that they do not become a hazard lying on the ground
- wear a pocketed apron for holding small tools to avoid stooping to retrieve them from the ground
- use a weeding box on wheels with a long handle
- take care with pushing. Use a lightweight wheelbarrow. Brace the back when lifting the handles
- take care with pulling, especially when pulling up stubborn roots. Again, brace the back
- avoid carrying heavy bags, such as compost. Lift them carefully onto and off the wheelbarrow
- when digging, use the legs for leverage, not the back. Take special care with digging holes or trenches because of the twist in the bent position as the earth is shifted. Move the earth only a short distance
- *restore the lordosis every 10 minutes*. Do not stoop to do something, then remain in the stooped position because the back is aching.

Ironing

Adjust the ironing board to the right height for either sitting or standing (Fig. 15.2). A high stool is useful during periods of back pain. Use a small footstool to change position and relieve pressure on the lumbar spine. Iron for short periods only.

Kitchen work

- Worktops should be the right height (Fig. 15.1).
- Equipment should be arranged so that the cooker and sink are close together or, ideally, at right angles to each other, to minimize the carrying distance of heavy saucepans.
- Cookers. If the oven is low, do not stoop to get to it; squat in front in a stable position. When purchasing free-standing cookers, avoid the drop-fronted variety because the door, which is not intended to support a load, is an obstacle to easy removal of dishes from the oven as it prevents squatting directly in front of the oven (Fig. 15.8).
- Washing machines, dishwashers and low cupboards, etc. The principle of avoiding stoop by using the knees applies to everything.
- Sit on a high stool for lengthy preparations. If having to stand to cut up vegetables or prepare food for long, stretch and move the back frequently, especially the thoracic spine.

- Keep a pair of steps handy for reaching into high cupboards.

Manual work

Although manual work is usually performed by fit people it exacts a heavy price in back problems (see Chapter 14).

- There are some insurmountable problems such as how to protect the back when lifting objects into or out of a narrow trench beneath the feet, the type of job service engineers have to cope with when laying pipes in narrow channels below ground level. There is no clever answer except to squat as close to the ground as possible, brace the back and straighten the legs. Ideally, the job should be done by two or more people or hoists and pulleys should be used.
- Pneumatic drill working involves both the stoop posture and the vibrational stress. Stand with a wide, firm base, knees slightly bent and back firmly braced, taking frequent breaks with change of position and back arch.
- The danger moments of manual work: twisting while in the stoop position; bending whilst carrying; poor lifting techniques, attempting to lift too heavy a weight; remaining stooped for hours without restoring the lordosis.
- After work, when fatigued, take care not to stand badly or slouch in floppy chairs. Lying prone on the floor, or in any comfortable position, for 10 minutes can be restorative.

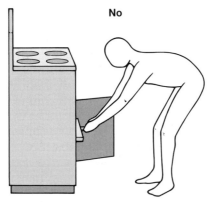 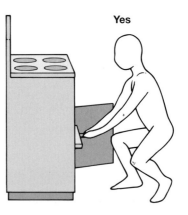

Figure 15.8 Reaching into low cupboards.

no   yes

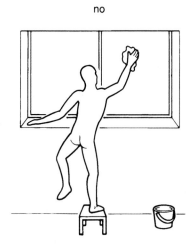
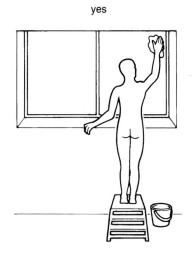

Figure 15.9 Reaching up.

Reaching

Painting and decorating, construction work, cleaning windows, hanging curtains, reaching into high cupboards, pruning trees, picking fruit, etc. all entail reaching above the head and reaching sideways. Stand firmly and symmetrically balanced, directly beneath the job (Fig. 15.9). Use a firm stepladder, trestle or table to stand on.

Stooping for small activities

These are the moments when people are often caught out, when performing automatically to accomplish insignificant objectives such as tying shoe laces, picking up a small object, bending to alter a power point switch, packing or unpacking a suitcase. It is important for people to train themselves to bend into a squat or half-kneel position whenever they perform *any* action below knee level. This must become a habit (Fig. 15.10).

Vacuuming or sweeping

- Buy lightweight equipment of the right height and size.
- While vacuuming, slacken the knees, keep one foot in front of the other and bend

No   Yes   Yes

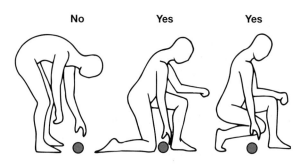

Figure 15.10 Picking up small objects.

forwards at the hips with back braced. Use small, relaxed arm movements. An upright cleaner is less stressful than a cylinder. Restore the lordosis frequently. Avoid vacuuming the stairs with an upright cleaner; always use the attachments.
- When sweeping, pushing away is less stressful than sweeping towards you but change direction frequently, sweeping in all directions. Restore the lordosis regularly.

Washing

Stooping over a bath to wash hair or over a basin to brush teeth are particularly difficult positions with a problem back. Either bend the knees, possibly propping them against the bath, or sit on a stool in front of the bath or wash basin.

Patient advice 15.1 Back care after stooping
• Avoid walking around in the stoop position. • Straighten up immediately and restore the lordosis even if it aches to do so. This can prevent the ache from becoming a major pain. • Change from stoop to arch every 5 minutes if having to remain in that position.

The early morning stoop is often a catalyst for the start of back trouble, especially if warning twinges of pain have been occurring (Patient advice 15.1).

GENERAL RULES FOR POSTURE AND THE USE OF TOOLS

• Avoid storage in awkward places.
• Use long-handled tools wherever possible.
• All mobile objects should have good castors.
• Posture should be adapted at all times to avoid stress, by using the legs and stabilizing the back.
• Avoid maintaining any position or activity for long.
• Change position and move around at frequent intervals.
• Always restore the lordosis *immediately* after completing a stoop action or a lift, or at intervals if the action is prolonged.

SEXUAL INTERCOURSE

Sexual intercourse is a naturally perfect activity for the lumbar spine, providing rhythmical, therapeutic pelvic tilts. However, it can be acutely disturbing when in a painful back episode.

Advise patients to discuss their pain with their partners to try to work out positions that are helpful and satisfactory for them both. Fear of pain and fear of failure can wreak havoc upon a sexual relationship; the situation needs infinite patience and understanding.

There are numerous different positions to try, the basic rule being that the partner in pain should be the least active. Possibly start by the painful partner adopting the most comfortable position and the other trying to adapt round it (Herbert 1994).

Possible position:

• one partner lying down, the other sitting upright astride
• one partner on a chair, the other sitting on the lap
• both lying on the side, face to face with legs intertwined
• both lying on the side, back to front.

Recommend the NBPA book *Sex and back pain* (Herbert 1994) (see Further reading).

REFERENCES

Bauer W, Wittig T 1998 Influence of screen and copy holder positions on head posture, muscle activity and user judgement. Applied Ergonomics 29(3): 185–192.
Bork B E, Cook T M, Rosecrance J C et al 1996 Work-related musculoskeletal disorders among physical therapists. Physical Therapy 76(8)
Boyling J D 1996 The 1996 Olive Sands Memorial Lecture. Work related upper limb disorders. In Touch 81: 2–6
Boyling J D 1997 Ergonomics and the management of pain. In: Wells P, Frampton V, Bowsher D (eds) Pain management by physiotherapy. Butterworth Heinemann, Oxford
Boyling J D, Palastanga N (eds) 1994 Grieve's modern manual therapy, 2nd edn. Churchill Livingstone, Edinburgh
Cohen M L, Arroyo J F, Champion G D, Browne C D 1992 In search of the pathogenesis of refractory cervicobrachial pain syndrome. Medical Journal of Australia 156: 432–436
EEC 1990 Official journal of the European Communities.

No. L 156/17 and 18, EC90/269/EEC, 21 June
Elvey R L, Quinter J L, Thomas A N 1986 A clinical study of RSI. Australian Family Physician 15(10): 1314–1315, 1319, 1322
Gassett R S, Hearne B, Keelan B 1996 Ergonomics and body mechanics in the workplace. Orthopedic Clinics of North America 27(4): 861–879
Gifford L 1992 Personal communication
Glazer A, Glazer L 1991 Sitting and the VDU directives. Legislation and recommendations in seating. In Touch 61: 32–33
Grant R, Jull G, Spencer T 1997 Active stabilisation training for screen based keyboard operators – a single case study. Australian Physiotherapy 43(4): 235–242
Greening J, Lynn B 1998 Vibration sense in the upper limb in patients with repetitive strain injury and a group of at-risk office workers. International Archives of Occupational and Environmental Health 71: 29–34
Griegel-Morris P, Larson K, Mueller-Klaus K, Oatis C A 1992

Incidence of common postural abnormalities in the cervical, shoulder, and thoracic regions and their association with pain in two age groups of healthy subjects. Physical Therapy 72(6): 425–430

Health and Safety Commission (HSC) 1998 Manual handling in the health services. HMSO, London

Health and Safety Executive (HSE) 1998a Musculoskeletal disorders in supermarket cashiers. HMSO, London

Health and Safety Executive (HSE) 1998b A pain in your workplace. HMSO, London

Health and Safety Executive 1999 Working with videos. HMSO, London

Helliwell P S 1996 Diagnostic criteria for upper limb disorders. Ergonomics and occupational health: the management of musculoskeletal disorders. Meeting organised by the Ergonomics Society, London, 3rd December

Herbert P T 1994 Sex and back pain. National Back Pain Association, Teddington

Kember J 1997 Focal dystonia in a musician. Manual Therapy 2(4): 221–225

Kember J M 1998 The physical therapist's contribution: neck and shoulders. In: Winspur I, Wynn Parry C B (eds) The musician's hand: a clinical guide. Martin Dunitz, London

Mandal A C 1984 The correct height of school furniture. Physiotherapy 70(2): 48–53

Mierzejewski M, Kumar S 1997 Prevalence of low back pain among physical therapists in Edmonton, Canada. Disability and Rehabilitation 19(8): 309–317

Mottram S 1997 Dynamic stability of the scapula. Manual Therapy 2(3): 123–131

National Back Pain Association (NBPA) 1998 The guide to the handling of patients, 4th edn. NBPA in collaboration with the Royal College of Nursing, London

Pheasant S 1991 Ergonomics, work and health. Macmillan, Basingstoke

Scheer S J, Mital A 1997 Ergonomics. A focused review. Archives of Physical Medicine and Rehabilitation 78: S36-S45

Turner B 1998 Prevention of work related musculoskeletal disorders (WMSD): an evidence based approach. In Touch 87: 11–15

FURTHER READING

Health and Safety Executive (HSE) 1999 A pain in your work place. Ergonomic problems and solutions. Health and Safety Executive, Sheffield

Herbert L 1994 Sex and back pain. National Back Pain Association, Teddington

16

How to cope with an acute attack

Impatience with illness and injury is a healthy and natural reaction. Most patients want to resume normal living very quickly and are often bewildered by the strange, uncontrollable forces which dominate their bodies. They are uncertain about the way to handle pain, afraid of doing something that makes things worse and frustrated because the injury 'should be better by now'. As a result either pain avoidance strategies begin or they struggle on, trying to function 'normally' but not necessarily correctly and so irritate and prolong the injurious process (Evans 1980).

ACUTE BACK PAIN

The approach to acute back pain should be that of the detective searching for clues and we should encourage this approach in a positive, practical sense in our patients. The first significant question is 'What provoked this pain?' Then, 'Was the onset gradual or sudden?' If gradual, 'Have any daily activities been different from usual?' If sudden, 'What was I doing when it happened?' or 'What did I do the day before?'

If there has been no obvious traumatic event, the analysis can be difficult: an apparently unimportant twinge of back pain while decorating followed by a long car drive at the weekend could well be a trigger, or an evening spent sitting in the cinema after a heavy day's work and a fast game of squash could be a reason for waking the next morning unable to move.

Discovering the causative factor can supply the danger situations to avoid and recognizing the sequence of events can provide the patient with valuable education for future back care.

After any injury, if pain is disabling and unrelenting or if a neurological deficit is added to referred pain, further investigations should be made.

PATIENT SELF-MANAGEMENT

If there appears to be an inflammatory element to the pain, the back should be treated like any soft tissue injury with ice, rest from full activity and possibly antiinflammatory medication. If the pain appears to be mechanical, then positional back care can be the most valuable beginning.

Application of ice

If ice is to be used, it should be administered as soon as possible after injury; measures taken within the first 15–20 minutes can make a difference of days or weeks to the length of rehabilitation (Knight 1989). The patient is unlikely to have one of the commercially produced ice packs at home but frozen peas are a good substitute and are readily available to most people. They are preferable to ice cubes, being more malleable and more comfortable. Added to which, it has been found that melting ice has a greater cooling effect than cooled gel packs (McMaster et al 1988). The patient needs to be advised about application (Patient advice 16.1).

There is no proof that ice is beneficial after the first 48 hours, when any swelling will have decreased; however, if it continues to give relief, advise less frequent use for longer application times (Black 1992). Ice should not be used on patients with vascular problems or any patient with a recent history of heart disease, nor should it be used on those who have diminished skin sensation (Major 1992).

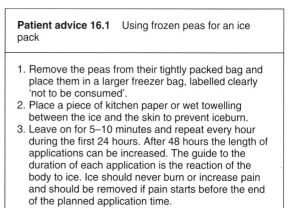

Patient advice 16.1   Using frozen peas for an ice pack

1. Remove the peas from their tightly packed bag and place them in a larger freezer bag, labelled clearly 'not to be consumed'.
2. Place a piece of kitchen paper or wet towelling between the ice and the skin to prevent iceburn.
3. Leave on for 5–10 minutes and repeat every hour during the first 24 hours. After 48 hours the length of applications can be increased. The guide to the duration of each application is the reaction of the body to ice. Ice should never burn or increase pain and should be removed if pain starts before the end of the planned application time.
4. Replace the peas in the freezer after use.

Rest

The quantity of rest required depends on the degree of injury and the severity of pain. It can vary from merely avoiding provocation to implementing complete bed rest but the latter should be very rare.

The effects of bed rest have received considerable investigation and it is clear that prolonged rest is actually deleterious, possibly leading to later chronicity. Within a week or two of inactivity, there is a decrease in strength, endurance, flexibility, coordination and fitness. Protracted rest leads to a catabolic state with general malaise, eventually leading to demineralization of bone and 3% loss of muscle per day (Nachemson 1983, Deyo et al 1986, Twomey & Taylor 1991, Waddell 1998). Deyo et al (1986) found that 2 days bed rest was as beneficial as 7 days in cases of straightforward acute low back pain without discogenic or pain referral complications.

Criteria for bed rest

The criteria for rest in acute pain are based upon the severity of symptoms and the inability to relieve pain. Patients should be encouraged to continue living as normally as possible with avoidance of provocative activities such as prolonged sitting, prolonged standing, long periods of driving, all manual work or sport and, with the full implementation of back care,

---

Patient advice 16.2   Prone lying

- Explain that when one lies supine, gravity pulls the lumbar spine into flexion.
- When one lies prone on the floor, gravity pulls the spine into a natural lordosis (not on the bed as the 'give' of the springs may increase extension).
- If it is painful to lie this way, do not use it.
- If it relieves pain, use it for 5 minutes every hour.

Patient advice 16.3   Resting in acute pain

Resting *does not mean*:
- slouching on the settee whilst craning the neck round to watch TV
- sitting slumped in a chair for hours
- sitting slumped in a chair with both feet up on a stool
- sitting propped up in bed on a pile of cushions.

Resting *does mean*:
- finding and using positions of relief in the horizontal position – prone, supine and side lying
- changing these positions every half an hour
- interspersing lying with moving around and sitting for meals.

---

there should be daily improvement. Only if pain is unremittingly severe, if there is acute leg pain referral or if symptoms are unmistakably deteriorating such that no relief can be found in any upright position should bed rest be advised.

'Bed rest', however, must be *correct rest*, combined with as much change of position or movement as the pain will allow, either in bed or on the floor, whichever gives greatest relief. Rest that is inadequate is worse than careful activity because it makes the sufferer feel that the injury is probably being provoked further:

> 'I've rested for a whole week and my pain is still as bad as ever!'
> 'How did you rest?'
> 'Oh, I lay on the settee' or 'I sat reading all day'!

The body should be completely supported horizontally, lying supine, prone or side lying, with frequent changes of position. Patients rarely try prone lying and it should be suggested to them with full instruction about the criteria (McKenzie 1981) (Patient advice 16.2). If prone lying helps, encourage use of it for 5 minutes every hour, but warn not to use it if it exacerbates pain. A discogenic problem can improve dramatically if treated this way during the first week.

Any position which reduces pain should be adopted frequently; any position which increases pain should be avoided. But *movement is essential* (Williams & Sperryn 1979, Nachemson 1983, Maitland 1986) (Patient advice 16.3). Gentle movements within the limits of pain actually reduce pain and enhance the healing process.

Figures 16.1–16.5 show possible ways of resting when in acute pain.

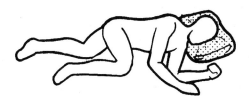

Figure 16.1   Lie on one side (usually the pain-free one) with both legs bent up and a pillow between the knees.

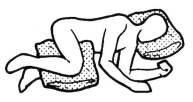

Figure 16.2   Lie on the pain-free side with the painful leg bent up, resting on the bed.

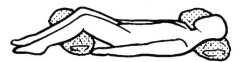

Figure 16.3   Lie supine with a pillow under both knees.

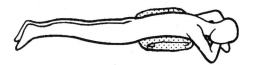

Figure 16.4   Lie prone with or without a pillow under the abdomen.

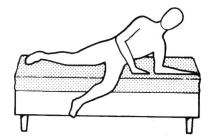

Figure 16.6   Roll onto one side (preferably the pain-free one) with both legs towards the edge of the bed; raise onto one elbow.

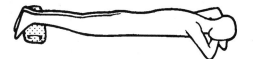

Figure 16.5   Lie prone with or without a pillow under both ankles.

Advise against staying in any position for long periods. Change positions frequently but give the back time to relax in each position before moving out of it.

Resting with referred pain

It is important to explain that the leg pain is coming from the back and there is nothing wrong with the leg itself, so thought has to go into the position of the back combined with the position of the leg. For example, suggest Figure 16.2.

Explain the possible provocative positions for leg pain: sitting with both legs on a stool or with the legs out straight in the bath or propped up in bed. Sitting is best avoided if pain is severe but whenever used, the knees should be bent with both feet on the floor. Substitute a shower for the bath or kneel in the bath. Heat or massage to the leg may feel soothing but it will not help to reduce the pain; the very action of bending forward into flexion to rub the leg may in fact exacerbate the pain.

If leg symptoms persist with paraesthesia or anesthesia, a doctor should be consulted.

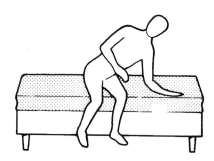

Figure 16.7   Push up with your arm into the sitting position while dropping both legs over the side of the bed.

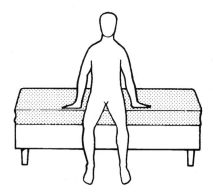

Figure 16.8   Sit for a moment and try to straighten up as much as possible.

Rising from bed in acute pain

Figures 16.6–16.9 show how to rise from bed when in acute pain.

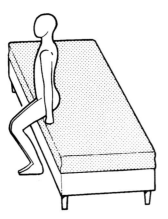

Figure 16.9 Slide to the edge of the bed with both feet tucked well in. Brace the back, edge well forwards and straighten the knees.

Putting on shoes and socks in acute pain

Simple tasks like putting on shoes and socks create a major difficulty. Suggest lying supine, bending one knee up at a time so that it is possible to reach a foot to put the sock on while the back remains supported on the bed.

Rising from sitting in acute pain

Rising from sitting when in acute pain is a time when it is not only permissible but actually necessary to use arm support. Advise the patient to edge to the front of the chair with the back straight, put both hands on the arms of the chair, get the weight of the body as far forwards over the feet as possible, remaining upright, then push with both arms and straighten the legs, keeping the back braced.

ANTIINFLAMMATORY MEDICATION

In the presence of acute pain it is important to limit C-fibre input and prevent summation of pain accompanied by alteration of dorsal horn activity. For this reason, pain of an inflammatory nature can benefit from the administration of antiinflammatory medication.

Non-steroidal antiinflammatory drugs (NSAIDs), of which there are a large selection, have three therapeutic actions: against pain, against inflammation and against fever (Melzack & Wall 1996, Thompson 1997). Their predominant action is to inhibit the synthesis of chemical pain mediators, in particular the prostaglandins. NSAIDs should be taken *regularly*, not merely as analgesics, and analgesics can be added if necessary. In cases where bleeding is suspected, antiinflammatory drugs are contraindicated for 48 hours after injury as they can delay the clotting process.

Antiinflammatory steroids (corticosteroids) are extremely effective in reducing the inflammatory reaction when injected into the site in the first 3 or 4 days after injury, but there are reservations about their effect upon the healing process (Evans 1980).

Recovery

Three to five days after injury all patients should have reduced pain. If not or if there is continuing limb referral, a reassessment should be made.

In simple back pain the repair process should now be aided by gently increasing movement without retraumatizing the injury until a fully pain-free situation is achieved. Encourage the patient to recognize the parameters of the pain, learn how far movement can take place in each direction without increasing it, then use all the pain-free range as normally as possible, thus avoiding pain without fearful 'pain avoidance'. Advise rest after work initially and avoidance of unnecessary social engagements, for example sitting in a theatre for several hours.

A variety of factors influence the rate of recovery, including the general health of the patient, the anatomy of injured tissue, the blood supply to the tissue and the severity of the injury (Sullivan 1994). On assessment, pain at rest, pain on palpation, pain with gentle stress, swelling and discomfort are all clinically informative. Transversus abdominis facilitation should be an early therapeutic instruction, progressing to trunk stabilization when appropriate. Mobilization should be added slowly, increasing the range of movement as the pain recedes. Tissues can be gently stressed once constant pain is eliminated and when movement no longer gives lingering pain. Pain should be the guide for the progression of exercises, the important criterion being whether any slight pain experienced during a movement gets worse on repetition of that movement or lingers afterwards. Avoid increasing pain by progressing too quickly.

Gradually increase the magnitude, duration and frequency of repeated active movement, progressively stressing ligamentous tissue (Sullivan 1994). Although injured tissue never returns to its original texture, careful stretching remodels the collagen of scar tissue and should be performed, with attention paid to the sensations in the area, until previous range is achieved (Evans 1980).

Encourage swimming (avoiding the poorly performed breast stroke) and the gradual increase of walking, both in speed and length, progressing to a rehabilitation programme if necessary.

The average back injury takes 3–6 weeks to recover but in severe cases, if there has been extensive tissue damage or discogenic involvement, it can take 6–12 months. Tissue damage can result in tissue shortening, scarring, limited neural dynamics, a decrease in joint mobility and proprioception, dysfunctional movement and muscle imbalance. Therapy should be able to address and treat most of these problems; however, it is essential for patients to understand that back pain of this kind is not a disease and full recovery is very much their responsibility (see 'Treatment of acute pain' in Chapter 10). A severe back injury may require a full warm-up regime with stretches prior to undertaking any sporting activities for the rest of life (Williams & Sperryn 1979).

Emotional recovery from back pain is as important as the physical recuperation. It is essential for patients to feel that they have 'got over' their injuries, that there is no longer a 'weakness' remaining. Whilst any uncertainty exists, a vulnerability will be present which may lead to pain avoidance, possible reinjury, chronic pain and disability.

THE USE OF CORSETS

There is no evidence to show that lumbar corsets or supports are beneficial or effective for treating patients with LBP or that they limit movement (Koes & Van Den Hoogen 1994). They have only a behavioural effect in that they remind the patient not to move that part of the body (Bogduk & Mercer 1995). In this respect, lumbar supports have some value for patients who must continue with normal daily activities even when they should not be doing so, such as a mother with a young family. Lumbar supports then act as a reminder to avoid stooping and to think of back care. It is important that corsets should not become a habit and they should be discarded as soon as the acute phase is over (Hayne 1984).

REFERENCES

Black N 1992 Personal communication

Bogduk N, Mercer S 1995 Selection and application of treatment. In: Refshauge K, Gass E (eds) Musculoskeletal physiotherapy. Butterworth Heinemann, Oxford

Deyo R A, Diehl A K, Rosenthal M 1986 How many days of bed rest for acute low back pain? New England Journal of Medicine 315: 1064–1070

Evans P 1980 The healing process at cellular level: a review. Physiotherapy 66(8): 256–259

Hayne C R 1984 Ergonomics and back pain. Physiotherapy 70(1): 9–13

Knight K L 1989 Crycotherapy in sports injury. In: Grisogono V (ed) Sports injuries. Churchill Livingstone, Edinburgh

Koes B W, Van Den Hoogen H M M 1994 Efficacy of bed rest and orthoses of low back pain. A review of randomised clinical trials. European Journal of Physical Medicine and Rehabilitation 4: 86–93

McKenzie R A 1981 The lumbar spine: mechanical diagnosis and therapy. Spinal Publications, Waikanae, New Zealand

McMaster W, Liddle S, Waugh T 1988 Laboratory evaluation of various cold therapy modalities. American Journal of Sports Medicine 6: 291–294

Maitland G D 1986 Vertebral manipulation, 5th edn. Butterworths, London

Major K 1992 Principles of treatment following joint examination and assessment. In: Tidswell M E (ed) Cash's textbook of orthopaedics and rheumatology for physiotherapists. Mosby Yearbook Europe, London

Melzack R, Wall P 1996 The challenge of pain. Penguin Books, Harmondsworth

Nachemson A 1983 Work for all: for those with low back pain as well. Clinical Orthopaedics and Related Research 179: 77–85

Sullivan M S 1994 Lifting and back pain. In: Twomey L T, Taylor J R (eds) Physical therapy of the low back. Churchill Livingstone, Edinburgh

Thompson J 1997 Pharmacology of pain relief. In: Wells P, Frampton V, Bowsher D (eds) Pain management by physiotherapy. Butterworth Heinemann, Oxford

Twomey L T, Taylor J 1991 Age-related changes of the lumbar spine and spinal rehabilitation. Physical and Rehabilitation Medicine 2(3): 153–169

Waddell G 1998 The back pain revolution. Churchill Livingstone, Edinburgh

Williams J G P, Sperryn P N 1979 Sports medicine. Edward Arnold, London

FURTHER READING

Forster A, Palastanga N 1995 Clayton's Electrotherapy. Theory and practice, 10th edn. Baillière Tindall, London

Palastanga N 1997 Heat and cold. In: Wells P, Frampton V, Bowsher D (eds) Pain management by physiotherapy. Butterworth Heinemann, Oxford

17

Exercise

DEFINING EXERCISE

Physical exercise can be defined as an exertion of the body in the form of organized play or specific movement which should improve musculoskeletal function, gain in skill at every performance, promote fitness and be pleasurable to perform.

Exercise is necessary because:

• it creates strong, healthy bones, actually promoting growth in the young and helping to avoid osteoporosis in the elderly (Peterson & Renstrom 1992, RCP 1999)

• it aids coordination and balance (Buchner et al 1993)

• it maintains joint and soft tissue mobility and midrange repetitive movements enhance the nourishment of specific tissues, especially the discs (Thomason 1979, Waddell 1998)

• it strengthens body musculature and bone density and increases metabolic activity (Jones & Round 1995, HEA 1997)

• it increases stamina and there are strong indications that regular physical activity may prevent cardiovascular disease (Peterson & Renstrom 1992, HEA 1992). Coronary heart disease (CHD) is the single most common form of death in the UK and lack of fitness has been found to be as important a risk factor for CHD as hypertension, raised blood cholesterol or smoking (DoH 1992)

• it reduces pain through several local and general physiological effects, for example by stabilizing the motion segment and by increasing the level of endorphins (McArdle et al 1991, Cailliet 1995, Richardson & Jull 1995)

• it enhances psychological well-being (HEA 1997).

Physical activity is usually associated with youth but recent evidence points to an even greater importance for older people. The loss of capacity and ability is often regarded as the hallmark of ageing but an even more important effect is the loss of the body's ability to respond to challenge. Not only can exercise prevent many of the problems that hitherto have been assumed to be the normal concomitants of ageing, but it can also improve fitness and lead to the ability to increase performance level (Muir Gray 1987).

SPORT

Sport is now accepted as an integral part of keeping fit. The days are long gone when natural endowment alone was enough to secure success in sport (McIntosh 1979). Training and practice are now a vital part of club activities for competitive sport and they are an important part of sport for pleasure in order to protect the body from injury. Training is necessary to improve or maintain physical capacity or endurance; practice requires the repetition and betterment of techniques (McIntosh 1979). Irregular participation in sports activities ignoring any regular training or keep fit sessions is a dangerous practice.

Predisposing factors for back injury in sport

Flexion/extension stress

Some sports include sustained positions in flexion or extension (for example, speed skating in flexion, gymnastics in extension) or high-velocity thrusts into extension often followed by flexion (for example, serving in tennis, bowling in cricket, javelin throwing, high jump, wind surfing). These positions and movements can bring about substantial structural changes in the joints and soft tissues of the lumbar spine in adolescents and young people. Care should be taken not to overload a young spine (Twomey et al 1988, Liston 1994).

Sustained flexion. This induces all the previously discussed tissue stresses and changes: damage to the intervertebral disc by deformation and fluid loss, damage to the facet joint cartilage and capsules with stress on the spinal ligaments and tissue adaptation (Radin & Paul 1972, Adams & Hutton 1983, Twomey & Taylor 1991, Herbert 1995).

Loaded extension or high-velocity movements into extension. These can damage the posterior annulus of the disc and, by impacting the facet joints, may increase the risk of weakening the pars interarticularis, especially in young people whose bones are still developing (Twomey et al 1988, Liston 1994).

Prevention. Ensure good postural alignment, with optimum muscle length, flexibility of soft tissues and correct functional movement.

Contact sports

As contact sports contain all the hazards of accident and impact, they should be avoided during periods of back pain.

Sports with excessive vibration

Sports such as motor racing and cross-country motor cycling provide vibration in sustained flexion, the motor cyclist having the added stress of handling a heavy vehicle. Contrary to some belief, there is no evidence that jogging is disadvantageous to the lumbar spine except in those with already damaged backs; it could even be useful for postural back pain (Twomey 1992).

Prevention. Regular fitness training should be maintained with back care advice, such as restoring the lordosis on standing after a period of driving.

Sports with vertebral compression thrust

These sports include water-ski jumping, ski jumping and sports which involve high-impact landing. Research done on water-ski jumping found an alarming number of spinal injuries occurring in young jumpers, some only 13 years old (Stubbs 1982). The report suggests an urgent review and limitation of jumping for adolescents, possibly by reducing the jump heights or the boat speed or by restricting the event to people over 16 years old (Stubbs 1982). In healthy adult spines, although the 'landing' force far exceeded the 'take-off' force, it did not appear to be intense enough to cause injury.

Every sport has its risk element; the aim of investigating these is not to deter people from participating but to make the activity safer (Stubbs 1982).

Water sports

Swimming is the ideal sport for back sufferers. The movement can be varied with frequent changes of stroke; swimming can be performed as gently or as energetically as desired and can be used aerobically by speeding up the pace. Patients must be warned that breast stroke with the head held in extension can exacerbate neck and arm pain.

Aquarobics are particularly beneficial, especially for the elderly, and offer a mode of good all-round rehabilitation (Baum 1998).

THERAPEUTIC EXERCISES

Richardson & Jull (1995) point out that therapeutic exercise encompasses several strategies (Box 17.1). Therapists have to be quite specific about the aims of exercise and muscle reeducation. Training effects are seen only in the particular training exercise, with minimal carry-over into other tasks, and exercise at a fixed muscle length and/or speed benefits the muscle function only at that length and speed (Lamb & Frost 1993).

Box 17.1 Therapeutic exercise

Therapeutic exercise can be used:
- for pain relief
- for functional rehabilitation of the muscle system
- to improve joint and muscle flexibility
- to enhance cardiovascular fitness.

Box 17.2 The ultimate functional goal of therapeutic exercises

- To reprogramme poor movement patterns
- To improve functional performance

Exercises must also be patient specific, based on biomechanic and neurophysiologic principles, and have individual functional goals (Bookhout 1996) (Box 17.2). Patients develop particular patterns of movement in response to their individual stresses and postures and no two patients are the same (Goldby 1996).

The normal muscle system provides stability and protection to articular structures, minimizes joint displacement, aids stress absorption and prolongs cartilage serving time (Baratta et al 1988). Segmental stabilization is provided by osseous, ligamentous and muscle restraints (Panjabi 1992). Early preprogrammed recruitment before action, together with co-contraction of agonists and antagonists, provide joint support (Hodges & Richardson 1996). Transversus abdominis (TA) and lumbar multifidus (LM) are the most important components of the local stability system, while other primary muscles involved in perturbations of the lumbar spine are the internal obliques, the diaphragm and the pelvic floor. The external obliques and rectus abdominis are primarily active during lumbar spine flexion/extension, but influence IAP, the obliques working with erector spinae control rotation (Richardson & Jull 1995, Allison et al 1998).

After injury, weakness in muscle and subtle movement in the motion segment's neutral zone may increase (Panjabi 1992). Tonic muscle fibres are affected by disuse and by both reflex and pain inhibition associated with lumbar pain. LM becomes dysfunctional after episodes of LBP and the recovery is not automatic after resolution of the pain (Richardson & Jull 1995, Hides et al 1994, 1996). Other muscles involved in the control of the lumbopelvic area also appear to be vulnerable to loss of their supporting roles: gluteus maximus (compared with other hip flexors), gluteus medius (compared to other hip abductors) and iliopsoas (compared to other hip flexors) (Richardson & Jull 1994).

Without assessment, it is impossible to say which exercises should be used for rehabilitation. The exercises here are a selection of those that are frequently used and are depicted partly as an aid to help a patient understand the movement. No exercise should be performed simply because it appears here. The relationship between exercise and pain is confusing for patients and they need guidance (Patient advice 17.1). They also need encouragement about the need to move (Patient advice 17.2).

McKenzie (1981) worked out a principle of examination of spinal problems, using repeated movements which are in themselves diagnostic; the exercises can then be used therapeutically.

His principles are described in three books: one for therapists (see Further reading) and two for patients: *Treat your own back* and *Treat your own neck*, published by Spinal Publications.

Exercises for pain relief

The aim is a programme for co-contraction of TA and LM whilst maintaining the spine in a neutral position. Functional demands for the need for stabilization indicate that isometric exercises for the local muscles, with low-level tonic contraction, held for 10 seconds and repeated as many times as possible throughout the day, are most beneficial (Richardson & Jull 1995).

These exercises start in the positions described in Figures 17.1–17.5. Progression of the exercise should start with minimal external loading and progress by combining dynamic functional exercises for other parts of the body (Figs 17.6 & 17.7) (Comerford et al 1998).

Facilitation and training of transversus abdominis

This is a difficult exercise to initiate, especially for a person with strong rectus abdominis and external obliques, who has done 100 sit-ups every morning! Teaching it needs time and patience.

Describe TA and its anatomical connection with LM: that they co-contract on activation of TA and it is important to activate them both for stabilization of the motion segment.

Setting transversus abdominis (TA) (Fig. 17.1).

• The patient should be in a comfortable side lying position with the upper arm resting on the

---

> **Patient advice 17.1** Exercise and pain
>
> *Stabilizing exercises*
> • There should be no pain in the performance of any exercise.
>
> *Mobilizing exercises*
> If there is:
> • sharp, severe or lasting pain during any exercise – *stop and do not repeat it*
> • slight end-of-range pain with no after effect – the exercise can be continued. The ROM should increase, with less pain
> • pain after performing an exercise:
>   1. if muscular, the exercise can be repeated but not progressed until reaction ceases
>   2. if a slight increase of the patient's pain, depending on severity and length of lingering, repeat less vigorously or with fewer repetitions or stop.
> Always **stop** if limb pain increases.
>
> *Always*
> • Introduce one new exercise at a time so that the effect of each exercise can be monitored.
> • Do not repeat any exercise which gives lasting pain after performance.

> **Patient advice 17.2** Movement and pain
>
> • Mid range gentle movements actually reduce pain.
> • Movement improves the nutrition of all structures of the motion segment.
> • Activation of large muscle groups increases the level of endorphins in cerebrospinal fluid, which in turn reduces levels of pain sensitivity.

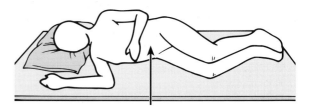

Figure 17.1 Setting transversus abdominis (TA). Initial training.

body, the fingers resting over the diaphragm and the fifth finger just under the ribs.

- Ask the patient to pull in the abdomen; this will invariably elicit either abdominal hollowing, rib flaring, breath holding or abdominal bracing, all of which are common substitution strategies for correct TA facilitation. Explain the incorrect points about any of these actions and point out the movement occurring under the fifth finger, which must be avoided.
- Explain that what is required is a very small, isolated, perfect contraction of TA while the diaphragm area under the hand remains relaxed and goes on moving gently as the patient breathes normally.
- Describe how activating the pelvic floor first helps to trigger TA.

Then, possibly with the therapist's hand on the patient's abdomen, just over/below the umbilicus, teach the correct TA setting.

1. Relax, feel the movement of your diaphragm under your hand.
2. Gently pull in your pelvic floor – did you feel the tiny movement in your lower tummy?
3. Good, now relax again. Next time when you tighten your pelvic floor, try to feel your lower tummy tighten and hold it in while you go on gently breathing.
4. So, keep breathing gently, tighten the pelvic floor, feel your tummy tighten and gently try to pull it in just a little bit more. Good, hold it in; let your diaphragm relax more and more as you keep your lower tummy in and count to 10 slowly.
5. Repeat this contraction 10 times and do the exercise every evening lying in bed.

Setting TA in sitting (Fig. 17.2). Repeat the same instructions for TA setting in sitting, with one hand on the diaphragm and one on the lower abdomen. Explain that the patient should repeat this whenever they are sitting, for example while watching TV, sitting in a car or pausing at work in the office.

When the patient is able to perform this accurately, add the facilitation of LM to the movement.

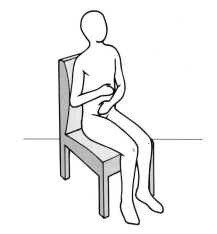

Figure 17.2   Setting TA in sitting.

Facilitation and training of multifidus

Describe multifidus as deep triangles of muscle that run down and out from the spinous processes. Describe an isometric contraction as the concept of a muscle swelling without moving the body (Comerford et al 1998).

Setting lumbar multifidus (LM) (Fig. 17.3). Sitting with the spine in neutral alignment, place the fingers/thumbs on either side of the vertebrae and let them sink into the muscle. Lean forwards from the hips, keeping the spine in neutral and feel the muscle tension. Return to the upright

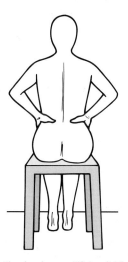

Figure 17.3   Setting lumbar multifidus (LM). (Reproduced with permission from Comerford et al 1998.)

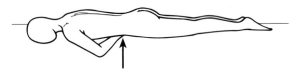

Figure 17.4 Setting TA/LM in prone lying.

position and feel the muscles relax. Try to swell the muscle when sitting upright.

Setting LM by using expiration. At the end of full expiration multifidus is strongly facilitated. Ask the patient to maintain the contraction and keep tension in the muscles as they breathe in again and continue holding the muscle tension with relaxed breathing for 10 seconds. Repeat 10 times.

Similar activation of multifidus can be performed in prone lying, by swelling the muscle against thumb/finger contact.

TA/LM setting in prone lying (Fig. 17.4). In prone lying with the patient's hands under the abdomen, ask the patient to draw the lower stomach gently away from the hands and hold for 10 seconds. Repeat 10 times.

The patient's hands can be replaced by pressure biofeedback for more accurate monitoring. Inflate to 70 mmHg of pressure, which should reduce by 6–10 mmHg on contraction of TA (Richardson & Jull 1995).

Setting TA/LM in four-point kneeling (Fig. 17.5). This is a slightly more difficult position in which to contract TA, but it is visually instructive. Ask the patient to adopt the four-point kneeling position in front of a mirror. Maintain the neutral position of the back with no anterior or posterior pelvic tilt. Draw in the lower abdomen as in the previous exercises, make sure the diaphragm and the obliques do not contract and keep the pelvis still. Continue gentle breathing with a

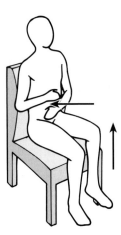

Figure 17.6 Adding limb load to TA/LM in sitting.

relaxed diaphragm while holding in TA. Hold for 10 seconds; repeat 10 times.

Functional rehabilitation of the muscle system

Adding limb load

Adding limb load to TA/LM in sitting (Fig. 17.6). Sitting upright in a chair, with the spine in neutral, draw in the lower abdomen as before, activating LM at the same time. Slowly lift one knee about 3 inches and hold for 10 seconds. Repeat with the other knee, alternately five times.

Crook lying, adding limb load to TA/LM (Fig. 17.7). Start in crook lying with hands under lumbar spine to monitor movement or use pressure biofeedback. Draw in the abdomen. There should be no change in pelvic tilt and only a very slight increase in pressure on the hands. Slowly lift one foot off the floor, bringing the thigh to the

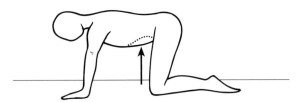

Figure 17.5 Setting TA/LM in four-point kneeling.

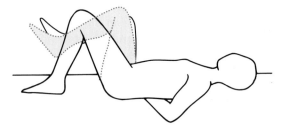

Figure 17.7 Adding limb load to TA/LM setting. (Reproduced from Comerford et al 1998.)

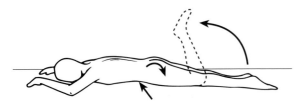

Figure 17.8 Pelvic stabilization using prone knee flexion.

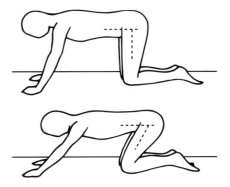

Figure 17.10 Pelvic stabilization in backward rocking. (Reproduced with permission from Comerford et al 1998.)

vertical position and then lift the second foot off the floor and bring it up beside the first. Hold this position, with no change in lumbar pressure on the hands, and then slowly lower one foot to the floor and bring it back again. Repeat with the other foot, slowly alternating the positions for 10 seconds so long as stability is maintained. Then lower both legs back to crook lying. Repeat 10 times.

Trunk stabilization

Pelvic stabilization using prone knee flexion (Fig. 17.8). In prone lying, draw in TA and contract the glutei. Hold this position and slowly bend one knee. Correct any tendency towards hip flexion or pelvic rotation. Stop at the point where the pelvis is likely to 'give'. Hold 10 seconds. Repeat alternately five times.

Single leg stand (Fig. 17.9). Standing in front of a mirror, imagine the trunk to be a rectangle,

a line across the shoulders and one across the ASISs forming the top and bottom of a 'box'. Activate TA/LM with no alteration of pelvic tilt. Keeping the 'box' absolutely steady, transfer the weight onto one leg and slowly lift the other foot off the ground. Notice any rotation on the standing leg, increased pelvic anterior/posterior tilt, hip hitch or trunk side flexion. Correct any dysfunction. Hold 10 seconds and repeat alternately five times. Progress to raising the thigh to the horizontal position with knee relaxed at 90° flexion.

Pelvic stabilization in backward rocking (Fig. 17.10). With patient in four-point kneeling with spine and pelvis in neutral alignment, stabilize the back. Slowly rock the hips back towards the heels, maintaining the neutral position of the spine. The neutral lumbar lordosis should be maintained, without going into flexion, until a position of 120° of hip flexion is reached. Stop at the point before the lumbar spine 'gives'. Repeat slowly five times.

Flat back forward bend (Fig. 17.11). Standing upright, set TA/LM, bend forwards from the hips maintaining a flat back to about 50° forward flexion. The spine should not 'give' into flexion, extension or rotation at any point. Repeat slowly five times. If control is poor, the upper body and trunk weight can be supported initially by resting the arms on a table, stabilizing the back and moving into the upright five times. Progress to the unsupported position as soon as stability can be maintained.

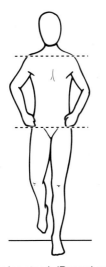

Figure 17.9 Single leg stand. (Reproduced with permission from Comerford et al 1998.)

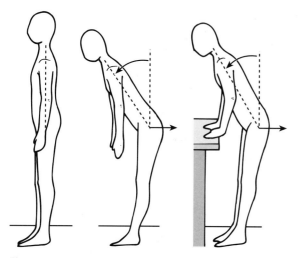

Figure 17.11 Flat back forward bend. (Reproduced with permission from Comerford et al 1998.)

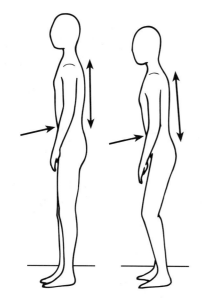

Figure 17.12 Standing two-knee bend. (Adapted from Sahrmann 1993.)

Standing two knees bend (Fig. 17.12). Standing with feet absolutely parallel, 10 cm apart, in correct posture, set TA/LM, pelvis in neutral. Bend both knees slowly forwards. There should be no alteration of pelvic tilt and the knees should not adduct with medial femoral rotation or increased foot pronation; a plumb line dropped from the patella should fall over the second toe. Repeat, maintaining trunk stabilization, bending

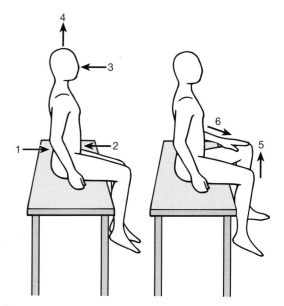

Figure 17.13 Trunk stabilization with resistance.

both knees towards the middle toe. Hold for 10 seconds; repeat 10 times (adapted from Sahrmann 1993).

Trunk stabilization with resistance (Fig. 17.13). Sit on a table, with the back supported in neutral. Set TA/LM. Lift the left knee from the table, resisting the movement with the left hand. The trunk should remain completely stabilized. Hold

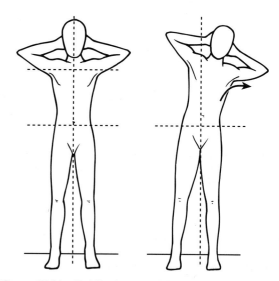

Figure 17.14 Stabilization in side flexion. (Reproduced with permission from Comerford et al 1998.)

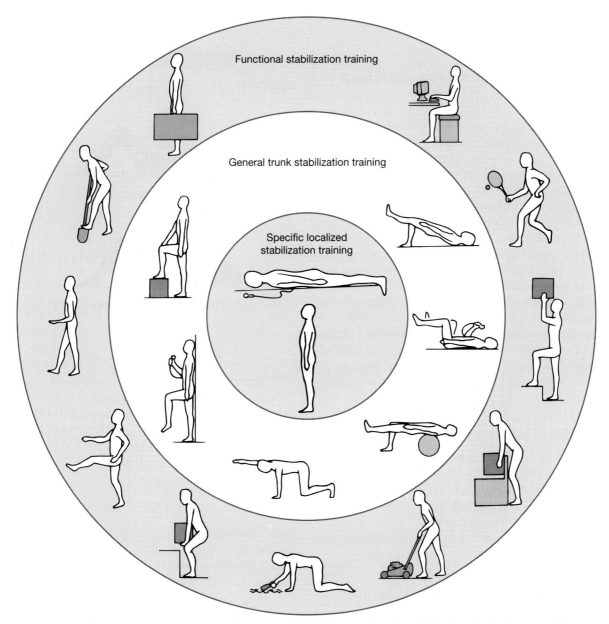

Figure 17.15 A diagrammatic representation of the stages of development of active stabilization of the lumbar spine. (From The lumbar spine. Stabilization training and the lumbar motion segment. Monograph no. 1, 1995. Australian Journal of Physiotherapy (ed. Sharpe M). With kind permission of authors and publisher.)

for 10 seconds. Repeat alternately five times (Braggins 1994).

Stabilization in side flexion (Fig. 17.14). Stand with feet apart, hip flexors unloaded, the back flattened onto the wall and fingers touching the sides of the head. Side-flex, keeping the pelvis level and maintaining contact with the wall. There must be no lumbar extension or anterior pelvic tilt, no pelvic or trunk rotation and no lateral tilt or shift of the pelvis.

Progress to using stabilization in all functional movements (Fig. 17.15).

Other abdominal muscle exercises

Abdominal bracing (Fig. 17.16)

This manoeuvre utilizes the intraabdominal pressure mechanism to stabilize and protect the lumbar spine during lifting moments in the stoop lift (Kennedy 1990). In crook lying or in standing, hands on hips just above the iliac crests, with fingers able to palpate the lateral abdominal muscles, breathe out and contract the abdominal muscles by tightening at the side under the fingers. Hold them tight and go on breathing. *Do not* pull them in by hollowing the abdomen and *do not* push the abdomen out. The oblique abdominal muscle should do the work, not the rectus abdominis. The movement should be comparable to a 'forcing' movement but the glottis should not be closed; air must be expelled easily and freely. There should be no feelings of head pressure during the movement (Kennedy 1990).

Abdominal hollowing (Fig. 17.17)

Using the oblique abdominals in crook lying, hollow or suck in the abdomen, allowing the ribs to 'flare' slightly. *Do not* lift the ribs; relax the chest and continue to breathe naturally while holding the contraction. Hold for a count of 10 seconds and repeat 10 times (Braggins 1994).

Pelvic tilt with abdominal hollowing (Fig. 17.18)

Using rectus abdominis in crook lying, pull in the abdomen until the lumbar spine is flat against the floor, in a posterior pelvic tilt. Hold for a count of 10 seconds while breathing normally, then relax. Repeat 10 times (Braggins 1994).

Abdominal curl-up (Fig. 17.19)

Crook lying with pelvic posterior tilt, slowly raise the head and both shoulders from the

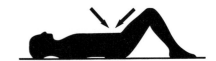

Figure 17.16   Abdominal bracing.

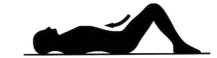

Figure 17.17   Abdominal hollowing.

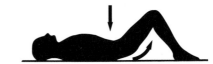

Figure 17.18   Pelvic tilting with abdominal hollowing.

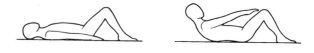

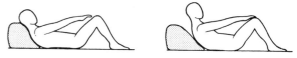

Figure 17.19   Abdominal curl-up.

floor, sliding both hands up the thighs and flexing the trunk. Hold for 10 seconds, then uncurl slowly, *maintaining the posterior pelvic tilt*. Repeat 10 times (Braggins 1994).

Contracting the oblique abdominals by resisting hip flexion (Fig. 17.20)

In crook lying, pull the left knee up towards the right shoulder, place the right hand on the knee and resist the movement. Hold 10 seconds, then relax slowly. Repeat five times with each leg. Increase the degree of resistance as the muscle strength increases. Do not stabilize with the opposite foot or allow substitution (Braggins 1994).

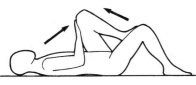

Figure 17.20 Contraction of the oblique abdominal muscles by resisting hip flexion.

Improving joint and muscle flexibility

Many of the mobilizing exercises here use movements of both flexion and extension alternately. If stiffness is the main problem rather than pain, use both movements as described. If one of these movements gives pain, do not push into it; use the pain-free movement while just moving slightly into the other in a pain-free range. The exercises listed below in each section begin with easier movements and progress towards the more difficult. Start with the minimum number of repetitions and increase as movement permits.

Flexion/extension of lumbar spine

Passive lumbar flexion (Fig. 17.21). In crook lying, pull both knees up towards the chest, clasp a hand round each knee and pull up to the chest, allowing the buttocks to leave the floor. Lower back to the floor (McKenzie 1981). Repeat regularly 5–10 times.

Passive lumbar extension (Fig. 17.22). In prone lying, place both hands on the floor by the shoulders and push with both arms, *passively* raising the shoulders off the ground as high as possible without pain, if possible until both arms are straight. It is *essential* that both legs, glutei and back remain completely relaxed while the arms raise the shoulders. Lower back to the starting position; repeat 5–10 times (McKenzie 1981).

Active lumbar flexion/extension (Fig. 17.23). Sitting on a stool, perform gentle pelvic rock into posterior then anterior tilt, maintaining stabilization of the thoracic spine.

Flexion/extension of thoracic spine

Active thoracic flexion/extension (Fig. 17.24). Sitting with both hands placed lightly behind the head, stabilize the lumbar spine, slump the thoracic spine into flexion with the elbows dropped forwards, then straighten up, opening the elbows and finally arching the thoracic spine into extension with the elbows pressed back towards each other. Repeat 3–5 times slowly.

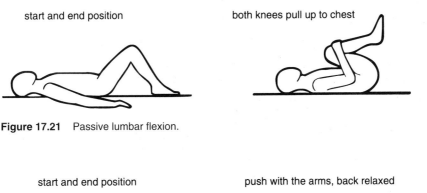

start and end position

Figure 17.21 Passive lumbar flexion.

both knees pull up to chest

start and end position

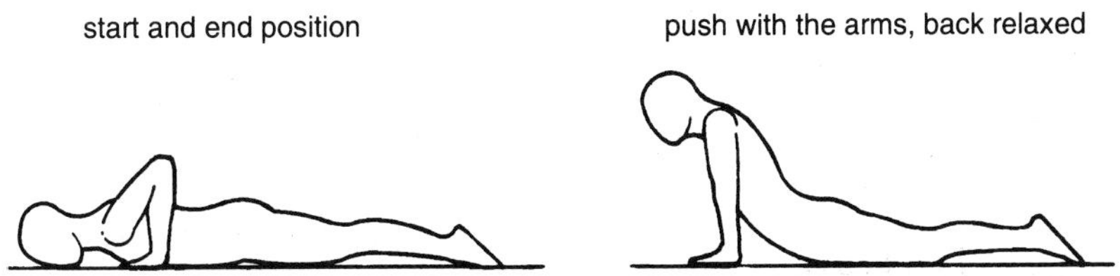

Figure 17.22 Passive lumbar extension.

push with the arms, back relaxed

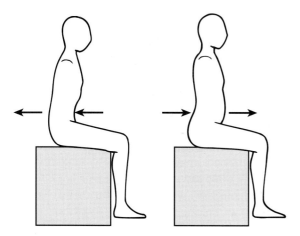

Figure 17.23   Active lumbar flexion/extension.

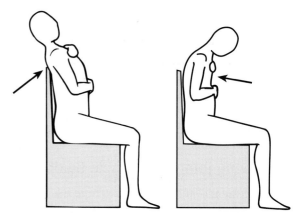

Figure 17.25   Thoracic flexion/extension, using the back of a chair.

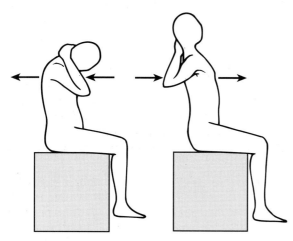

Figure 17.24   Active flexion/extension of thoracic spine.

Thoracic flexion/extension using the back of a chair (Fig. 17.25). Sitting on a chair with the backrest level with the bottom of the scapulae, place the fingers of one hand at the top of the sternum and the fingers of the other hand on the navel, flex the thoracic spine so that the top hand approaches the lower hand, then arch back over the back of the chair so that both hands separate as far as possible. Repeat 3–5 times.

Thoracic spine flexion/extension in squat-kneel (the sphinx) (Fig. 17.26). Kneeling, sitting back on both heels and resting on both elbows, flex the thoracic spine, tucking the head down, then extend the thoracic spine and raise the head. Repeat five times. Moving the elbows further forwards or further back towards the knees can alter the segmental level of thoracic movement.

Exercises for rotation

Double-knee rolling (Fig. 17.27). In crook lying, roll both knees as far as is comfortable one way and then the other. Use a small range to start with and gradually increase with pain reduction. Repeat 10 times.

Single-knee rolling (Fig. 17.28). Lying with one knee bent and foot on the floor, the other leg straight, roll the bent knee over the straight leg,

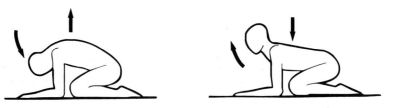

Figure 17.26   Thoracic spine flexion/extension in squat kneel.

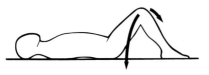

Figure 17.27   Double-knee rolling.

press it towards the floor and bring it up again. Repeat 4–6 times. Repeat with the other leg. This is a sacroiliac stretch, therefore use with caution.

   Passive/active rotation in sitting (Fig. 17.29). Sit on a straight-backed chair. Turn the shoulders to the right, place the right hand behind the chair and with the left hand holding the side of the backrest, pull with the hands to increase rotation. Perform the movement with no hand pull for active work. Then repeat to the left.

   Rotation in sitting with change of arm position (Fig. 17.30). Sitting on a stool:

- for rotating the *upper thoracic spine* – leave the arms hanging by the side and turn slowly round to the left and then to the right as far as possible. Repeat six times
- for rotating the *midthoracic area* – repeat this with elbows bent and hands touching the shoulders
- for rotating the *lower thoracic spine* – repeat the same movement with both arms stretched above the head (Comerford 1993).

Exercises for the cervical spine

   Upper cervical flexion (Fig. 17.31). In crook lying, lengthen the head up the floor with a feeling of holding the position of a head-nod. This exercise should use the upper cervical flexors and lower cervical extensors but there should be no active chin retraction. Hold 5–10 seconds, repeat 3–10 times.

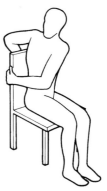

Figure 17.29   Passive/active rotation in sitting.

   When this can be performed, progress to a 'nod' in which the forehead lifts with no chin protrusion (lower cervical flexion), raising the back of the head *just off* the floor. Hold for 3–10 seconds, repeat 5–10 times.

   Correction of the forward head posture (Fig. 17.32). Sit or stand with posture corrected. Move the head forwards a little way as if smelling a flower, then retract the chin away from a 'bad smell'. This should be a horizontal movement of the chin, avoiding any upward or downward movement.

   Lower cervical extension with scapulae setting (Fig. 17.33). Lie face downwards at the end of the plinth or firm bed with the chin hanging over the end. Keeping the face parallel to the floor, retract the chin; hold it retracted then set both scapulae by gently stretching the clavicles back and down. Hold 5–10 seconds. Repeat 3–5 times.

   Stronger upper cervical flexion correction (Fig. 17.34). Sitting on a stool against a wall or standing with the feet 20 cm from the wall, shoulders and arms relaxed, gradually pull the upper thoracic spine back against the wall. Hold

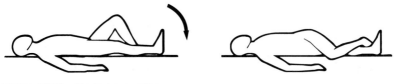

Figure 17.28   Single-knee rolling.

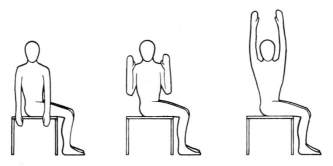

Figure 17.30 Rotation in sitting with change of arm position.

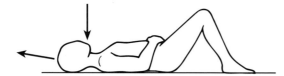

Figure 17.31 Upper cervical flexion.

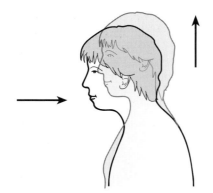

Figure 17.32 Correction of the forward head posture.

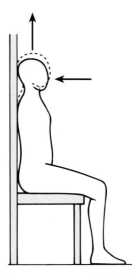

Figure 17.34 Stronger upper cervical flexion.

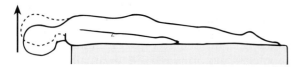

Figure 17.33 Lower cervical extension with scapulae setting.

it firmly there, keeping the chin in neutral. Stretch the back of the head up the wall, using upper cervical flexion. Keep shoulders and arms relaxed. Finally lengthen both clavicles out and down (scapulae setting using lower trapezius). Hold for 10 seconds. Repeat 3–5 times. Do not substitute with chin retraction or shoulder retraction.

Exercises for the back and hip extensors

Gentle back extension (Fig. 17.35). In prone lying with a pillow under the abdomen, raise the head and shoulders just up from the floor, not above the level of the hips. Hold for 20 seconds. Repeat 3–6 times.

Strong back extension (Fig. 17.36). In prone lying with both arms by the side, lift the head and shoulders and both legs off the ground at the same time, but lift only as high as is comfortable. Hold for 5 seconds, then lower. This is a strong exercise and should not be done unless the person is ready for it. Repeat 3–5 times.

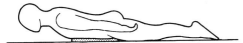

Figure 17.35 Gentle back extension.

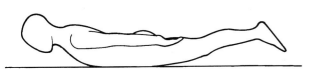

Figure 17.36 Strong back extension.

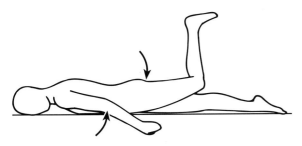

Figure 17.37 Hip extension (gluteus maximus) with back stabilization. (Reproduced with kind permission from Comerford et al 1998.)

Hip extension with back stabilization (Fig. 17.37). In prone lying, bend one knee to 90°, lift the knee off the floor 2–3 inches, maintaining a neutral lumbopelvic position, hold for 10 seconds and repeat 10 times. There should be no strong hamstring work, no hyperextension, pivot or rotation of the lumbar spine.

Shoulder and hip extension with back stabilization (Fig. 17.38). In prone kneeling with neutral back position, lift the right arm forwards and the left leg back to the horizontal. Hold for 10 seconds and lower. Repeat with the other arm

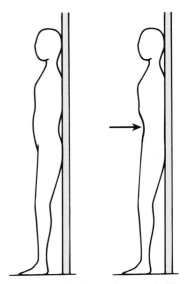

Figure 17.39 Lumbar flexion against a wall. (Reproduced with permission from Comerford et al 1998.)

and leg 3–4 times. This exercise can be used initially with only the arm or only the leg movement. There should be no pelvic rotation and no lumbar hyperextension with any limb movement.

Lumbar flexion

Lumbar flexion against a wall (Fig. 17.39). Stand with the feet 20 cm from the wall, feet wide apart and knees relaxed. Contract the abdominal and gluteal muscles to flatten the back against the wall. Hold for 20–30 seconds. Repeat 5–10 times.

Lumbar flexion in four-point kneeling (Fig. 17.40). In four-point kneeling, contract the gluteal and abdominal muscles to posterior tilt

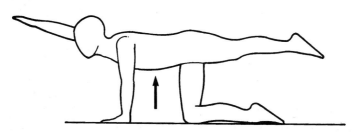

Figure 17.38 Shoulder and hip extension with back stabilization.

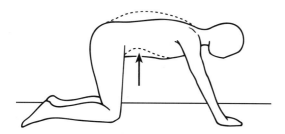

Figure 17.40 Lumbar flexion in four-point kneeling. (Reproduced with permission from Comerford et al 1998.)

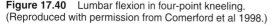

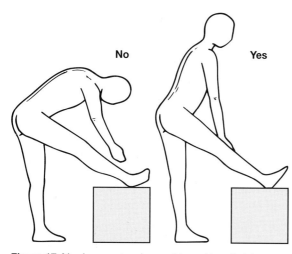

Figure 17.41 Incorrect and correct hamstring stretch.

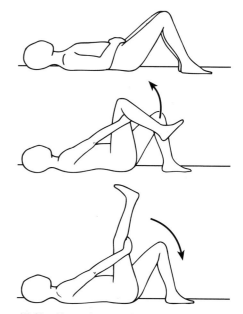

Figure 17.42 Hamstring stretch with thigh support.

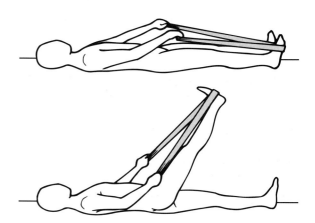

Figure 17.43 Hamstring stretch using a strap.

the pelvis, flex the lumbar spine and then the thoracic spine. Hold for 20–30 seconds and repeat 3–5 times.

Hamstring stretches

Incorrect and correct hamstring stretch (Fig. 17.41). In the 'No' position, the stretch is taking place in the lumbar and especially the thoracic spine. In the 'Yes' position, lumbar extension is maintained and forward flexion occurs only at the hip joint. Place one heel on a stool, stabilize the lumbar spine and lean forwards from the hip maintaining the lordosis. Hold for 20 seconds and repeat 3–5 times.

Hamstring stretch with thigh support (Fig. 17.42). Lying supine, bend one knee to the vertical position, place both hands around the thigh and straighten the knee slowly. Hold for

20–30 seconds and repeat 3–5 times with each leg.

Hamstring stretch with a strap (Fig. 17.43). Lying supine holding a strap extending around the foot of one leg, slowly raise the leg by pulling on the strap until a stretch position is reached. Hold for 20 seconds and repeat 3–5 times.

Hamstring stretch in sitting (Fig. 17.44). Sitting on a table, stabilize the lumbar spine so that it is firmly held in the normal lordosis. Slowly

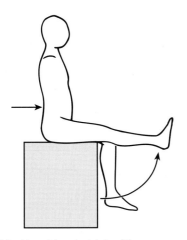

Figure 17.44   Hamstring stretch in sitting.

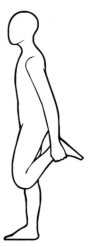

Figure 17.46   Rectus femoris stretch in standing.

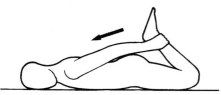

Figure 17.45   Rectus femoris stretch prone.

straighten one leg and hold it straight whilst maintaining the stabilized position of the back. Hold for 10–20 seconds and repeat alternately 3–5 times. Do not let the lumbar spine 'give' when the leg is extended. This can be used as a combined stabilizing lumbar spine and stretching hamstring movement which can be especially useful for teenage LBP rehabilitation.

Rectus femoris stretch

Rectus femoris stretch prone (Fig. 17.45). In prone lying, bend the right knee, bringing the heel towards the buttocks. Pull the leg up further either by gripping the ankle with the right hand or by hooking a towel or belt round the ankle. Hold for a count of 10–20 seconds and repeat 3–5 times with each leg.

Rectus femoris stretch in standing (Fig. 17.46). Standing on one leg, bend the other knee, bringing the foot up behind. Grasp the ankle with the hand and pull the heel towards the buttocks. Actively contract the abdominals and gluteal

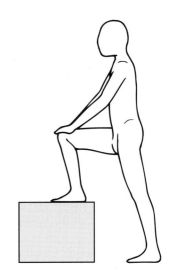

Figure 17.47   Gastrocnemius, soleus and anterior hip stretch.

muscles to posterior pelvic tilt and pull the leg into hip extension. Hold for 10–20 seconds and repeat 3–5 times.

Gastrocnemius/soleus/anterior hip stretch (Fig. 17.47). This position can be used for three stretches. Stand with one leg behind you, foot flat on the floor and the other foot up on a stool.

1. Lean forwards onto the front leg, pushing the foot into dorsiflexion to stretch soleus, allowing the rear knee to relax.

2. With the rear leg stretched well back and foot flat on the floor, lean forwards onto the front leg, stretching the rear ankle gastrocnemius.

3. With the left leg stretched well back, on the ball of the foot, lean onto the right leg, stretching the left hip flexors. Repeat with the right leg stretched back.

In each case hold the stretch for 10–20 seconds and repeat 3–5 times.

Rectus femoris, iliopsoas/anterior hip capsule and tensor fascia latae/iliotibial band test stretch

Test. The patient assumes tight crook lying with their feet at the end of the plinth. The therapist stands on the right side of the patient and places the left hand under the patient's lumbar spine. The patient pulls the left knee up towards the chest until the lumbar spine is flat on the plinth and holds the knee with both hands. The therapist holds the right thigh at 90° hip flexion with the knee at 90° flexion, thigh adducted to the midline. The therapist passively lowers the right test leg down towards the plinth, keeping the femur in the body midline until either the lumbar spine extends or the thigh is flat on the couch.

If the lumbar spine 'gives', the patient should actively stabilize the lumbar spine while the test is repeated. Test both legs. However, *if the patient cannot stabilize the lumbar spine the test should not be performed.*

Result. For all muscles to have good length, the thigh should rest in the body midline position, flat on the plinth with knee flexed to 90°.

If the thigh cannot lie on the plinth with the lumbar spine flat, something is short. To test for short muscle:

1. extend the knee with the thigh adducted to the midline; if the thigh lowers, rectus femoris is short
2. abduct the thigh with the knee at 90° flexion; if the thigh lowers, TFL/ITB is short
3. keep the knee extended and abduct the thigh; if the thigh lowers, iliopsoas is short or anterior hip capsule is tight. The capsular

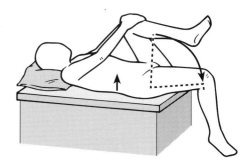

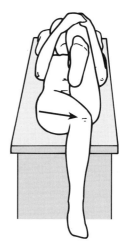

Figure 17.48   TFL/ITB stretch. (Reproduced with permission from Comerford et al 1998.)

end-feel is short, tight and springy; the iliopsoas end-feel is larger and bouncy with recoil (Comerford et al 1998).

Treatment.

• Rectus femoris stretch – use exercises shown in Figures 17.45 or 17.46.

• TFL/ITB stretch (Fig. 17.48). For right TFL treatment, in tight crook lying at the end of the couch, pull the left knee up and hold it at the point of lumbar flattening. Stabilize. Lift the right knee to 90° hip flexion with knee relaxed. Maintaining a flat lumbar spine, slowly lower the right leg with knee relaxed, brushing the left foot to maintain adduction to the midline. At the point where the leg hangs, actively adduct the leg under the left foot and hold for 20–30 seconds. Repeat 3–5 times.

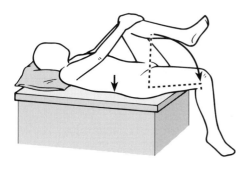

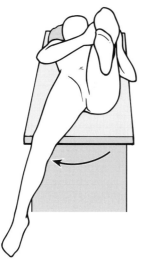

Figure 17.49   Iliopsoas/anterior hip capsule stretch.
(Reproduced with permission from Comerford et al 1998.)

- Iliopsoas/anterior capsule stretch (Fig. 17.49). Repeat the action but lower the leg towards abduction to slacken off TFL/ITB. Hold for 20–30 seconds as above.

Hip and sacroiliac problems can be provoked by these exercises *so care must be taken* (Comerford et al 1998).

Exercises for cardiovascular fitness

In 1992 the Health Education Authority started a campaign to encourage cardiovascular activity in order to improve fitness countrywide. For people who have no medical reason to contra-indicate it, they recommend any activity which slightly increases the heart and respiratory rate, even if it means merely walking fast round the block for 20 minutes, five times a week.

Typical aerobic activities are swimming, walking, running, skipping, cycling (including the static bike), the treadmill and any other gymnasium activity which stimulates the cardio-vascular system.

- The exercise or activity should be performed for between 15 and 45 minutes, 3–5 days a week but adequate rest periods are essential between bouts of training (Kisner & Colby 1988).
- A good warm-up before starting is essential. This should include stretching and slow speed movements, gradually increasing the rate and effort until the person feels ready for action.
- Good equipment is important; for example, good shoes or the right length of skipping rope.
- The environment is also important. Running on soft ground in the countryside is preferable to running on hard pavements in town.
- Strain or overuse of muscles should be avoided. This can occur if too much is done too often. In endurance training, quantity should always be measured in relation to time and speed.

CLASSES FOR REHABILITATION, FITNESS AND FLEXIBILITY

The effects of static and dynamic exercises on patients with CLBP were compared and dynamic exercises were found to be statistically more effective than static exercise in the restoration of function (Goldby 1996). It is feasible to suggest that dynamic exercise may address neural control mechanisms resulting in the normalization of movement patterns (Goldby 1996). Strong aerobic activity also increases the output of endogenous opioid peptides. For this reason it is important for patients to continue with some form of rehabilitation after treatment ceases.

Keep fit

Keep fit classes of all kinds operate throughout the country offering different forms of training. They vary in standard and regime provided. The classes range from traditional keep fit to aerobic classes. There are many special classes for the older person. The teacher should be fully qualified.

Yoga

Yoga is a classical Indian discipline whose origin dates back thousands of years, but which has become widely popular in the West as a practical approach to achieving physical and mental health. Physically, yoga involves a series of stretching postures which increase the mobility of the body by taking the joints and tissues into their full range in careful, unstressed movements. Mentally, the poses themselves become meditative through the quiet focusing of the mind on the activity of the body. By extending the consciousness into the cells of the body which are habitually unaware, yoga unites mind and body. The word *yoga* itself means yoke or union.

Pilates

Pilates also offers both a mental and physical training. It relies on strengthening the postural muscles (particularly transversus) which stabilize the torso, realigning the body by correcting muscle imbalance. Pilates avoids the muscle and ligament damage sometimes associated with other fitness regimes and plays a key role in many injury rehabilitation programmes in dance, sport and general practice (see Useful addresses).

Swimming

Discussed on page 211, swimming is the ideal activity for rehabilitation, fitness and maintaining flexibility.

EXERCISES TO AVOID

These three exercises, two for the back and one for the neck, are unacceptable.

- Lying supine, lifting both legs together at the same time.
- Lying supine, sit-ups with straight legs.

These two exercises are only acceptable if performed under expert training and supervision to achieve correct trunk stabilization first (Comerford et al 1998).

- Neck-circling exercise. This exercise, which is often used in keep fit classes of all kinds, screws the cervical spine round in a complicated range of combined movements which stress the joints quite unproductively and provide no beneficial effect.

Acknowledgement

I would like to thank Mark Comerford and Kinetic Control Ltd for permission to use text and illustrations from their publications.

REFERENCES

Adams M A, Hutton W C 1983 The effect of posture on the fluid content of lumbar intervertebral discs. Spine 8(6): 665–671

Allison G, Kendle K, Roll S et al 1998 The role of the diaphragm during abdominal hollowing exercises. Australian Physiotherapy 44(2): 95–102

Baratta R, Solomon M, Zhou B H et al 1988 Muscular activation. The role of the antagonist musculature in maintaining knee stability. American Journal of Sports Medicine 16(2): 113–122

Baum G 1998 Aquarobics. The training manual.

W B Saunders, Philadelphia

Bookhout M R 1996 Exercise and somatic dysfunction. Manual Medicine 7(4): 845–862

Braggins S 1994 The back: functions, malfunctions and care. Mosby Yearbook Europe, London

Buchner D M, Cress E M, Wagner E H et al 1993 The Seattle FISCIT/Move It Study. Journal of the American Geriatrics Society 41: 321–322

Cailliet R 1995 Low back pain syndrome. F A Davis Co, Philadelphia

Comerford M 1993 Personal communication

Comerford M, Kinetic Control Ltd 1998 Dynamic stability and muscle balance of the lumbar spine and trunk. Course notes

Department of Health (DoH) 1992 The health of the nation: key area handbook – coronary heart disease and stroke. DoH, London

Goldby L 1996 Exercises for low back pain. British Journal for Therapy and Rehabilitation 3(11): 612–615

Health Education Authority (HEA)/Sports Council 1992 Allied Dunbar national fitness survey. HEA, London

Health Education Authority (HEA) 1997 Young people and physical activity. A literature review. HEA, London

Herbert R 1995 Adaptations of muscle and connective tissue In: Refshauge K, Gass E (eds) Musculoskeletal physiotherapy. Butterworth Heinemann, Oxford

Hides J A, Stokes M J, Saide M, Jull G A, Cooper D H 1994 Evidence of lumbar multifidus muscle wasting ipsilateral to symptoms in patients with acute/subacute low back pain. Spine 19(2): 165–172

Hides J A, Richardson C A, Jull G A 1996 Multifidus muscle recovery is not automatic after resolution of acute, first-episode low back pain. Spine 21(23): 2763–2769

Hodges P W, Richardson C A 1996 Inefficient muscular stabilization of the lumbar spine associated with low back pain. Spine 21(22): 2640–2650

Jones D A, Round J M 1995 Skeletal muscle in health and disease. Manchester University Press, Manchester

Kennedy B 1990 An Australian programme for management of back problems. Physiotherapy 66(4): 108–111

Kisner C, Colby L A 1988 Therapeutic exercises. Foundations and techniques. F A Davis, Philadelphia

Lamb S, Frost H 1993 Exercise – the other root of our profession. Physiotherapy 79(11): 772

Liston C B 1994 Low back pain: physical treatment in children and adolescents. In: Twomey L T, Taylor J R (eds) Physiotherapy of the low back. Churchill Livingstone, Edinburgh

McArdle W D, Katch F I, Katch V L 1991 Exercise physiology, energy, nutrition and human performance, 3rd edn. Lea and Febiger, Philadelphia

McIntosh P C 1979 Sport in society. In: Williams J G P,

Sperryn P N (eds) Sports medicine, 2nd edn. Edward Arnold, London

McKenzie R 1981 The lumbar spine. Mechanical diagnosis and therapy. Spinal Publications, Waikanae, New Zealand

Muir Gray J A 1987 Exercise and ageing. In: Macleod D, Maughan R (eds) Exercise, benefits, limits and adaptations. E & F N Spon, New York

Panjabi M 1992 The stabilizing system of the spine. Part II Neutral zone and instability hypothesis. Journal of Spinal Disorders 5: 390–397

Peterson L, Renstrom P 1992 Sports injuries. Martin Dunitz, London

Radin E L, Paul I L 1972 A consolidated concept of joint lubrication. Journal of Bone and Joint Surgery 54-A(3): 607–615

Richardson C A, Jull G A 1994 Rehabilitation of active stabilisation of the lumbar spine. In: Twomey L T, Taylor J R (eds) Physical therapy of the low back. Churchill Livingstone, Edinburgh

Richardson C A, Jull G A 1995 Muscle control – pain control. What exercises would you prescribe? Manual Therapy 1: 2–10

Royal College of Physicians (RCP) 1999 Osteoporosis. Clinical guidelines for prevention and treatment. RCGP, London

Sahrmann A S 1993 Diagnosis and treatment of movement system imbalances associated with musculoskeletal pain. Washington University School of Medicine, course notes

Stubbs D A 1982 Back problems in work and leisure. Physiotherapy 68(6): 174–176

Thomason F 1979 Joints. In: Williams J G, Sperryn P N (eds) Sports medicine. Edward Arnold, London

Twomey L 1992 Personal communication

Twomey L T, Taylor J R 1991 Age-related changes of the lumbar spine and spinal rehabilitation. Critical Reviews in Physical and Rehabilitation Medicine 2(3): 153–169

Twomey L T, Taylor J R, Oliver M J 1988 Sustained flexion loading, rapid extension loading of the lumbar spine, and the physical therapy of related injuries. Physiotherapy Practice 4: 129–137

Waddell G 1998 The back pain revolution. Churchill Livingstone, Edinburgh

FURTHER READING

Baum G 1998 Aquarobics. The training manual. W B Saunders, Philadelphia

Comerford M, Kinetic Control Ltd 1998 Dynamic stability and muscle balance of the lumbar spine and trunk. Kinetic Control, course notes

McKenzie R 1981 The lumbar spine. Mechanical diagnosis and therapy. Spinal Publications, Waikanae, New Zealand

18

Treatments available

Although the aim of back care is to encourage patients to administer their own pain management, pain relief frequently requires help from other sources. These sources include pain modulation in various ways, by medication, by techniques such as physical therapies and alternative therapies or by diagnostic investigation through a range of procedures (Box 18.1) (Baxter 1988, Thompson 1997).

MODULATION OF PAIN BY MEDICATION

The benefit from and use of any medication is entirely dependent upon the cause and severity of the pain. Drugs can be used to affect pain at a wide range of sites along the sensory pathways, ranging from action against the pathological process producing pain to interrupting the nociceptive input or modulation of the cerebral

---

Box 18.1   Pain modulation

Pain can be modulated by various means.
- Removing the peripheral stimulus by ice, NSAIDs and corticosteroids.
- Interrupting the nociceptive input with local anaesthetics or NSAIDs.
- Enhancing the nociceptive inhibitory mechanism by massage or mobilization, TENS, vibration, heat (C fibres), ice (A-delta fibres), acupuncture (A-delta fibres).
- Modulating the central perception of pain by opioid analgesics.

Box 18.2 Primary analgesics

Non-opioid or non-narcotic analgesics
1. Analgesics with no antiinflammatory action, e.g. paracetamol
2. Non-steroidal antiinflammatory agents (NSAIDs), e.g. aspirin, ibuprofen, voltorol, etc.
3. Slow-acting antirheumatic drugs, e.g. gold, sulphasalazine or other immunosuppressants

Opioid or narcotic analgesics
1. Morphine and codeine – derived from the opium poppy
2. Opioids, e.g. pethidine – chemically produced drugs possessing morphine-like activity

---

response at the emotional level (Baxter 1988, Thompson 1997). Only those more commonly used in the treatment of back pain are discussed here (Box 18. 2).

Non-opioid and opioid analgesics

Non-opioid or non-narcotic analgesics

Non-narcotic analgesics can be divided into three groups (Box 18.2). Their main action is on the injured tissue and they are thus described as peripherally acting compounds. Many of these peripherally acting medications possess analgesic, antipyretic and antiinflammatory properties, although paracetamol is minimally antiinflammatory (Sunshine & Olson 1989). The antiinflammatory drugs constitute a mixed group of compounds differing in chemical structure but sharing certain pharmaceutical and therapeutic actions (Conaghan & Day 1995, Melzack & Wall 1996, Thompson 1997).

Mechanical pain, triggered by a non-inflammatory reaction, does not respond to antiinflammatory medication and NSAIDs should not be used in these conditions (Melzack & Wall 1996). However, in most traumatically induced episodes there is an element of inflammation and NSAIDs can be of value in reducing pain and alleviating muscle spasm, thus assisting sleep. Sleep is both psychologically and physiologically important for the process of healing and nourishment of tissues.

When NSAIDs are necessary, they should not be used like 'painkillers'. This is a common mistake; patients take them sporadically then claim they are having no effect. Patients should be advised to use them as prescribed on the packet, taking them regularly with food, for at least 1 week to ascertain their effect. If they are obviously helping they should be continued for 2–3 weeks or until the inflammatory element has subsided.

Opioid or narcotic analgesics

The narcotic analgesics consist of opiates and opioids. These drugs modulate the central perception of pain and are used in more chronic situations (Thompson 1997).

Antiinflammatory steroids or corticosteroids

Glucocorticosteroids are produced naturally in the body by the cortex of the adrenal gland. Cortisol (or hydrocortisone) is the main glucocorticoid produced in humans (Conaghan & Day 1995).

Corticosteroids are used medicinally for three purposes (Conaghan & Day 1995, Thompson 1997):

- replacement therapy (for example, in Addison's disease)
- antiinflammatory and immunosuppressive therapy (for example, in rheumatoid arthritis)
- palliative medicine (for example, in cerebral oedema) or locally by injection for nerve compression.

Steroids are potent reducers of tissue swelling but their long-term use can lead to osteoporotic changes in bone or local tissues.

Antidepressants and muscle relaxants

Antidepressants and muscle relaxants have been used successfully since the 1950s for the management of chronic pain and the analgesic efficacy is independent of whether the patient is depressed or not. It seems likely that the beneficial effect is from activation or reinforcement of pain-controlling systems in the brain or spinal cord which depend on certain neurotransmitters, such as noradrenalin. Imipramine and amitriptyline are known to have an effect on chronic pain (Melzack & Wall 1996, Thompson 1997).

The minor tranquillizers, such as diazepam (Valium) and librium, are usually ineffective in treating chronic pain and may even increase both depression and pain (Melzack & Wall 1996). Diazepam has useful muscle relaxant properties and for this reason can be of value in cases of extreme protective spasm (Baxter 1988).

MANIPULATIVE THERAPIES

Manipulative therapies using touch and mobilization stimulate the nociceptive system via the A-beta fibres and so modulate pain by closing the gate.

Physiotherapy

Physiotherapy is a health care profession which emphasizes the use of physical approaches in the prevention and treatment of disease and disability (CSP 1991). Over 60 years ago, Dr J B Mennell, physical medicine consultant at St Thomas' Hospital, was the first to advocate physical treatment by movement, manipulation and massage (Mennell 1934) and for the first time manipulation was formally included in the physiotherapy curriculum at St Thomas'. Later, in the 1950s, Dr J Cyriax devised a system of assessing and diagnosing musculoskeletal disorders and treating these by manipulation and movement (Cyriax 1984). Prior to that there was minimal specialization, and in the musculoskeletal field physiotherapy consisted of heat, massage and exercises.

Physiotherapy has again changed dynamically since the late 1960s. Greg Grieve (1988) and Geoff Maitland (1991, 1992) pioneered the way into a new approach to musculoskeletal assessment and treatment. As always, new ideas stimulate further investigation; new techniques relating to vertebral mobilization (for example, Grant 1988, Edwards 1992) and soft tissue treatments (for example, Palastanga 1991, Weintraube 1991) are constantly

developing. Neural tissue has been looked at in completely new ways (Elvey et al 1986, Butler 1991) as have muscle function and dysfunction (Richardson et al 1992, Kendall et al 1993, Sahrmann 1993, Comerford et al 1998). Now Gifford (1999) is opening doors into a deeper and broader understanding of pain mechanisms.

Prior to 1977, treatment could only be carried out with medical diagnosis and referral by a doctor. Health circular HC (77) 33 issued by the DHSS in 1977 removed this requirement (Bithell 1992). Now physiotherapy analysis takes into account the patient's current psychological, cultural and social factors and is based on an examination and assessment. The aim is to identify and diagnose the specific components of dysfunction responsible for the patient's physical problems (CSP 1991).

The history of the patient's injury or problem, including the past history of previous ailments, is followed by a meticulous objective examination to identify any neuromusculoskeletal dysfunction. The assessment should lead to a clinical diagnosis and a plan of treatment. Treatment consists of mobilization or manipulation of the joints and/or soft tissue, muscle stabilization, the restoration of pain-free neurodynamics, soft tissue stretching, traction, postural correction and any electrical treatment the physiotherapist may deem applicable. The patient's working posture is discussed and advised upon. Treatment includes a programme of exercises to reinforce progress that has been made and to try to prevent further recurrence.

For 2–3 years after qualifying, physiotherapists work in general hospitals gaining experience in all fields. They then choose one of the following specialities and focus on that area with ongoing postgraduate training: paediatrics, respiratory care, care of the elderly, neurology, orthopaedics, sports injuries or musculoskeletal conditions. They may continue to work in the National Health Service or in private practice.

Osteopathy

Osteopathy started in the USA in 1892. Since then it has flourished in the USA, Britain and parts of Europe (Belshaw 1987). It is the science of human mechanics, a system of diagnosis and manual treatment which places its main emphasis on the structural and mechanical problems of the body. Osteopaths are concerned with the biomechanics of the body and the maintenance of proper mechanical function. Central to osteopathic concept is that much of the pain and disability affecting people stems from abnormalities in the function of the musculoskeletal system rather than from any identifiable pathology. Impaired function in one part of the musculoskeletal system can exist without symptoms but may throw considerable strain onto another part of the body (Fielding et al 1990).

Treatment uses predominantly gentle manual methods of articulatory techniques and soft tissue stretching and a diagnostic procedure similar to a conventional medical examination but with particular attention to detailed assessment of the patient's musculoskeletal system. Osteopaths treat tension headaches, neck and shoulder pain, joint strains in all parts of the body, pains and discomfort associated with pregnancy and sports injuries (Fielding et al 1990).

Registered osteopaths are members of the General Council and Register of Osteopaths and have the letters MRO after their name.

Chiropractic

Chiropractic is a profession which specializes in the diagnosis and treatment of conditions which are due to mechanical dysfunction of the joints and their effects on the nervous system. The term is derived from the Greek words *chiero* (hand) and *praktos* (to use), meaning treatment by hand or manipulation.

Chiropractors will take a thorough case history and carry out a full neurological and orthopaedic examination. They may also take X-rays to check for any abnormalities or conditions which will show if another form of treatment would be more appropriate. The chiropractor then carries out a detailed analysis of how the individual bones, joints and muscles move, in order to identify the specific problem area (Bennett 1992).

Chiropractors use their hands to adjust the joints of the spine and extremities with the aim of improving mobility and relieving pain. This treatment is known as 'adjustment' or 'manipulation' and allows the body's own healing powers to improve health and well-being (BCA 1999).

The British Chiropractic Association is the representative body for the profession and maintains a register of fully qualified chiropractors who have the letters BCA after their name.

SENSORY MODULATION OF PAIN

Transcutaneous electrical nerve stimulation

Transcutaneous electrical nerve stimulation or TENS is a pulsed electrical current which is used for pain relief. It is based on the gate control theory (p. 105) and stimulates the A-beta fibres, thus closing the gate of pain perception (Lewith 1984, Garrison & Foreman 1994, Frampton 1997). The apparatus consists of a small box about 8 cm square from which two or four leads carry the current to rubber electrodes placed on the skin. It is used for long-standing severe pain (particularly in acute nerve root lesions), chronic pain, postherpetic neuralgia, phantom limb pain and during labour (Thomson et al 1991, Melzack & Wall 1996).

Acupuncture

Acupuncture is an old and well-tried treatment of pain used for thousands of years in China. It is now being used more and more widely in the Western world and many chartered physiotherapists are also acupuncturists (Melzack 1989, Alltree 1997).

Special needles are inserted at strategic places and vibrated to produce a sensory input; electrical currents are sometimes passed through the needles as added stimulation. Its effect is based on the gate control theory and investigation by Melzack found that the precise factor is the intense degree of stimulation, the site of the stimulation being less important than the output (Melzack 1989).

Traditional acupuncture selects points on the basis of traditional diagnosis but 'classical' acupuncture uses traditional points in conjunction with Western diagnosis (Alltree 1997). Trigger point acupuncture involves the needling of trigger points in muscles in order to deactivate and relieve pain referred by them. There are conflicting reports on the neurophysiology of acupuncture due to the many methods of point selection.

In the periphery, needling stimulates A-delta mechanoreceptors. At the spinal level, enkephalinergic interneurones of A-delta fibres inhibit pain transmission. A-delta input continues via the spinothalamic tract to the thalamus, with a major collateral branch to the periaqueductal grey matter. This then produces descending inhibition (Alltree 1997). Acupuncture analgesia is mediated by a change in body fluid, stimulating endogenous endorphin release in the cerebrospinal fluid. It also has an effect on the autonomic nervous system and is used in treating sympathetic maintained pain (Alltree 1997).

Acupuncture is used in a wide range of painful conditions, including a variety of soft tissue and degenerative disorders. Neuropathic pain, including neuralgia and phantom limb pain, may respond and pain clinics use acupuncture for chronic pain refractory to other forms of treatment (Alltree 1997). Acupuncture should not be seen as a treatment of 'last resort' but should be considered alongside other modalities from the onset of treatment. See Alltree (1997) for further reading.

OTHER ELECTRICAL MODALITIES
Therapeutic ultrasound

Ultrasound is a high-frequency mechanical wave or vibration, above the audible range of sound, requiring an elastic medium through which to travel (Kitchen & Partridge 1990). It is generated by a piezo-electric or quartz crystal called a transducer. The crystal is housed in a small torch-like casing or even a smaller pencil-shaped instrument. It had been thought that therapeutic ultrasound required a frequency between 0.75 and 3 MHz but now kilohertz ultrasound is available (Dyson et al 1999). The MHz devices require a gel or water to aid transmission but the KHz machine

is more simple. It is the absorbed energy that produces the biological effect (Dyson et al 1999).

Ultrasound is mostly without sensation but warmth can be felt, depending upon the type of current used. The biological results of ultrasound are due to thermal or non-thermal effects such as cavitation, acoustic streaming and the production of standing waves (Dyson & Suckling 1978, Low 1997).

Thermal effects

As a result of heating and metabolic changes, there will be an increase in blood flow, dilation of blood vessels and more rapid exchanges across capillary walls and cell membrane (Low 1997). Heating fibrous tissue such as tendons, ligaments and joint capsules, or scar tissue, can cause an increase in their extensibility. Thus ultrasound coupled with active movement or passive stretching can lead to an increase in joint or tissue mobility (Low 1997).

Non-thermal effects

The vibration of the current oscillates the particles in the fluid content of the tissue cells, stimulating the release of chemical mediators which accelerates the healing process (Kitchen & Partridge 1990).

Ultrasound speeds up the healing process and is used to treat many conditions from open wounds, for example leg ulcers, to sprains and sports injuries, traumatic bruising, postoperative scarring and muscle spasm; in fact, wherever there is local tenderness, swelling and inflammation (Dyson et al 1999). When applied to a nerve, it is believed to raise the pain threshold in the territory of that nerve, probably due to modulation of C fibres (Bogduk & Mercer 1995). It will not help mechanical pain.

Interferential

Interferential is an electrical stimulation using two medium-frequency currents to produce a low-frequency effect within the body. It is applied with two or four pads which can be of the suction type or flat pads encased in wet foam rubber. By varying the frequency of the current, it is possible to treat muscular and all types of neural tissue, motor, sensory, sympathetic and para-sympathetic. It is believed to improve deep venous and lymphatic circulation (Bogduk & Mercer 1995). It is used for the treatment of pain, swelling, inflammation, muscular reeducation and for conditions which require an increase of circulation (Major 1992).

Laser

'Laser' is an acronym for Light Amplification by Stimulated Emission of Radiation. Specific sub-stances are stimulated electrically to emit a narrow beam of radiation which produces differing energy levels (laser energy). Laser is used for tissue repair, wound healing and pain relief. The effects spread from one cell to another and therefore to surrounding tissue (Thomson et al 1991, Low 1997). Laser is also used in operative techniques.

Short-wave diathermy or pulsed electromagnetic energy

Short-wave diathermy (SWD) or pulsed electro-magnetic energy (PEME) is an oscillating electro-magnetic field which affects the molecules in the tissues. Heat is generated in unpulsed SWD and used to treat both deep and superficial tissue. It is now used more frequently in its pulsed form for pain relief in acute soft tissue lesions, obtaining a marked reduction in local swelling; it is also used in wound healing (Thomson et al 1991).

ALTERNATIVE THERAPIES

Feldenkrais

Feldenkrais is a gentle non-invasive method of movement reeducation, making changes by using the transformational abilities of the nervous system (McCrea 1993). The reeducation is based on changing habitual patterns of movement by learning to move in non-habitual ways. The lessons give increasingly complex demands of coordination, balance, fine adjustments of intention and impulse. The learning process becomes automatic (Luypers 1990).

Alexander technique

The principal aim of the Alexander technique is to help people learn how to 'use' themselves better. It is a method of psychophysical education which is claimed to work at a fundamental level, affecting how we think, react, support our bodies and move. Clients are referred to as pupils or students since they work with the teacher rather than passively receive treatment. Using methods of changing from sit to stand, crawling or walking, pupils are taught how to free the neck and lengthen and widen the back throughout all movements (Trevelyan 1993).

INVESTIGATIVE PROCEDURES
Radiography or X-ray

X-rays are a non-invasive tool in which a beam of radiation is passed through the body region to form an image on photographic film which shows shadows of the bones, but X-rays do not show the condition of the more important soft tissues (Porter 1986, Mourad 1991). They show fractures, degenerative changes, disc narrowing, osteophytes, Schmorl's nodes, bony anomalies, such as spondylolisthesis, and bony diseases. Oblique views can show the sizes of the inter-vertebral foramina.

Conventional X-ray tomography

This technique utilizes conventional X-ray tubes and image receptors which are capable of moving relative to each other so as to blur out all structures except those at a chosen level (Bigg-Wither & Kelly 1995). Before the advent of CT and MRI scans (see below), this technique was used fre-quently in bone imaging and chest X-rays and although less utilized now, it is useful when metal implants preclude CT imaging or there is a con-traindication for MRI examination (Bigg-Wither & Kelly 1995).

Computed tomography (CT) scan

CT scan is a non-invasive technique now widely used to diagnose lesions in the spine. With the use of high-resolution scanning, cross-sectional views of the spine are made; it is now possible to demonstrate soft tissue shadows and the nature of the soft tissue can be assessed with reasonable accuracy. By rotating the patient on the examination table, it is possible to study the effect of movement upon the facet joints and the lateral canals (Kirkaldy-Willis & Tchang 1988, Eisenstein 1992).

CT scans are used for diagnosis in disc lesions, spinal stenosis and associated compression of neural structures, complex fractures, shoulder instability and in the evaluation of joint problems, bone tumours or chronic osteomyelitis (Bigg-Wither & Kelly, 1995).

Magnetic resonance imaging (MRI)

MRI is a non-invasive procedure in which very high magnetic forces are sent through the body to alter the alignment of hydrogen ions in the nuclei of cells. When irradiation stops, the nuclear atoms return to their original position, emitting the absorbed energy as signals that are stored by computer and projected as images (Mourad 1991). It has proved to be a useful adjunct to the CT scan. It provides markedly improved soft tissue contrast resolution of discs and neural elements, as well as the capability of imaging in multiple planes. The improved soft tissue resolution shows clear differentiation between structures such as disc material, neural elements, intraspinal haematoma and spinal tumours (Heithoff 1988).

Ultrasound imaging

Ultra high-frequency sound waves (5–10 MHz) are propagated into the tissues using a transducer placed on the skin (Bigg-Wither & Kelly 1995). By reflecting and transmitting the sound waves through different tissues, the depth of a structure can be determined and an image formed.

Myelography or radiculography

Myelography is contrast radiography. It has now been replaced by the CT scan but when this is unavailable, myelography is still used. A water-soluble contrast medium is injected into the spinal canal, filling the subarachnoid space of the thecal sac and nerve root sleeves and so outlining the contour of the thecal sac, nerve roots and spinal cord. X-rays are then taken of the spine. With modern contrast agents and fine-gauge needles, there are significantly fewer reactions than in the days when oil-based contrast media elicited side-effects such as nausea, vomiting, headaches, arachnoiditis and disorientation (Bigg-Wither & Kelly 1995).

Myelograms show disc herniation within the confines of the spinal canal and anterior or anterolateral defects within the vertebral column but they never demonstrate disc herniation in the lateral nerve canal. Tumour, neurofibromas and extradural abscesses are clearly shown (Kirkaldy-Willis & Tchang 1988).

Discography

Discography involves injecting a contrast medium into the disc, under X-ray guidance, in order to fill the area of the nucleus. The amount of injection material required to fill the nucleus depends on the state of the disc. The grossly degenerate disc has virtually no limit to the volume that can be injected (Porter 1986). The discs are then X-rayed. The radiological appearances of normal and degenerate discs are quite characteristic. The outline of the degenerate nucleus is irregular and the 'tissue sequestrum' can be identified (Porter 1986). Patients may experience pain during discography.

Radionuclide or radioisotope bone scan

This involves an intravenous injection of a tracer substance which localizes in bony tissue. The scan detects altered physiology by concentrating in areas of increased vascularity and areas of increased bone turnover. The emitted variation is recorded by a gamma camera adjacent to the body. These scans are useful for locating cancer, infection and inflammation (Eisenstein 1992, Bigg-Wither & Kelly 1995).

Facet arthrography

Facet arthrography is a technique for evaluating internal derangements of joints by injecting a contrast agent into a joint, followed by radiographic examination. These can be plain X-rays or CT scans. Arthrography is used less since the advent of more sophisticated imaging techniques.

Electromyography

Electromyography is used to diagnose either motor or sensory neural impairment. Routine nerve conduction studies are often normal in patients with nerve root lesions although they do help to exclude other conditions such as neuropathy which may confuse diagnosis. Electromyography, an electrical test, shows fibrillation potentials and motor unit changes in denervated muscle; the distribution of abnormalities may help to localize the lesion to a particular root. The EMG is negative in patients whose symptoms are due to irritation of the dorsal roots (Kirkaldy-Willis & Tchang 1988).

SURGERY

In general, surgery is used to treat pain when the causal lesion is known and can be removed or treated. Types of surgical procedures vary from removal of part of the disc to spinal fusion (Eisenstein 1992) and now microsurgery and endoscopic laser techniques are becoming more widespread (Knight et al 1998). Descriptions of these operations are beyond the scope of this book and it is hoped that with back care followed religiously, this step need never be taken.

REFERENCES

Alltree J 1997 Acupuncture. In: Wells P E, Frampton V, Bowsher D (eds) Pain management by physiotherapy. Butterworth Heinemann, Oxford

Baxter R 1988 Drug control of pain. In: Wells P E, Frampton V, Bowsher D (eds) Pain. Management and control in physiotherapy. Heinemann Medical Books, Oxford

Belshaw C 1987 Osteopathy. Is it for you? Element Books, Shaftesbury, 1987

Bennett M 1992 Chiropractic. What is it and how does it work? British Chiropractic Association, Reading

Bigg-Wither G, Kelly P 1995 Diagnostic imaging in musculoskeletal physiotherapy. In: Refshauge K, Gass E (eds) Musculoskeletal physiotherapy. Butterworth Heinemann, Oxford

Bithell C 1992 The Olive Sands memorial lecture: clinical diagnosis. In Touch 64: 31–34

Bogduk N, Mercer S 1995 Selection and application of treatment. In: Refshauge K, Gass E (eds) Musculoskeletal physiotherapy. Butterworth Heinemann, Oxford

British Chiropractic Association (BCA) 1999 Chiropractic – a great career. British Chiropractic Association, Reading

Butler D 1991 Mobilisation of the nervous system. Churchill Livingstone, Edinburgh

Chartered Society of Physiotherapy (CSP) 1991 Definition of physiotherapy. Curriculum of Study. Chartered Society of Physiotherapists, London

Comerford M, Kinetic Control 1998 Dynamic stability and muscle balance of the lumbar spine and trunk. Kinetic Control Ltd, Harrow

Conaghan P G, Day R O 1995 Physiology and clinical pharmacology: inflammation, pain and anti-inflammatory drugs and analgesics. In: Refshauge K, Gass E (eds) Musculoskeletal physiotherapy. Butterworth Heinemann, Oxford

Cyriax J 1984 Textbook of orthopaedic medicine, 11th edn. Baillière Tindall, London

Dyson M, Suckling J 1978 Stimulation of tissue repair by ultrasound: a survey of the mechanisms involved. Physiotherapy 64: 105–108

Dyson M, Preston R, Woledge R, Kitchen S 1999 Longwave ultrasound. Physiotherapy 85(1): 40–49

Edwards B C 1992 Manual of combined movements. Churchill Livingstone, Edinburgh

Eisenstein S 1992 Surgery for spinal disorders. In: Tidswell M E (ed) Cash's textbook of orthopaedics and rheumatology for physiotherapists. Mosby Yearbook Europe, London

Elvey R, Quinter J, Thomas A 1986 A clinical study of RSI. Australian Family Physician 15(2): 1314–1322

Fielding S, Mason G, Pattinson et al 1990 Osteopathy and medicine today. General Council and Register of Osteopaths, London

Frampton V 1997 Transcutaneous electrical nerve stimulation and chronic pain. In: Wells P, Frampton V, Bowsher D (eds) Pain management by physiotherapy. Butterworth Heinemann, Oxford

Garrison D W, Foreman R D 1994 Decreased activity of spontaneous and noxiously evoked dorsal horn cells during transcutaneous electrical stimulation (TENS). Pain 58: 309–315

Gifford L 1999 Topical issues in pain. Physiotherapy Pain
Association Yearbook 1998–1999. NOI Press, Falmouth,
Adelaide

Grant R 1988 Dizziness testing and manipulation of the
cervical spine. In: Grant R (ed) Physical therapy of the
cervical and thoracic spine. Churchill Livingstone,
Edinburgh

Grieve G G 1988 Common vertebral joint problems, 2nd edn.
Churchill Livingstone, Edinburgh

Heithoff K B 1988 Magnetic resonance imaging of the
lumbar spine. In: Kirkaldy-Willis W H (ed) Managing low
back pain, 2nd edn. Churchill Livingstone, Edinburgh

Kendall F P, McCleary F, Provance P C 1993 Muscle testing
and function, 3rd edn. Williams and Wilkins, Baltimore

Kirkaldy-Willis W H, Tchang S 1988 Diagnostic techniques.
In: Kirkaldy-Willis W H (ed) Managing low back pain.
Churchill Livingstone, Edinburgh

Kitchen S S, Partridge C J 1990 A review of therapeutic
ultrasound. Physiotherapy 76(10): 593–600

Knight M T N, Vajda A, Jakab G V, Awan S 1998 Endoscopic
laser foraminoplasty on the lumbar spine – early
experience. Minimally Invasive Neurosurgery 41(1): 1–14

Lewith G T 1984 Transcutaneous electrical nerve stimulation
for pain relief. World of Medicine 15 January: 225–229

Low J 1997 Electro-therapeutic modalities. In: Wells P E,
Frampton V, Bowsher D (eds) Pain management by
physiotherapy. Butterworth Heinemann, Oxford

Luypers W F 1990 The Feldenkrais approach. New Zealand
Journal of Physiotherapy August: 11

McCrea B 1993 The Feldenkrais method. Physiotherapy in
Sport XVIII(3)

Maitland G D 1991 Vertebral manipulation, 6th edn.
Butterworths, London

Maitland G D 1992 Peripheral manipulation, 3rd edn.
Butterworths, London

Major K 1992 Principles of treatment following joint

examination and assessment. In: Tidswell M E (eds)
Cash's textbook of orthopaedics and rheumatology for
physiotherapists, 2nd edn. Mosby Yearbook Europe,
London

Melzack R 1989 Folk medicine and the sensory modulation
of pain. In: Wall P D, Melzack R (eds) Textbook of pain,
2nd edn. Churchill Livingstone, Edinburgh

Melzack R, Wall P 1996 The challenge of pain. Penguin
Books, Harmondsworth

Mennell J P 1934 Physical treatment by movement,
manipulation and massage. A Churchill, London

Mourad L A 1991 Orthopedic disorders. Mosby Yearbook,
St Louis

Palastanga N 1991 Connective tissue massage. In: Grieve G
(ed) Modern manual therapy. Churchill Livingstone,
Edinburgh

Porter R W 1986 Management of back pain. Churchill
Livingstone, Edinburgh

Richardson C, Jull G, Toppenberg R, Comerford M 1992
Techniques for active lumbar stabilisation for spinal
protection: a pilot study. Australian Physiotherapy
38(2): 105–112

Sahrmann S 1993 Muscle imbalance. Course notes

Sunshine A, Olson N 1989 Non-narcotic analgesics. In: Wall
P, Melzack R (eds) Textbook of pain. Churchill
Livingstone, Edinburgh

Thompson J W 1997 Pharmacology of pain relief. In:
Wells P E, Frampton V, Bowsh D (eds) Pain management
by physiotherapy. Butterworth Heinemann, Oxford

Thomson A, Skinner A, Piercy J 1991 Tidy's physiotherapy,
12th edn. Butterworths, London

Trevelyan J 1993 Alexander technique. Nursing Times
89 (49): 50–52

Weintraube A 1991 Soft tissue mobilisation. In: Grieve G (ed)
Modern manual therapy. Churchill Livingstone,
Edinburgh

FURTHER READING

Dyson M 1987 Mechanisms involved in therapeutic
ultrasound. Physiotherapy 73(3): 116–120

Dyson M, Preston R, Woledge R, Kitchen S 1999 Longwave
ultrasound. Physiotherapy 85(1): 40–49

Kitchen S, Bazin S 1995 Clayton's Electrotherapy, 10th edn.
W B Saunders

Kitchen S S, Partridge C U 1991 A review of low laser
therapy. Physiotherapy 77(3): 161–167

Low J, Reed A 1990 Electrotherapy explained: principles and
practice. Butterworth Heinemann, Oxford

Useful addresses

Arachnoiditis Self-help Group (ASHG)
1 Luton Court
Broadstairs
Kent LT10 2DE

Arthritis and Rheumatism Council for Research
Copeman House
St Mary's Court
St Mary's Gate
Chesterfield
Derbyshire S4I 7TD
Tel: 01246 558033

Back Care (previously known as National Back Pain Association)
16 Elmtree Road
Teddington
TW11 0AB
Tel: 0181 977 5474

Body Control Pilates Association
17 Queensberry Mews West
South Kensington
London SW7 2DY
Tel: 0171 379 3734

British Chiropractic Association
Blagrave House
17 Blagrave Street
Reading RG1 1QB
Tel: 0118 950 5950

Chartered Society of Physiotherapy
14 Bedford Row
London WC1R 4ED
Tel: 0171 242 1841 or 0171 306 6620

Department of Movement Science
University of Liverpool
Liverpool L69 3BX
Tel: 0151 794 2000

Disabled Living Foundation
Equipment Centre and Information Service
380–384 Harrow Road
London W9 2HU
Tel: 0171 289 6111

Ergonomics Research Unit
Robens Institute
University of Surrey
Guildford
Surrey GU2 5HX
Tel: 01483 300 800

Ergonomics Society
Devonshire House
Devonshire Square
Loughborough
Leics LE11 3DW
Tel: 01509 234904

Exercises Association of England
Unit 4
Angel Gate
City Road
London EC1 2PT
Tel: 0171 278 0811

Feldenkrais Method
Feldenkrais Guild
PO Box 370
London N10 3XL

General Osteopathic Council
Osteopathy House
176 Tower Bridge Road
London SE1 3LU
Tel: 0171 357 6655

Health Education Authority (HEA)
St Peter's Street
London SW1 P2HW
Tel: 0171 222 5300

Health and Safety Executive (HSE)
Sovereign House
110 Queen's Street
Sheffield S1 2ES
Tel: 0114 291 2300

Health and Safety Laboratory
Sutherland House
Queen's Street
Sheffield S3 7HQ
Tel: 0114 289 2000

Her Majesty's Stationery Office (HMSO)
49 High Holborn
London WC1V 6HB
Tel: 0171 600 5522

Human Performance Laboratory
Royal Free Hospital School of Medicine

Pond Street
Hampstead
London NW3
Tel: 0171 794 0500

Institute for Occupational Ergonomics
University of Nottingham
Nottingham NG7 2RD
Tel: 01159 515151

Keep Fit Association
Francis House
Francis Street
London SW1P 1DE
Tel: 0171 233 8898

Kinetic Control
3rd Floor
Hygeia Building
66 College Road
Harrow
Middlesex HA1 1BE
Tel: 0181 324 1687

National Osteoporosis Society
PO Box 10
Radstock
Bath BA3 3YB
Tel: 01761 471771

Rambler's Association
1–5 Wandsworth Road
London SW8 2XX
Tel: 0171 582 6878

Royal College of General Practitioners
14 Prince's Gate
London SW7
Tel: 0171 581 3232

Royal College of Physicians of London
11 St Andrew's Place
London NW1 4LE
Tel: 0171 935 1174

Scoliosis Society of the UK
2 Ivebury Court
323–327 Latimer Road
London W10 6RA
Tel: 0181 964 5343

Sleep Council
High Corn Mill
Chapel Hill
Skipton BD23 1NL
Tel: 01756 792327

Society of Teachers of the Alexander Technique
10 London House
266 Fulham Road
London SW10 9EL
Tel: 0171 351 0828

Patient handouts

CHAPTER CONTENTS

INTRODUCTION TO HANDOUTS

The following handouts on particular elements of back care are provided for therapists to photocopy and, where appropriate, to give to their patients. The selection has been made on the basis of frequency of use within my own practice and the relative importance of the information contained as messages for the public in general. The handouts are:

- Posture in sitting.
- Posture in carrying.
- School pupils' posture.
- VDU work station posture.
- Pause exercises for workers in static postures.
- Teaching transversus abdominis.
- Hamstring stretches.
- A quartet of mobilizing exercises.

As we know, no back care advice can be universally applicable, for example, the handouts given for advice on maintaining the lordosis in sitting would not be suitable for someone with a spondylolisthesis. However, for the average joint-stressed or discogenic back, supporting the lumbar spine in sitting is vitally important and is often overlooked by leg pain sufferers who sit every evening with a flexed lumbar spine and their feet up on a stool, possibly thus maintaining their pain. This should be routinely checked and corrected for anyone with leg pain.

The growing incidence of teenage back pain is a subject that involves us all, so the handout on school bags and school pupils' posture is worth passing on to any parent as an adjunct to their own postural advice.

VDU stations and the correct working posture should be discussed at the very first assessment, even if the patient uses a computer for only a short period each day. However, for the person with upper limb disorders, pause exercises need to be carefully chosen and these, as it states at the top of the page, are intended as a 'preventative measure', not for general use with arm pain.

The three exercise handouts are self-explanatory:
1. Teaching the recruitment of TA is almost routine.
2. Hamstring stretches, so often incorrectly performed, need to be used accurately
3. The four mobilizing exercises are a quartet that can often help with elderly stiff backs, patients who are not likely to be able to get into a regime of swimming, Yoga or Pilates but who are happy to do something each day. They can be used where applicable after careful introduction and assessment of the effect of each exercise.

PATIENT HANDOUTS

POSTURE IN SITTING

Remaining in one position for longer than half an hour is stressful for the back. Try to change position frequently.

Chairs should support your body in a good position. You can never sit well in the chair on the left below as the seat is too deep and you need several cushions to support your back. When you buy a chair, make sure that the depth of the seat is shorter than the length of your thigh so that you can get your hips right back in the chair with your feet comfortably on the floor. The back of the chair should be at an angle of about 110–115° so that it holds your back in a good upright position.

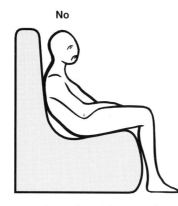

No

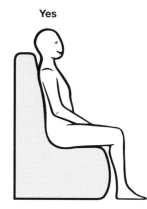

Yes

If you need to sit with your feet up on a stool, make sure you have a reclining chair. If you sit in a normal chair with your feet up, your back is forced to slump. You can actually prolong back pain or leg pain by sitting in this position. For the same reason, you should not sit propped up in bed watching TV – lower the pillows and raise the TV.

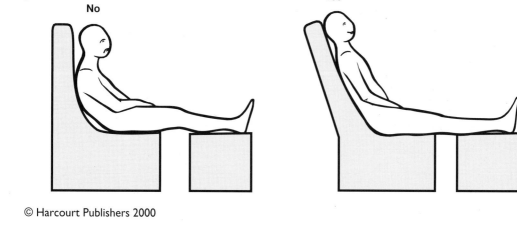

No

Yes

If you move around a lot, take a cushion with you for your back or a wedge-shaped cushion to sit on. The wedge-shaped cushion is also good to use in the car.

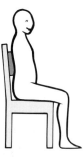

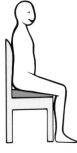

Back cushion

Wedge-shaped cushion

Avoid sitting slouched in a chair to read, try to have the book propped up in front of you with your back supported in a good position.

No

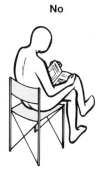

Yes

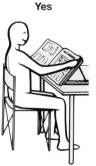

In the car, the seat must be at a comfortable distance from the pedals with your legs as straight as you can *safely* drive. The back of the seat must be brought up to an almost upright position, about 95–100° angle, so that your arms are comfortably relaxed in a slightly bent position, with the head rest immediately behind your head. When you buy a car make sure the height inside allows you to look out of the windscreen with your back upright and your head held straight, not in a slumped position with your chin poking forwards.

No   **Yes**

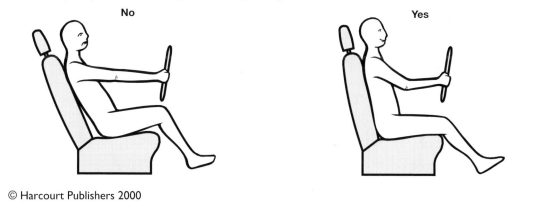

POSTURE IN CARRYING

Do not carry too heavy a weight.

Do aim to be balanced so that your body is straight, neither twisting nor leaning to one side: carry two bags instead of one or put all your belongings into a good backpack.

If the weight is excessive, use a trolley.

School pupils

Try to minimize the number of books you carry around. Do not carry in any way which distorts your body. Do use a small load in each hand or carry the weight clasped close to you. Use a backpack or sling a satchel across from the opposite shoulder.

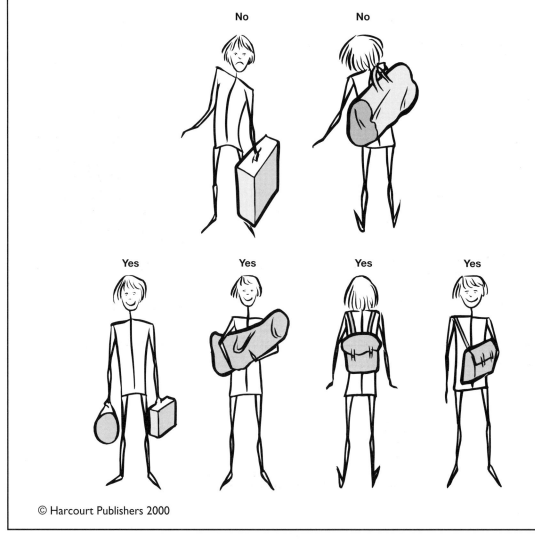

SCHOOL PUPILS

Sitting at a desk, the chair should be the right height to have both feet on the floor without the chair pressing into the backs of your thighs. The desk should be high enough so that your elbows can rest on it without causing your back to slump into a rounded curve. Ideally, the desk should slope upwards slightly.

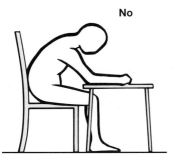

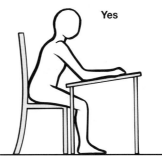

Avoid sitting for hours watching TV with your legs crossed and your back slumped or with your back slouched in any position.

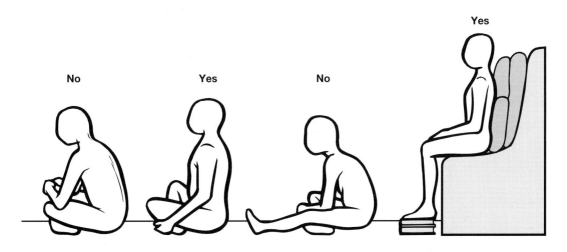

Try lying on your tummy with your head supported in your hands for some of the time while you read or watch TV.

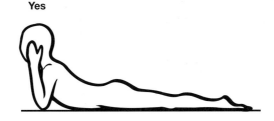

WORK-RELATED POSTURE

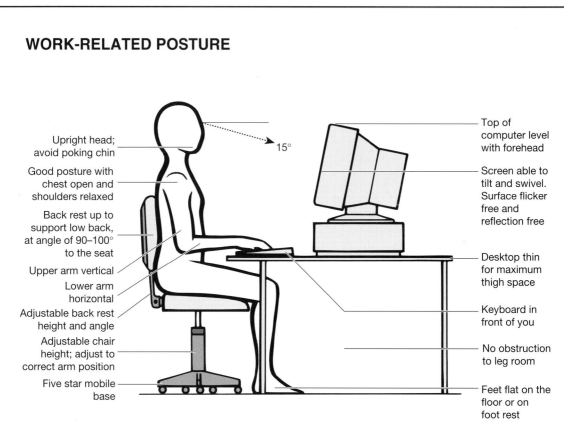

Upright head; avoid poking chin

Good posture with chest open and shoulders relaxed

Back rest up to support low back, at angle of 90–100° to the seat

Upper arm vertical

Lower arm horizontal

Adjustable back rest height and angle

Adjustable chair height; adjust to correct arm position

Five star mobile base

15°

Top of computer level with forehead

Screen able to tilt and swivel. Surface flicker free and reflection free

Desktop thin for maximum thigh space

Keyboard in front of you

No obstruction to leg room

Feet flat on the floor or on foot rest

Glasses

Do not use bifocals for computer work. Get specially focused reading glasses or discuss with your optician. Bifocals cause you to tip your head back when you look at the screen; this is bad for your neck and can create neck and/or arm pain.

Telephone

Do not hold the phone between ear and shoulder.

Pause exercises for computer or checkout workers

As a preventive measure, do one or two of the following exercises whenever you pause for thought. Movement is essential.

NB: If you already have neck and arm pain or have any other relevant medical condition, seek medical advice first.

Do not do any of these exercises if they give pain in your neck or arms.

1. Sit with your hands placed lightly behind your neck. Round your back, dropping your elbows down and your head towards your abdomen. Straighten up, opening out your elbows and really arch your upper back, pressing both elbows backwards.
2. Bend the right ear to the right shoulder, stretching the left side of the neck. Repeat to the left.
3. Sit up straight. Reach your nose forwards as if you were smelling a flower, then pull your head back, stretching the back of your neck, but do not press your chin down.
4. Sit up straight, arms relaxed. Pull in your spine between your shoulder blades, so that your upper back straightens and your chest moves forwards. Retract your head with your chin in neutral (not stuck up in the air or pressed in). Then lengthen your collar bones, opening the front of your chest.
5. Clasp both hands in front of you, turn them inside out, keep your elbows straight and stretch both arms up above your head, stretching up and back towards the ceiling.
6. Touch your right shoulder with the right hand, straighten out the arm sideways, palm facing up, then point the hand towards the floor, palm facing away from you. Repeat 3–5 times. Do not jerk the movement or overstretch. Repeat with the other arm.
7. Stand with arms by your side, the backs of your hands towards your side and your wrist bent up away from you. Lift your arm sideways, up and down five times. Repeat with the other arm.
8. Put your palms together in front of you with your elbows held out sideways: press the palms together, stretching the front of your wrists. Touch your chest with the tips of your fingers and then point the tips away from you, fast. Repeat the movement quickly.
9. Get up frequently and walk around the room. Every time you rise from sitting, arch your back and stretch.

TRANSVERSUS ABDOMINIS EXERCISE

You have five abdominal muscles. The most important one for you is called transversus abdominis. Transversus runs across the front of your lower abdomen round to the spine at the back and connects with an important back muscle called multifidus. These muscles often weaken after an episode of back pain. Contracting transversus helps to activate multifidus and also helps to flatten the bulge at the bottom of your tummy. Sit-ups will never do this, even if you do 100 a day!

Contracting your pelvic floor muscles (as if you were trying to stop passing water) helps to activate transversus.

Lying on your side in bed

1. Rest your top arm on your body with your hand over the area of your diaphragm, just under your ribs. Let your abdomen relax so that the whole area hangs down. Feel your diaphragm moving gently as you breathe.
2. Relax. Feel the regular, gentle rhythm of your diaphragm and try not to hold your breath.
3. Think of the area of your abdomen below your navel (transversus): contract your pelvic floor and then gently pull in transversus.

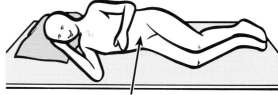

4. Keep transversus held in and check that your diaphragm is still relaxed and moving gently as you hold in the lower area. Hold at least 10 seconds.
5. Now relax it all and feel transversus letting go. Repeat 10 times.

Sitting in a chair

Whenever you are sitting, watching TV, pausing for thought at the office or at any time, rest one hand on your diaphragm and one hand on your lower abdomen. Relax. Feel your regular breathing with the top hand, then gradually pull in your lower abdomen and feel it moving away from your lower hand. Make sure your diaphragm is relaxed and that it is moving in and out as you hold in transversus. Hold for 10 seconds and repeat 10 times.

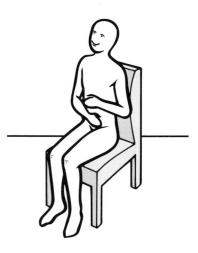

Try to hold in transversus hundreds of times a day when you are standing, walking or just moving about your work, so that you train it to stay contracted.

STRETCHES

All stretching exercises must be performed carefully using a slow, held stretch. *Never* jerk or bounce into a stretch.

Hamstring stretches are often incorrectly performed. They should never be done with a rounded back. Here are three alternative hamstring stretches:

1. Lie on your back with both knees bent and feet on the floor. Pull one knee up towards you and hold the thigh with your hands; straighten the knee until the hamstrings pull gently and hold 20–30 seconds. Let the knee bend. Repeat five times. Repeat with the other leg.

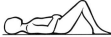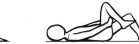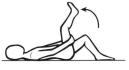

2. Sit on a table with both legs hanging down. Make sure your back is held in its natural arch and hold this position all the time. Slowly straighten one leg, keeping the thigh on the table, until the hamstrings pull gently. Hold 20–30 seconds. Do not pull so hard that your back is forced to round. Repeat with alternate legs 3–5 times.

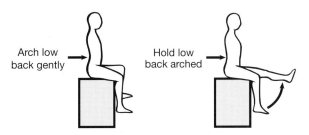

Arch low back gently → 　　　Hold low back arched →

3. Stand by a firm, knee-high stool or bench. Place the heel of one foot on the stool and place both hands on the knee of the raised leg. Lean forwards at the hips, *keeping the back straight*, with the lumbar curve held in its natural position until you feel the hamstrings pull. Hold 20–30 seconds. Repeat 3–5 times. This exercise is often wrongly performed by bending the back and reaching forwards with the arms.

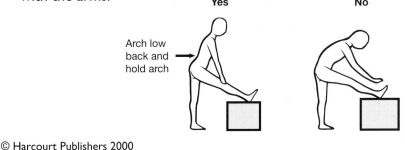

Yes　　　　**No**

Arch low back and → hold arch

252

GENTLE MOBILIZING EXERCISES

If you have a bad back *do not* do these exercises unless advised by a therapist.
Do not do any of them if they give pain.

1. Lie on the floor with both knees bent and feet on the floor. Roll both knees
   from side to side a few degrees, gradually increasing the roll as the days pass
   until your knees touch the floor on either side. Repeat 6–10 times.

2. Lie on the floor, pull one knee up towards your chest while you push the other
   leg straight down onto the floor. Repeat with the other leg, alternately three
   times each.

3. Lie on the floor with both knees bent and feet on the floor. Pull both knees
   gently up towards your shoulders, using your hands to help the pull up. Replace
   your feet on the floor. Repeat 5–10 times with a free-flowing movement, no
   jerk or rock.

4. Lie on the floor with both knees bent and feet on the floor. Lift your buttocks
   off the floor so that your hips are high and your body is straight, then tighten
   your abdomen and buttocks at the same time. Hold the position for a count
   of 10. Repeat three times.

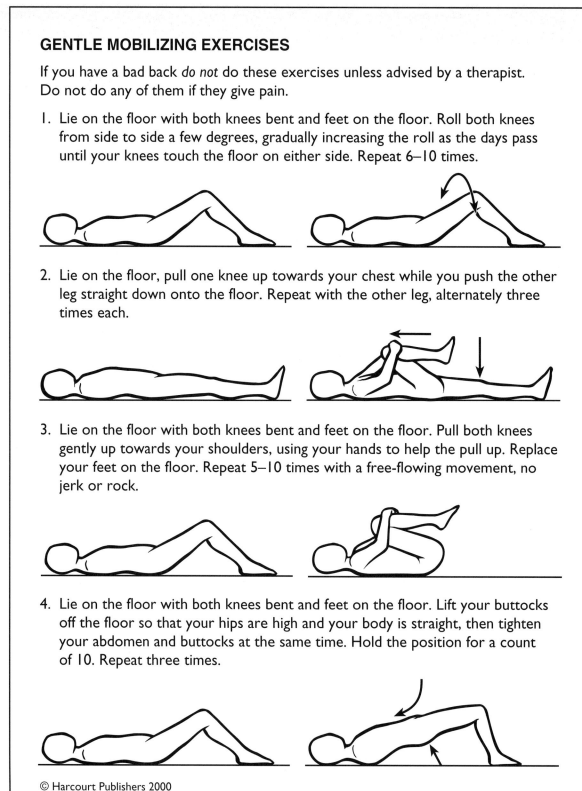

Index

Numbers in **bold** refer to tables or illustrations